C0-BQG-023

Aging and
Environmental Toxicology

The Johns Hopkins Series in Environmental Toxicology
Zoltan Annau, Series Editor

Neurobehavioral Toxicology, edited by Zoltan Annau

Monitoring the Worker for Exposure and Disease: Scientific, Legal, and Ethical Considerations in the Use of Biomarkers, Nicholas A. Ashford, Christine J. Spadafor, Dale B. Hattis, and Charles C. Caldart

Variations in Susceptibility to Inhaled Pollutants; Identification, Mechanisms, and Policy Implications, edited by Joseph D. Brain, Barbara D. Beck, A. Jane Warren, and Rashid A. Shaikh

The Toxicity of Methyl Mercury, edited by Christine U. Eccles and Zoltan Annau

Lead Toxicity: History and Environmental Impact, edited by Richard Lansdown and William Yule

Toxic Chemicals, Health, and the Environment, edited by Lester B. Lave and Arthur C. Upton

Aging and Environmental Toxicology

Biological and Behavioral Perspectives

Edited by Ralph L. Cooper
Chief, Endocrine/Gerontology Section, Reproductive Toxicology Branch
Developmental Toxicology Division, Health Effects Research Laboratory
U.S. Environmental Protection Agency, Research Triangle Park, N.C.

Jerome M. Goldman
Project Supervisor, Reproductive Toxicology Group
NSI Technology Services, Environmental Sciences
Research Triangle Park, N.C.

Thomas J. Harbin
Clinical Psychologist, Gullick and Associates, Fayetteville, N.C.

The Johns Hopkins University Press
Baltimore and London

© 1991 The Johns Hopkins University Press
All rights reserved
Printed in the United States of America

The Johns Hopkins University Press, 701 West 40th Street, Baltimore, Maryland 21211
The Johns Hopkins Press Ltd., London

∞
The paper in this book meets the minimum requirements of American National Standard
for Information Sciences—Permanence of Paper for Printed Library Materials, ANSI
Z39.48-1984.

The research described in chapters 1, 6, 8, and 9 has been reviewed by the Health
Effects Research Laboratory, U.S. Environmental Protection Agency, and approved
for publication. Approval does not signify that the contents necessarily reflect the views
and policies of the agency, nor does mention of trade name or commercial products
constitute endorsement or recommendation for use.

The views of Richard M. Lewis in Chapter 5 do not purport to reflect the views of the
U.S. Army or the Department of Defense.

Library of Congress Cataloging-in-Publication Data

Aging and environmental toxicology : biological and behavioral perspectives / edited by
Ralph L. Cooper, Jerome M. Goldman, and Thomas J. Harbin.
    p.   cm.—(The Johns Hopkins series in environmental toxicology)
    Includes index.
    ISBN 0-8018-4105-4 (alk. paper)
    1. Aging—Physiological aspects. 2. Toxicology. 3. Adaptation (Physiology). 4. Xeno-
biotics—Physiological effect. I. Cooper, Ralph L., 1942–   . II. Goldman, Jerome M.
III. Harbin, Thomas J., 1954–   . IV. Series.
    [DNLM: 1. Aging—physiology. 2. Environmental Exposure. 3. Hazardous Sub-
stances—adverse effects. 4. Nervous System—drug effects.]
QP86.A35915   1991
612.6'7—dc20
DNLM/DLC
for Library of Congress   90-5134 CIP

Contents

Contributors

Linda S. Birnbaum, Ph.D., Director, Environmental Toxicology Division, Health Effects Research Laboratory, U.S. Environmental Protection Agency, Research Triangle Park, N.C.

Edward J. Calabrese, Ph.D., Professor, School of Public Health, University of Massachusetts

Andrew T. Canada, Ph.D., Assistant Professor, Department of Anesthesiology, Duke University Medical Center

Joy Cavagnaro, Ph.D., Special Assisitant to the Director, Office of Biologics Research, U.S. Food and Drug Administration

Harvey Jay Cohen, M.D., Director, Chief of Geriatrics, and Professor of Medicine, Center for the Study of Aging and Human Development, Duke University Medical Center; and Director, Geriatric Research Education and Clinical Center, Durham Veterans Administration Medical Center

Jeffrey Crawford, MD., Assistant Clinical Professor, Division of Hematology and Medical Oncology, Center for the Study of Aging and Human Development, Duke University Medical Center; and Staff Physician, Geriatric Research Education and Clinical Center, Durham Veterans Administration Medical Center

Bruce Fishman, Ph.D., ENSR, Consulting and Engineering, Acton, Mass.

Barbara A. Gilchrest, M.D., Chair, Department of Dermatology, Boston University School of Medicine

Leon Earl Gray, Jr., Ph.D., Chief, Developmental Reproductive Biology Section, Reproductive Toxicology Branch, Developmental Toxicology Division, Health Effects Research Laboratory, U.S. Environmental Protection Agency, Research Triangle Park, N.C.

Christopher Lau, Ph.D., Pharmacologist, Developmental Toxicology Division, U.S. Environmental Protection Agency, Research Triangle Park, N.C.

Richard M. Lewis, Ph.D., Chemist, Division of Blood and Blood Products, Center for Biologics Evaluation and Research, U.S. Food and Drug Administration

Kenneth W. Lyles, M.D., Associate Professor of Medicine, Geriatric Research Education and Clinical Center, Durham Veterans Administration Medical Center; and Department of Medicine, Duke University Medical Center

S. Spence McCachren, M.D., Assistant Professor of Medicine, Divisions of Geriatrics and Hematology and Medical Oncology, Duke University Medical Center; and Geriatric Research Education and Clinical Center, Durham Veterans Administration Medical Center

Timothy F. McMahon, Ph.D., IRTA Fellow, Experimental Toxicology Branch, National Institute of Environmental Health Sciences, Research Triangle Park, N.C.

Gail R. Marsh, Ph.D., Associate Professor of Medical Psychology, Department of Psychiatry; and Senior Fellow, Center for the Study of Aging and Human Development, Duke University Medical Center

John D. Ranseen, Ph.D., Assistant Professor of Psychiatry and Adjunct Assistant Professor of Neurology and Psychology, University of Kentucky and Lexington Veterans Administration Medical Center

Gary S. Rogers, M.D., Assistant Professor of Dermatology and Surgery, Department of Dermatology, Boston University School of Medicine

Frederick A. Schmitt, Ph.D., Associate Professor of Neurology, Adjunct Associate Professor of Psychiatry and Psychology, and Center Associate, Sanders-Brown Center on Aging, University of Kentucky, and Lexington Veterans Administration Medical Center

Richard F. Walker, Ph.D., Assistant Director of Toxicology, Research and Development Division, SmithKline Beecham Laboratories, King of Prussia, Pa.

Aging and
Environmental Toxicology

Introduction: Assessing Environmental Influences on the Aging Process

Ralph L. Cooper, Ph.D.

Jerome M. Goldman, Ph.D.

Thomas J. Harbin, Ph.D.

The elderly population of the United States is growing much more rapidly than is the population as a whole. This growth is partly the result of enhanced fertility rates and increased infant survival and partly the result of significant improvements in nutrition, health care (e.g., vaccines and antibiotics), and personal life-style. Life expectancy in the United States is now nearly 70 years for men and 77 years for women, compared with 58 and 62, respectively, as recently as 1930 (Siegel and Taeuber, 1986). As the total population increased 11 percent in the 1970s, the population age 65 and older increased 28 percent and the population age 85 and older increased 59 percent. Individuals age 85 and over comprise the most rapidly growing of the four older age groups (55–64, 65–74, 75–84, and 85 and over), and this group is expected to triple between 1980 and 2020. Census projections for 2050 indicate that the proportion of the population age 65 and older will be almost twice as great as today—22 percent compared with 12 percent (Siegel and Taeuber, 1986).

The shifts in the age of the U.S. population have been accompanied by an increased awareness that the greater numbers of older people will present new social, economic, and political concerns. Indeed, these demographic changes have already had a tremendous impact on the systems for the provision of health care, because older people are more likely than other groups to need medical attention. Moreover, expanding research in basic gerontology and geriatric medicine has shown that elderly persons have an increased vulnerability to a number of stressors, including those imposed on them from the environment. However, the extent to which an elderly individual is more susceptible

1

to toxic effects following either acute or chronic exposure to potentially hazardous environmental compounds remains to be determined.

The demographic shift toward increased longevity has created a set of circumstances that, a priori, should result in increased concern for the health risk of the elderly population. Elderly individuals may be at increased risk to acute toxicant exposure because of the numerous changes in the body's protective mechanisms. Also, because the survival rate of such individuals in the environment is longer than had previously been possible, there is a more protracted period of lifetime exposure to chemicals than had been experienced in the past. There is also more time for the latent adverse effects from earlier lifetime exposures to manifest themselves, simply because these individuals are living longer and there is sufficient time for possible cumulative effects to emerge. Furthermore, cohorts reaching age 65 and older in the 1990s will be exposed to vastly different life-span environments than those who reached 65 in the 1960s. This is compounded by the fact that there is an ever-growing number of chemical agents discharged into our environment that could have potentially adverse health effects. Finally, because of the longer life span, there is an increased possibility for the interaction of different toxicants, or of drugs and toxicants, to become manifest.

Although all of the aforementioned possibilities exist and are factors potentially leading to significant health risks, our limited knowledge precludes setting forth, at the present time, any specific guidelines or statements that would be applicable to aged individuals as a special subpopulation. Epidemiological approaches can continue to clarify the relationships between aging and disease states or environmental insult, identifying increased risk of mortality or morbidity in this population from a variety of external influences. For example, substantial epidemiological data and experimental animal data have implicated the ultraviolet portion of sunlight in the premature aging of the skin. Fair-skinned people living in areas of high insolation (solar intensity) and having extensive vocational or recreational sun exposure are affected earliest and most severely (see Chapter 4). Extensive epidemiological data support a causal role of photoaging in a large percentage of basal and squamous cell carcinomas (Urbach, Epstein, and Forbes, 1974).

There is also a clear relationship between age and environmental factors such as smoking in the loss of lung function. Equally clear is an important correlation between lung dysfunction and mortality from all causes. Yet, the evidence of implicating ambient concentrations of air pollutants in the decline of lung function with age is controversial (U.S. Environmental Protection Agency, 1986), although the potential impact of environmental exposures, either outdoor or indoor, on susceptible people is real and deserves further study.

It has also been suggested that environmental factors play an important role in the development of aging disorders such as cataracts (National Research Council, 1987). Cataract incidence is extraordinarily high in Tibet and Nepal, and a threefold difference in prevalence of cataract has been reported among different climatic zones in northern India. Also, there are apparent differences in the incidence of cataracts between the population of India and the United States (National Research Council, 1987). However, before these regional differences in age-related diseases can be attributed to environmental factors, a number of confounders (e.g., diet and genetic factors) must be addressed.

A similar dilemma exists in the interpretation of the epidemiological data indicating a higher incidence of breast cancer in women in the San Francisco Bay Area than in Slovenia, Yugoslavia, or Osaka, Japan (Petrakis, Ernster, and King 1982).

Thus, with the evident increased diversities in biological and sociopsychological histories, minimizing the confounding variables in the construction of epidemiological studies presents a formidable challenge. Nevertheless, such studies in conjunction with clinical evidence and toxicological experimentation in the aging animal can provide valuable information on the interaction between exposure to environmental factors and the reduced adaptive capabilities of the elderly population. Only then can the impact of age be placed in the proper perspective. Such information is vital for the creation of appropriate policies to address the emerging problems associated with aging and environmental toxicity.

Insults from our environment may take many forms. In contrast to the obvious effects of the physical trauma of accidents, environmental hazards may be much more subtle in nature. An incredibly broad range of physicochemical insults is present in the environment. These can be studied at a number of different levels, ranging from the molecular to the organ system, in order to characterize the particular mechanisms involved and establish the functional impact of the effect. Moreover, individual organ systems exhibit both differential sensitivities to various forms of insult and considerable overall variation in their relative susceptibility to damage. This presents a considerable challenge in any comprehensive presentation of the influence of environmental agents on the aging organism.

This book brings together a distinguished group of scientists with diverse research interests who have in common an abiding interest in the processes of aging and the relationship of these processes to an organism's interactions with its environment. The environmental hazards addressed by these contributors include a variety of distinct types of exposure that may be present throughout the life span, ranging from various kinds of chemical insult to the physical trauma of sensory bombardment.

Chapters 1 through 3 address the broader molecular/biochemical aspects of xenobiotic metabolism, free radical production, and adverse health outcomes. These fundamental mechanisms underlie the organ and functional systems discussed in subsequent chapters. It could be argued that the older person would be more sensitive to the adverse health effects of an environmental toxicant because of the numerous physiological changes in absorption, metabolism, distribution, and elimination that have been identified in this age group. Furthermore, the homeostatic mechanisms involved in fending off such insults change with age. It would follow, therefore, that acute exposure should have a greater impact on the older organism. On the other hand, if a compound has to be transformed into a reactive metabolite, and metabolic capability is compromised in the elderly, then perhaps their risk to exposure may be reduced compared with that of young adults. In Chapter 1 McMahon and Birnbaum discuss these issues and the potential impact that diferences in xenobiotic distribution and metabolism may have across the life span.

A parallel issue concerns the age-related increases in the metabolic production of free radicals. In Chapter 2, Canada and Calabrese introduce the topic of free radicals and the age-related erosion of the systems that protect the organism from those reactive metabolites generated by a variety of pharmacological and environmental agents (including ozone and NO_2). McCachren, Crawford, and Cohen in Chapter 3 extend the discussion of xenobiotic metabolism to include the induction of neoplastic changes in the aging organism. This theme is carried over in Chapter 4 by Rogers and Gilchrest in their discussion of the well-established relationship between exposure to ultraviolet radiation and skin cancer. Here the extent of exposure is influenced by pollutant emissions that cause global or regional atmospheric alterations.

Even those stimuli that normally bombard our physical and chemical senses can at times be hazardous. For example, there is an association between hearing loss and exposure for prolonged periods to high-intensity sound at a particular frequency or mix of frequencies. However, as discussed by Marsh in Chapter 13, the extent to which age-related alterations in the functioning of other sensory systems is attributable to environmental factors remains to be determined.

With advancing age, the functional changes in a variety of systems are compromised, leaving the organism more vulnerable to insult and less capable of adapting to physical and chemical stressors. There are well-described alterations in immune function in elderly individuals. Indeed, some research suggests that the aging process itself represents an immunological phenomenon. Lewis and Cavagnaro discuss the possible role of environmental toxicants in the age-related changes in immune function in Chapter 5. Cardiovascular aging continues to receive a great deal of attention because of the number of deaths related to cardiac failure and vascular insufficiency. A summary of the effects of pharmacological agents and environmental toxicants on the aging cardiovascular system is presented by Lau in Chapter 6. The loss of bone mass and disturbances in bone metabolism are other significant debilitating processes present in elderly individuals. In Chapter 7, Lyles discusses age-dependent alterations in bone metabolism and the potential role that environmental toxicants may play in causing skeletal disease.

The endocrine and nervous systems are responsible for the integration and coordination of numerous physiological processes. Consequently, these systems are critical to the maintenance of homeostasis and the overall health of the organism. Both systems rely on cell-to-cell communication and therefore share certain physiological attributes. The cells of the nervous and endocrine systems must synthesize and release their respective chemical messengers, which then travel varying distances to the receiving cells. The receiving cells must possess the appropriate receptors to recognize the chemical messenger and be capable of responding appropriately to the stimulus. Basic research in gerontology has shown that functional alterations in both the nervous and endocrine systems can occur at each of these various steps in cell-to-cell communication. Similarly, research in toxicology has shown that environmental compounds may affect one or more of these stages. These issues are discussed in detail by Goldman and Cooper in Chapter 8, addressing the effects of environmentally induced alterations in endocrine function, and by Walker and Fishman in Chapter 10, discussing the action of xenobiotics on the aging central nervous system.

A loss in the integrative function of the neuroendocrine system would have obvious consequences on the brain's ability to process information, and subsequently on the behavior of the individual. Age-related alterations in brain function are of great concern because such changes can result in marked alterations in personality, that which constitutes the uniqueness of each individual. Such changes become even more tragic when the extremes are reached, such as the behavioral alterations observed in the patient with Alzheimer's disease. Chapter 11 by Harbin and Chapter 12 by Schmitt and Ranseen represent two different approaches used to study the way in which xenobiotic exposure may modify function of the central nervous system and behavior in the aged population.

One additional issue in geriatric toxicology is how exposure to xenobiotics during development and/or adulthood may influence the rate of aging. In Chapter 9, Gray provides several examples in which changes within a number of physiological systems are irreversibly altered if the organism is exposed to xenobiotics at certain critical times during development. This is an important issue, because it is often difficult to identify the connection between the exposure and its resultant adverse effect given the long latency between the two events.

This book is not intended to be an encyclopedic compendium of facts documenting the responses of elderly persons to environmental agents. Rather, it provides the reader with different perspectives on the principal issues in aging and environmental toxicology, along with various insights into problems associated with this growing area of scientific concern. Also, in many cases the authors present examples of current and proposed research approaches that should prove useful for investigators concerned with proper assessment of contemporary issues such as radon, indoor air quality, acid aerosols, and the contamination of food products by pesticides. The consensus of the contributors is that an enormous amount of research is still needed before any definitive statements can be made about the risks associated with aging and environmental toxicity. It is hoped that this book will serve to increase a general awareness of the multiplicity of issues in aging and environmental toxicity and at the same time stimulate scientific concerns about the importance of these issues to the field of toxicology.

References

National Research Council. 1987. *Aging in Today's Environment*. Washington, DC, National Academy Press.

Petrakis, N. L., Ernster, V. L., and King, M. C. 1982. Breast. In Schottenfeld, D., and Fraumeni, J. F. (Eds.), *Cancer Epidemiology and Prevention*. Philadelphia, W. B. Saunders, pp. 855–870.

Siegel, J. S., and Taeuber, C. M. 1986. Demographic perspectives on the long-lived society. *Daedalus* 115:77–117.

Urbach, F., Epstein, J. H., and Forbes, P. D. 1974. Ultraviolet carcinogenesis: Experimental, global and genetic aspects. In Pathak, M. A., Harber, L. C., Seiji, M., and Kukita, A. (Eds.), *Sunlight and Man: Normal and Abnormal Photobiologic Responses*. Tokyo, University of Tokyo Press, pp. 259–283.

U.S. Environmental Protection Agency. 1986. *Air Quality Criteria for Ozone and Other Photochemical Oxidants* (EPA/600/8-84-029AF). Research Triangle Park, NC, U.S. Environmental Protection Agency, Environmental Criteria and Assessment Office.

Age-Related Changes
in the Disposition and Metabolism
of Xenobiotics

Timothy F. McMahon, Ph.D.
Linda S. Birnbaum, Ph.D.

In modern industrial society, there is the potential for human beings to be exposed to a variety of toxicants, discharged into the environment from industrial and chemical manufacturing processes (e.g., dioxins and polyhalogenated biphenyls), present naturally (e.g., radon and ultraviolet light), or given as therapeutic agents (e.g., antineoplastic drugs). The study of the effects on human health of environmental toxicants has been the subject of extensive scientific research, insofar as many of these compounds have been associated with cancer development in humans as well as laboratory animals (Williams and Weisburger, 1986). A central question arising from such studies is the effect of exposure to these compounds on human health over a lifetime, that is, the effects of exposure as they relate to aging. This question is particularly important, because the proportion of the American population age 65 and older is increasing. Thus, regulatory decisions governing the limits of exposure to environmental toxicants should take into consideration the elderly population, who have been shown to manifest increased sensitivity to environmental toxicants (National Research Council, 1987).

Aging was recognized as a significant variable in exposure to xenobiotics in humans as early as 1945 by Stern, Hinds, and Askonas, who noted that elderly humans had an impaired ability to convert benzoic acid to the glycine conjugate hippuric acid. In experimental animals, Kato and co-workers (1964) were first to demonstrate a decreased activity of the hepatic mixed function oxidase system in old rats, introducing the possibility that animals might serve as a model for the study of age-related changes in drug disposition. Since these initial findings, there have been numerous studies aimed at characterizing age-related changes in drug disposition, the findings of which are now contained within several recent reviews Birnbaum, 1987, 1988; Loi and Vestal, 1988; Schmucker, 1985). Important findings include the following: (1) Several physiological and biochemical changes do occur with aging in the mammalian organism, resulting in altered disposition of drugs that may lead to enhanced sensitivity to pharmacological agents in elderly subjects. (2) The process of "normal" aging must be understood in the larger context of "biological" aging, which includes the effects of pathological states, genetic factors, and environmental exposures on the aging process. (3) Age-related differences in drug disposition cannot be due simply to anatomical and physiological changes that occur with "normal" aging (Loi and Vestal, 1988).

It may be speculated that any toxic substance to which people are exposed has the potential for producing an altered response in older humans. However, environmental toxicants, like pharmacological agents, comprise a diverse group of compounds with widely differing chemical and biological properties. Aging does not occur uniformly, especially among humans, which may lead to varied responses from exposure to environmental toxicants, similar to what has been observed with drugs (Loi and Vestal, 1988). Nonetheless, the study of the effects of aging on exposure to xenobiotics should be considered a significant area of research, because exposure to environmental toxicants may take place over an entire lifetime, in contrast to the typical exposure situation with pharmacological agents. Also, in light of the large body of evidence demonstrating altered biotransformation of drugs in aged subjects, it is possible that these changes in enzyme function can affect biotransformation of toxic chemicals, and thus alter the aged organism's susceptibility to exposure. Thus, not only will aging potentially result in alterations in the disposition and metabolism of xenobiotics that may influence toxicity, but these chemicals may have greater potential themselves for altering the aging process than conventional therapeutic agents (Anisimov, 1987). Thus, the purpose of this chapter is to review the available information regarding aging and disposition of environmental toxicants. This is approached by first considering age-related changes in the composition and activities of the xenobiotic metabolizing enzymes of a number of major organ systems. Although extensive work has been done on this subject in liver (for a review, see Birnbaum, 1987), evidence suggests that the biotransformation capability of extrahepatic organs such as the lungs, kidney, skin, and gastrointestinal tract also changes with age (Gram, 1980) and may contribute to the fate of xenobiotics to which the organism is exposed. Although the biotransformation capability of extrahepatic organs is usually limited compared with that of the liver, metabolism of xenobiotics in extrahepatic organs may have important toxicological consequences for that organ (Sipes and Gandolfi, 1986). Thus, age-related alterations in the biotransformation of xenobiotics may lead to changes in the organism's susceptibility to xenobiotic insult.

In contrast to the extensive data on drug disposition and aging (Schmucker, 1985), relatively little has been done with the disposition of environmental toxicants and aging (Birnbaum, 1988). However, dispositional studies on this topic are reviewed in this chapter, as well as studies of age-related changes in xenobiotic metabolizing enzymes that are relevant to this subject. The impact of exposure to environmental chemicals on the aging process is also discussed.

Age-Related Changes in Xenobiotic Metabolizing Enzymes

The hypothesis that age-related alterations in metabolism of drugs and xenobiotics may lead to an altered toxic response has received support in large part from in vitro studies examining the effects of age on the activity and specific molecular components of both the cytochrome P-450 dependent mixed function oxidase (MFO) system, as well as the properties of various Phase II enzymes, using either subcellular fractions or isolated cells from the livers of experimental animals. More recent work has directed attention to age-related changes in metabolism of drugs and xenobiotics in various extrahepatic organs (Gram, 1980) as well as changes in the phospholipid composition of cellular membranes, insofar as cell membrane changes may influence the activity of these enzymes, as well as cellular transport processes (Birnbaum and Baird, 1978). Metabolic activation and/or detoxification of xenobiotics can be considered one of the most important factors influencing the effects of age on susceptibility to xenobiotic insult. Although changes occurring with age in the absorption, distribution, and elimination of xenobiotics will influence the effective dose of xenobiotic reaching the target organ, it is the activity of enzymes responsible for xenobiotic and carcinogen metabolism that determines the level of reactive species produced. This is well illustrated in the area of chemical carcinogenesis through the now established hypothesis (as originally demonstrated by Miller and Miller, 1981) that the carcinogenicity of many compounds is the result of their biotransformation to more reactive species by enzymes present within the organism. This significant discovery has given added impetus to the examination of changes occurring with age in the activity of those enzymes responsible for such biotransformations. Much of what has been gained in this area has been from studies involving experimental animals as aging models. This review discusses results obtained from such studies and the possible implications for humans.

Liver

The majority of studies on aging and biotransformation have concentrated on changes occurring in the enzymatic components and activities of the liver, which is known to be the major site in many organisms for drug and xenobiotic biotransformation. There is evidence for changes in both the activity and content of MFO (Phase I) and Phase II biotransformation enzymes in the liver, as well as for some non-MFO pathways. Age-dependent changes in hepatic Phase I and Phase II biotransformation of drugs and xenobiotics in both humans and experimental animals have been studied extensively and are contained in recent reviews (Birnbaum, 1987; Loi and Vestal, 1988; Schmucker, 1985). Age-dependent alterations in the kinetics of ethoxyresorufin deethylation and aldrin epoxidation in hepatic microsomes (Wynne et al., 1987) as well as changes in the activities of some non-MFO enzymes (Rikans and Moore, 1987) have also been recently examined. The results of these numerous investigations in the liver have shown that age-dependent changes in the biotransformation of drugs and xenobiotics depend on species, strain, and sex of the organism, as well as the substrate. Thus, it is not possible to make broad generalizations concerning the susceptibility of the elderly to xenobiotic insult on the basis of changes in hepatic metabolism alone.

Extrahepatic Organs

There is a growing interest in extrahepatic sites of xenobiotic biotransformation, because xenobiotics can be selectively metabolized in extrahepatic organs to reactive species responsible for organ-specific toxicity. For example, the nitrosamines have been shown to be potent carcinogens for a number of organs, including esophagus, lung, and urinary bladder (Preussmann and Wiessler, 1987). In the esophagus, N-nitrosomethylbenzylamine can be metabolized to a methylating species by a form of cytochrome P-450 found in the esophagus (Preussmann and Wiessler, 1987), while the small intestine has been implicated in the generation of metabolites of N-nitrosodibutylamine that are carcinogenic for the urinary bladder (Richter, Zwickenpflug, and Wiessler, 1988). Extrahepatic sites of biotransformation may thus have toxicological consequences for particular organs and may also produce metabolites that are toxic to other organs.

Lung There have been few studies concerning aging and biotransformation of xenobiotics in lung tissue. The lung is itself an important route of exposure to xenobiotics, because not only can this organ be exposed to xenobiotics by inhalation, but it may also receive exposure from blood-borne metabolites as well. The high blood flow in this organ may also lead to rapid distribution of inhaled toxicants. In addition, the lung is known to contain at least 40 different cell types (Sorokin, 1970). This cellular heterogeneity may result in differential susceptibility of lung tissue to toxic insult, because of variation in the ability of cells to activate and detoxify xenobiotics (Baron et al., 1988).

The few studies on pulmonary xenobiotic metabolism and aging have, like those on the liver, demonstrated differing results. Rabovsky et al. (1984), using lung fractions from young and old male rats, demonstrated a 100 percent increase in the activity of aryl hydrocarbon hydroxylase in old rats. In contrast, Robertson and Birnbaum (1982) reported an 80 percent decrease in activation of the carcinogen 2-aminofluorene by liver microsomes from old rats to mutagenic metabolite(s) using the Ames test, but no effect of age in the activation of 2-acetylaminofluorene by pulmonary homogenates.

Studies of Phase II enzymes in lungs of aged animals are also limited. Using p-nitrophenol (PNP) as substrate, Borghoff and Birnbaum (1985) observed no effect of age on glucuronidation of this compound in lung microsomes from old male Fischer 344 rats. Extensive work by Spearman and Liebman (1983) examined age-related changes in the conjugation of styrene oxide, 1,2-epoxy-3-phenoxypropane, epichlorhydrin, 1,1,1-trichloro-2-propene oxide (TCPO), 1-octene oxide (OCTO), and cyclohexene oxide (CHXO) by glutathione-S-transferase (GST) in pulmonary cytosol from young (2–3 months), middle-aged (11–12 months), and old (23–24 months) male and female F344 rats. In contrast to liver, where substrate specific changes were noted with age, only decreases in OCTO and CHXO conjugation were observed with age in lung cytosol from old males and in OCTO conjugation from old females. Further studies (Spearman and Liebman, 1984a) with the isozyme-specific substrates 1-chloro-2,4-dinitrobenzene (CDNB), 1,2-dichloro-4-nitrobenzene (DCNB), p-nitrobenzyl chloride, and 1,2-epoxy-3-(p-nitrophenoxy)propane in the same tissues also revealed differential age- and sex-related changes in conjugation of these substrates in both tissues. The finding that aging results in differential changes toward isozyme-specific substrates for GST provides evidence for selective age- and sex-related, substrate-specific, and tissue-specific changes in pulmonary GST isozymes. Thus, it is extremely important that specific forms of enzymes involved in xenobiotic biotransformation be examined in aging studies.

The available information on lung biotransformation and aging indicates that, similar to the liver, the metabolic pattern observed with age depends on species of animal and substrate. However, these studies in laboratory animals may not be a good model for the changes that occur with age in this organ, for human lungs are constantly exposed to inhaled pollutants, which likely results in temporary or permanent alteration of biotransformation capability. As specific changes have been observed in inducibility of hepatic biotransformation enzymes in aged animals (Birnbaum, 1987), a similar situation in lung may have important toxicological consequences for inhaled xenobiotics.

Kidney The kidney has been studied for age-related changes in the activities of enzymes involved in the biotransformation of drugs and xenobiotics as well as the relationship of these changes to chemically induce nephrotoxicity. McMartin et al. (1980) examined the levels of cytochrome P-450 and NADPH cytochrome c reductase in kidneys from young and old Wistar rats. An age-related decline was observed in activity of both enzymes, as was a diminished induction of P-450 by β-naphthoflavone in old rats. It was suggested that the diminished induction of P-450 in old rats may have been due to a shift in isozyme composition with age.

A similar age-related decrease in renal P-450 levels was observed by Beierschmitt and Weiner (1986) in aged male Fischer rats. This decrease was observed concomitantly with a decrease in production of the reactive metabolite of APAP by renal MFO in aged rats. However, deacetylation of APAP to the nephrotoxic metabolite p-aminophenol (PAP) was unchanged with age. In contrast to the finding of McMartin et al. (1980), activity of NADPH cytochrome c reductase was found to be unchanged with age in this study, while renal activity of GST (employing CDNB as substrate) declined significantly in aged rats. Thus, an age-related change in the ratio of nephrotoxic metabolites of APAP produced by the kidney was observed, with production of PAP from APAP predominant in aged rats. It is possible that this alteration in production of nephrotoxic metabolites was a contributing factor to the increased nephrotoxicity of APAP observed in aged rats after in vivo administration (Beierschmitt, Keenan, and Weiner, 1986). Pharmacokinetic changes (such as increased delivery of APAP to the kidney) occurring with age were also suggested to play a role. However, increased susceptibility of older male Sprague-Dawley rats to salicylate-induced nephrotoxicity was not due to alterations in either metabolism or elimination of salicylate (Kyle and Kocsis, 1985). There was also no difference in the level of salicylate in kidneys of either 3- or 12-month-old rats.

Other data concerning age-related changes in activity of renal xenobiotic metabolizing enzymes are limited, and involve mainly the activities of Phase II pathways. Borghoff and Birnbaum (1985) observed an age-related decline in vitro of glucuronyltransferase activity in kidney microsomes from male Fischer rats using PNP as substrate, while activity of β-glucuronidase in this organ increased with age, suggesting a shift toward deglucuronidation with age in this organ. Kyle and Kocsis (1985) observed decreased production of salicyluric acid from salicylate in vivo in 12-month-old Sprague-Dawley rats as compared with 3-month-old rats, while McMahon, Diliberto, and Birnbaum (1989) did not observe any age-related decrease in formation of hippuric acid in vivo after oral administration of benzyl acetate to either male Fischer rats ages 4, 9, and 25 months or male C57BL/6N mice ages 13 and 25 months. The significance of these findings concerning glycine conjugation remains to be determined, because although the kidney is regarded as a prominent site of glycine conjugation in vivo (Huckle, Tait, and Millburn, 1981), this Phase II process involves activation of the substrate to an acetyl-CoA intermediate prior to reaction with glycine, and there is no clear evidence to indicate whether changes occur in either enzymatic step with age.

Skin   Metabolism of both endogenous substances and xenobiotics has been demonstrated in skin from experimental animals (Mukhtar, Athar, and Bickers, 1987; Storm, Stewart, and Bronaugh, 1988). Although no studies are presently available on age-related changes in skin metabolism, data are available on age-related changes in susceptibility of experimental animals to skin carcinogenesis. In general, the results of studies on aging and skin carcinogenesis in mice indicate that young (2–4 months) animals appear to be more sensitive to chemically induced skin carcinogenesis than mature (12–13 months) animals, and old (more than 20 months) animals display enhanced sensitivity compared with mature animals (Anisimov, 1987). It is possible that this pattern is related to changes that occur in the mitotic activity of skin with age, for cell proliferation and renewal in mouse skin is significantly decreased between 3 and 19 months of age (Cameron and Thrasher, 1976). Investigation of the relationship of this pattern to changes in skin metabolism of carcinogens might prove to be fruitful.

Intestines   Little data have appeared regarding the effects of age on the drug metabolism system of the gastrointestinal tract. In a study by Sun and Strobel (1986), microsomal fractions of liver, lungs, kidney cortex, and colon from male Sprague-Dawley rats ages 2, 4, 10, 24, and 78 weeks were examined for total cytochrome P-450 content, cytochrome P-450 reductase activity, and benzo(a)pyrene hydroxylase (BPOH) activity. In liver microsomes from 24- and 78-week-old rats,

BPOH activity was decreased 50 percent, whereas in colon microsomes, BPOH showed little change in activity with age. In addition, the induction of BPOH in liver by administration of phenobarbital/hydrocortisone showed a pattern with age similar to BPOH activity in liver microsomes from untreated rats, whereas in colon microsomes from 78-week-old treated rats BPOH activity increased 12-fold. Interestingly, the changes in BPOH activity observed with age in both liver and colon from phenobarbital/hydrocortisone-treated rats paralleled the alterations in content of the isozyme of P-450 responsible for benzo(a)pyrene metabolism in these organs, with an 80 percent increase observed in the level of this isozyme in the colon.

The work of McMahon, Beierschmitt, and Weiner (1987) extended these results by demonstrating that several Phase I biotransformation reactions in the large intestine (including BPOH, β-glucuronidase, and alcohol dehydrogenase) were maintained in male Fischer rats up to 24 months of age. Activity of BPOH was also found to be unchanged with age in the small intestine of these same rats.

Using human autopsy tissue 3–7 hr postmortem, Newaz, Fang, and Strobel (1983) examined the metabolism of 1,2-dimethylhydrazine (1,2-DMH) in microsomes isolated from ascending, transverse, and descending segments of human colon. Although the monooxygenase components of human colon were not characterized in this study, it was found that metabolism of 1,2-DMH was considerably higher in colon microsomes from older individuals and displayed a gradient of activity in all tissue samples, increasing from ascending to descending colon. The trend for increased colonic metabolism of 1,2-DMH in older humans and increased colonic BPOH activity in older rats (McMahon, Beierschmitt, and Weiner, 1987; Sun, Lau, and Strobel, 1986) is consistent with findings of an age-related increase in tumor incidence observed in the colon of both humans (Baranovsky and Myers, 1986) and animals (Anisimov, 1983), and suggests that age-related changes in biotransformation capability within the large intestine may be an important factor in the development of cancer in this organ.

Limited work has also appeared on age-related changes in the Phase II conjugation capacity of the gastrointestinal tract. Borghoff and Birnbaum (1985) found no effect of age on small intestinal glucuronyltransferase activity in male Fischer rats, while McMahon, Beierschmitt, and Weiner (1987) found significant age-related declines in the activities of colonic glucuronyltransferase (using PNP as substrate) and GST (using CDNB as substrate) in this same strain of rat. Weiner, McMahon, and Centra (1988) examined the Phase II metabolism of methylazoxymethanol (MAM) to a glucuronide conjugate using colon microsomes from various age groups of Fischer rats. MAM noncompetitively inhibited glucuronidation of 4-methylumbelliferone (4-MU), which rose significantly in 12- and 24-month-old rats. This increase in 4-MU glucuronyltransferase activity, which was postulated to be involved in detoxification of MAM, was associated with an age-related decrease in tumorigenicity of azoxymethane, the metabolic precursor of MAM. Because the gastrointestinal tract can be continually exposed to xenobiotics through ingestion, the increase in glucuronyltransferase enzyme activity with age might represent an adaptation of the large intestine to xenobiotic insult. No firm evidence exists for the conjugation of MAM by glucuronyltransferase. Thus, this line of inquiry requires further investigation.

Age-Related Changes in Enzymes Involved in Defense against Prooxidants

In addition to the numerous Phase I and Phase II biotransformation reactions among the various tissues and organs that are typically associated with activation and detoxification of xenobiotics, there is another important class of enzymes within the mammalian organism. These enzymes are involved with protecting cells and tissues against damage by prooxidants, that is, reactive oxygen metabolites or molecular oxygen generated from cellular metabolic processes or as a result of biotransformation of xenobiotics. These enzymes include catalase, superoxide dismutase (SOD), and glutathione peroxidase (GSH-PX). Because of the inherent reactivity of radical oxygen species, it is difficult to study their production directly. Thus, studies of the aged organism's ability to cope with oxidative stress have been inferred from examination of those enzymes involved in defense against such stress. Oxidative stress has been proposed to contribute to the process of aging itself (Emanuel, 1976), as well as the development of cancer (Cotgreave, Moldeus, and Orrenius, 1988). However, research in this area has not received a great deal of attention, and conflicting results have been obtained regarding the ability of aged organisms to cope with oxidative stress.

Radojicic et al. (1987) examined hepatic SOD activity in male Mill Hill hooded rats ages 3, 12, 18, and 30 months after pretreatment with either diethyldithiocarbamate (DDC), an inhibitor of SOD activity, or cycloheximide, alone and in combination with DDC. A significant age-related decline was observed in liver SOD in untreated rats age 30 months versus other age groups studied. Treatment with DDC produced significant inhibition of SOD activity in all age groups, but was greatest in 18- and 30-month-old rats, whereas cycloheximide in combination with DDC potentiated its effects in adult (12 months) but not old rats. From the additional observation that 30-month-old rats treated with DDC showed reduced incorporation of a labeled amino acid mixture into liver cytosol protein compared with 3-month-old rats, the suggestion was made that the capacity for liver SOD synthesis was reduced in old rats.

Imre and Juhasz (1987) examined the effect of H_2O_2 administration on the activities of hepatic SOD, catalase, and lipid peroxidation in female BALB/c mice ages 12 and 25 months. Whereas no age-related difference was noted in activity of SOD in untreated mice (in contrast to that observed by Radojicic et al., 1987), an age-related decline in catalase as well as lipid peroxidation capacity was observed in untreated 25-month-old mice. Administration of a high dose of H_2O_2 (0.5 percent in drinking water for 2 months) resulted in significantly greater inducibility of catalase and lipid peroxidation in 3-month-old mice compared with 25-month-old mice, suggesting a decline in inducibility of these enzymes in aged mice. However, SOD activity was found to be induced to a greater extent in 25-month-old mice than 3-month-old mice following this treatment. Inducibility of catalase and SOD by H_2O_2 may in part explain the increased catalase and GSH-PX activity found in heart mitochondrial preparations from 24-month-old male Wistar rats versus 3-month-old rats, inasmuch as aging may result in increased levels of H_2O_2 and lipid peroxides (Nohl, Hegner, and Summer, 1979).

The diminished inducibility of lipid peroxidation observed by Imre and Juhasz (1987) is interesting in light of work by Videla, Fernandez, and Valenzuela (1987), who demonstrated decreased thiobarbituric acid content (an index of lipid peroxidation) in 12-month-old Wistar rats in response to acute ethanol administration, a known inducer of hepatic lipid peroxidation. These studies would seem to suggest that although defense against oxidative stress is altered in the liver with aging, the oxidative activity of the liver is also diminished in older animals. However, Langaniere and Yu (1987) observed that enzymatically or nonenzymatically induced malondialdehyde production was 35–40 percent higher in hepatic mitochondria and microsomes from old Fischer rats compared with young adult rats. Thus, the question of a reduced capacity of aged organisms to adapt to oxidative stress as well as the possible age-related decrease in hepatic oxidative capacity is still unanswered.

The selenoenzyme GSH-PX has also been investigated for age-related changes in liver, kidney, heart, and large intestine of rats and mice. Selenium-dependent and -independent GSH-PX activity was observed to decline significantly in liver from middle-aged and old female Swiss-Webster mice (S. J. Stohs, unpublished data) as well as in old male C57BL/6J mice (Hazelton and Lang, 1985). In contrast, no significant changes were observed in either the relative amounts or the activities of both Form I (selenium dependent) and Form II (selenium independent) of this enzyme in kidney cytosol from older male Fischer 344 rats (Beierschmitt, 1986). However, kidney GSH-PX activity was observed to decline in old male C57BL/6J mice (Hazelton and Lang, 1985). In addition, a trend toward decreasing activity with age was observed in Form II of GSH-PX in large intestine of male Fischer rats (McMahon, Beierschmitt, and Weiner, 1987). The activity of Form II was also noted to be significantly lower than that of Form I in this organ. GSH-PX activity in heart mitochondria, by contrast, was found to increase in 24-month-old male Wistar rats as compared with 3-month-old rats (Nohl, Hegner, and Summer, 1979), and no selenium-independent GSH-PX activity was detected in this organ.

In addition to enzymatic defense against tissue oxidation, several small endogenous compounds may also serve as antioxidants, including the nucleophilic tripeptide glutathione (GSH), uric acid, and ascorbic acid. Changes with age in levels of GSH have been examined in liver of both rats and mice, with reports of either an increase (Birnbaum and Baird, 1979; Borghoff and Birnbaum, 1986) no change (Rikans and Kosanke, 1984; Spearman and Liebman, 1984b) or a decrease (Stohs and Lawson, 1986). Examination of GSH levels in extrahepatic tissues such as kidney (Beierschmitt and Weiner, 1986), colon (McMahon, Beierschmitt, and Weiner, 1987), lung, heart, brain, testis, and lens (Rikans and Moore, 1988) of rats has shown no significant age-related changes except in lens, where the concentration of GSH declined by almost 50 percent between 15 and 26 months of age in male Fischer rats. However, in mice, content of kidney, heart, small intestine, and blood GSH were reported to decline with age (Rikans and Moore, 1988). Thus, age-related changes in GSH content appear to be species- and tissue-dependent, similar to that found for metabolism of xenobiotics. A decrease in the level of GSH may make tissues more sensitive to injury by free radicals and reactive oxygen species, resulting in enhanced tissue damage (Stohs and Lawson, 1986). No studies are available on the enzymes of GSH synthesis in aged animals, although activity of gamma-glutamyl-transferase has been shown to increase markedly between 2 and 10 weeks in male Sprague-Dawley rats (Gregus, Stein, and Klaassen, 1987). Tissue concentrations of ascorbic acid have been reported to decline with age in liver, lung, and lens of aged Fischer rats, while the concentration of uric acid was reported to decline only in liver (Rikans and Moore, 1988). The concentration of uric acid rose with age in heart, kidney, and testis (Rikans and Moore, 1988).

Consequences of Aging and Exposure to Xenobiotics

The accumulated evidence on aging and exposure to environmental toxicants has led to the development and investigation of three major hypotheses: (1) Age-related alterations in the metabolism of xenobiotics might contribute to the increased incidence of cancer observed with age. (2) Certain other diseases associated with aging, such as atherosclerosis and rheumatoid arthritis, may be the result of the activation of toxic chemicals by cytochromes P-448. (3) Environmental toxicants (particularly carcinogens) may accelerate the aging process.

That age-related changes in activation and detoxification of chemical carcinogens might play a role in the increased incidence of cancer observed in the elderly was first tested by Baird and Birnbaum (1979), who examined the degree of reversion in *Salmonella typhimurium* induced by incubating benzo(a)pyrene and 2-aminofluorene with liver S9 fractions from senescent male CFN rats and C57BL/6J mice. S9 fractions from both senescent rats and mice were more effective in producing his^+ revertants than their younger counterparts, indicating increased production of mutagenic metabolites in older animals. Other studies using the Ames test (e.g., Birmbaum, 1987) have reported either decreases in mutagenicity with age or, in kidney and lung tissue extracts, no age-related change in carcinogen activation. Thus, Baird and Birnbaum (1979) reported an increase in 2-aminofluorene mutagenicity using liver homogenates from male Wistar rats, while Robertson and Birnbaum (1982) reported a decrease in activation of this carcinogen using liver extracts from female Long-Evans rats. This evidence would suggest that the changes in mutagenicity observed with age are dependent on the species and strain of rodent from which the liver fractions were made. Thus, age-related alterations in biotransformation of xenobiotics may under certain circumstances play a role in the increased incidence of cancer observed in elderly subjects.

While age-related changes in the metabolism of chemical carcinogens have been found to be only one facet of many contributing to the age-associated rise in tumor incidence, the relationship between biotransformation of toxic compounds and certain other disease states associated with aging has recently been explored (Ioannides and Parke, 1987). This hypothesis is based on evidence that cytochromes P-448 specifically oxygenate chemical carcinogens in sterically hindered positions, resulting in the formation of reactive intermediates that are poorly detoxified. In contrast, the oxygenation of substrates by cytochromes P-450 occurs at sterically unhindered positions, which results in conjugation and detoxification (Ioannides and Parke, 1987). Thus, damage to tissue resulting in carcinogenesis or other pathological states is most likely to result from activation via the cytochrome P-448 pathway.

The association of these disease states with cytochromes P-448 is supported experimentally by the work of Paigen et al. (1986), who demonstrated that an Ah-responsive strain of mouse, AKXL-38a, was more susceptible to 3-methylcholanthrene-induced atherosclerosis than an Ah-nonresponsive strain, AKXL-38. This susceptibility was found to segregate with the Ah locus, further establishing the role of cytochromes P-448 in the production of this disease. It would be of practical importance to determine age-related changes in cytochrome(s) P-448 and to identify potential high-risk populations or individuals if this hypothesis is to be substantiated.

The ability of carcinogens and other environmental toxicants to decrease the life span is a well-established phenomenon (Anisimov, 1987; Cory-Slechta, 1988; Massie, 1985) and has often been considered an acceleration of the aging process. When the experimental data concerning changes in biochemical parameters that occur with age are compared with those changes that take place as a result of exposure to xenobiotics, a close similarity is indeed found (Anisimov, 1987). This supports the idea that chemical carcinogens (and possibly other toxicants) may act in such a manner as to accelerate normal age-related changes in organ function. However, acceleration of aging may not occur under conditions of low-level exposure, as suggested from a study by Stenbeck, Weisburger, and Williams (1988) involving the lifetime treatment of mice with 2-diaminoethanol.

Age-Related Changes in Disposition of Xenobiotics

Organisms may come into contact with xenobiotics by similar routes as for drugs, that is, through ingestion, inhalation, or absorption through the skin. It is evident that age might alter the disposition and toxicity of xenobiotics through exposure by one or all of these routes, as has been clearly demonstrated for therapeutic agents (Loi and Vestal, 1988; Schmucker, 1985). In fact, there is evidence to indicate that certain physiologic properties of many of the organs and tissues relevant to xenobiotic exposure may undergo alterations such that older organisms face a different exposure situation than their younger counterparts. The relevance of this statement may be illustrated by mentioning certain "experiments of nature" in which large numbers of humans were accidentally exposed to one or more environmental toxicants. Of those exposed, it was found that elderly persons were the most susceptible to the adverse effects of these toxicants (National Research Council, 1987). Given the large number of pollutants and carcinogens present in the environment, it is important to assess the biological impact of exposure to these agents in elderly people.

In assessing the elderly population's susceptibility to xenobiotics, it is understood that aging is not a uniform process, even among inbred strains of laboratory animals. In addition, the inherent biological processes within the organism that change during the life span contribute only partly to the total process termed "aging." How the organism interacts with its environment as well as the exposure situations can affect the process of aging, because it is clear that the environment and the contaminants it contains have a major impact on the general health of the organism and, potentially, its life span.

Many studies are available on the developmental toxicity of a number of environmental compounds (Calabrese, 1986), and the following review of the disposition of environmental toxicants in aged subjects is limited only by lack of available data in this area. It is noteworthy that the majority of compounds investigated in old animals have demonstrated increased toxicity, similar to what has been found in humans. However, there is a need for future research in this area.

Environmental Pollutants

Polychlorinated dibenzo-p-dioxins, dibenzofurans, and biphenyls (PCB) are recognized as widespread environmental contaminants (Kimbrough, 1980) and have been the subject of extensive research because these compounds are among the most potent and/or persistent environmental toxicants known to humans (Williams and Weisburger, 1986). Yet the study of the relationship of aging to the disposition and toxicity of these agents has not been extensive, and only a few reports are available for review in this area.

Birnbaum (1983) examined the distribution and excretion of 2,3,6,2',3',6'-hexachlorobiphenyl (236; a readily metabolized PCB congener) and 2,4,5,2',4',5'-hexachlorobiphenyl (245; a poorly metabolized PCB congener) in senescent (24 months) Sprague-Dawley rats. When compared with earlier disposition data on the same compounds in young Sprague-Dawley rats (Matthews and Anderson, 1975; Matthews and Tuey, 1980) conducted at the same laboratory under identical conditions, both age groups readily metabolized and excreted the 236 isomer, whereas 245 was poorly metabolized and persisted in the tissues of both age groups. However, enhanced retention of metabolites of both 245 and 236 occurred in the muscle and skin of senescent animals. In addition, the percentage of the total dose of both PCB isomers was greater in senescent animals than the young at all time points following administration of the compounds, with 50 percent more of the dose of 236 in adipose tissue of senescent rats at the peak of 236 accumulation. Thus, senescent animals tended to excrete both PBC isomers more slowly than young animals and retain the metabolites in tissues to a greater degree. These changes were consistent with both an increased content of body fat and decreased tissue blood flow in senescent animals (Birnbaum, 1983).

The results of this study are in good agreement with prior work by Schumann, Fox, and Watanabe (1982) on the disposition of inhaled methyl chloroform when given repeatedly to mice and rats for 6 hr/day, 5 days/week, over a period of 16 months. Long-term exposure of mice and rats to methyl chloroform did not significantly alter the disposition of this compound when results were compared with acutely exposed age-matched controls. However, in comparison with acutely exposed young animals, old animals demonstrated significant increases in both body burden of methyl chloroform and decreased pulmonary elimination of this compound.

The results of these two studies may be indicative of physiologic alterations occurring with age, such that older animals are inherently more susceptible to the adverse effects of exposure to environmental toxicants. This is supported by the studies of both Chadwick and Copeland (1985) on the metabolism of lindane in various age groups of mice and Bell, Hitte, and Mazze (1975) on the disposition of methoxyflurane in rats. In both of these studies, the toxicity of these compounds was found to be greater in old animals as the result of alterations in disposition. Specifically, changes in percentage of body fat occurring with age were felt to be responsible for increased tissue storage and decreased elimination of lindane and methoxyflurane from older animals. It is conceivable that the disposition of other lipophilic xenobiotics may show a similar pattern in old animals.

The observation that lipophilic toxicants such as 2,3,7,8-tetrachlorodibenzo-p-dioxin (TCDD) and PCBs may be retained for a longer period of time in the tissues of older animals could affect the toxicity of these compounds. Thus, in a study by Lubet et al. (1986), the suppression of the plaque-forming response (a measure of immune competence) by acute administration of 3,4,5,3',4',5'-hexabromobiphenyl to B6C3F$_1$ mice was much more severe in old (72 weeks) than in young (8 weeks) mice. Given that thymic atrophy is known to occur naturally with age (Lubet et al., 1986), it might be expected that exposure of older individuals to polybrominated biphenyls and related compounds would cause more severe suppression of immune function, given the natural age-related decline in immune competence and the suspected age-related alterations in disposition of halogenated hydrocarbons.

The toxicological implications of enhanced retention of xenobiotics in older subjects may also be applied to the area of carcinogenesis.

For example, evidence from in vitro cell culture experiments as well as from examination of the mitotic and DNA synthesizing index in tissues of aged animals has shown that proliferative activity of many tissues declines with age (Anisimov, 1987). Proliferative activity of tissues is one of the leading factors responsible for tissue sensitivity to carcinogens, and there are ample data on the enhancement of carcinogenesis caused by stimulation of proliferation (Anisimov, 1987). Experiments performed in rat liver to assess age-related changes in response to proliferative stimulu have shown that this response appears to be diminished in old animals (Anisimov, 1987). This may explain in part the reduced incidence of liver tumors found in old (12–14 months) versus young (1 month) partially hepatectomized rats treated with 1,2-DMH. An age-related diminution of response to proliferative stimuli has also been found to occur in rat mesenterium, as well as in human lymphocytes in culture (Anisimov, 1987). However, some tissues in senescent individuals may demonstrate enhanced proliferative activity (Anisimov, 1987). Thus, an altered response to proliferative stimuli (such as carcinogens) may occur in older individuals, but further work is needed with specific tissues and carcinogens to determine the significance of these changes and their implications for chemically induced neoplasia in elderly persons.

In terms of age-related alterations in absorption of the dibenzo-p-dioxins and related compounds, Hebert and Birnbaum (1987) examined intestinal absorption of TCDD in male Fischer rats ages 13 weeks, 13 months, and 26 months using an isolated intestinal perfusion procedure. Although an increase was found in the relative weight of intestinal mucosa in the 26-month-old rats, there was no significant age-related difference in the intestinal absorption of TCDD when expressed as either nanogram of TCDD absorbed per gram of body weight per hour or as nanogram of TCDD absorbed per gram of intestinal dry weight per hour. However, in 13-week-old rats, the rate of absorption of 245 was found to be enhanced by simultaneous perfusion of TCDD. Because 245 is essentially completely absorbed even in the absence of TCDD (Hebert and Birnbaum, 1987), the effect of TCDD must be to increase the rate of intestinal absorption of 245. Thus, as concluded for other compounds that are absorbed by diffusion (Hebert and Birnbaum, 1987), aging has no significant effect on intestinal absorption of TCDD. In contrast, a decrease was found with age in the dermal absorption of 2,3,4,7,8-pentachlorodibenzofuran, a potent promoter of hepatic carcinogenesis (Banks, Brewster, and Birnbaum, 1990).

Only one study is available on age-related differences in toxicity of inhaled pollutants using old animals. Stiles and Tyler (1988) studied the influence of age on morphological changes in lungs of female Sprague-

Dawley rats ages 60 and 444 days exposed to 0.35 or 0.8 ppm ozone. Although the ozone-induced lesions were qualitatively similar in younger and older rats, there was a twofold difference in the proportion of lung involvement after similar exposures, with the larger proportion of lesions in younger rats. Several explanations were put forth to explain this difference, but the question of the relative susceptibility of various populations to ozone has not been adequately studied. In general, further investigation into the susceptibility of older animals to inhaled pollutants would seem warranted in light of recent evidence demonstrating a decreased antibody response in lungs of aged (22–26 monihs) male Fischer rats to challenge with influenza vaccine (Ganguly, Desai, and Khakoo, 1988).

Industrial Chemicals

Although there are a plethora of industrial chemicals present in today's environment, only limited work has addressed the toxicity of industrial chemicals in older animals. Ghanayem et al. (1987) examined the effect of age on toxicity and metabolism of ethylene glycol monobutyl ether (BE), a widely used industrial solvent that primarily affects the hematopoietic system of rats, resulting in acute hemolytic anemia. Pathological changes are also observed in liver and kidney as secondary effects. In this study, adult (9–13 weeks) male Fischer rats were found to be more sensitive to the hemolytic and secondary pathological effects of BE than young (4–5 weeks) rats. Examination of the kinetics of BE elimination in plasma of 3- and 12-month-old rats (Ghanayem et al., 1990) showed that half-life for BE was unchanged with age, but area under the curve and maximal plasma concentration were significantly higher for butoxyacetic acid, a toxic metabolite of BE, in 12-month-old rats. It was suggested that compromised urinary elimination rather than alterations in metabolism of BE was responsible for the alterations in kinetics observed in older rats. This phenomenon may explain the increased sensitivity of older rats to the hematotoxic effects of BE (Ghanayem et al., 1987).

The metabolism and toxicity of 4,4'-thiobis(6-t-butyl-m-cresol) (TBBC), a high-production-volume antioxidant used in the plastics and rubber industry, has also been investigated (Borghoff, Stefanski, and Birnbaum, 1988). TBBC is primarily conjugated with glucuronic acid (UDPGA) without prior oxidation, and was employed in this study to determine whether changes in conjugation and excretion of TBBC would alter the toxic response in older animals. Thus, glucuronidation of TBBC was assessed both in vivo and in vitro in male Fischer 344 rats ages 2.5, 16, and 26 months, and hepatic UDPGA levels were also measured. Toxicity was determined by administration of TBBC at 0.25

percent in feed to these same age groups of rats for 14 days. In vivo, the percentage of TBBC-derived radioactivity eliminated in feces declined in 26-month-old rats compared with 2.5- and 16-month-old rats. In addition, the percentage of an administered dose excreted as a monoglucuronide also declined as a function of age, which was in good agreement with an observed decline in TBBC glucuronidation in vitro in hepatic microsomes. There was no age-related change in toxicity to animals given TBBC in feed, with the exception that in 26-month-old rats, there was an increase in the incidence and severity of leukemia over the expected incidence. The apparent ability of TBBC to precipitate the onset of leukemia and/or shorten the latency period for development of this disease merits further investigation.

Anesthetics

As already mentioned, the disposition of methoxyflurane in old animals is altered such that this age group may be more susceptible to the nephrotoxic effects of this anesthetic. The toxicity of 2,2,2-trifluoroethanol (TFE), a metabolite of various anesthetics, also appears to be greater in old animals, as determined in a histological study by Kim and Kaminsky (1988) using 36-month-old male Wistar rats. In these animals, TFE was administered by intraperitoneal injection once a week for 5 weeks at a dose of 100 mg/kg of body weight. Compared with young rats (4–6 months), TFE produced more advanced degenerative changes in a number of organs of 36-month-old rats, including liver, testicle, stomach, kidneys, spleen, urinary bladder, and brain. However, there was no clear explanation for this age-related change in toxicity, and thus the delineation of the mechanism(s) of TFE-mediated toxicity requires further study.

Conclusions

Experimental evidence has shown that physiological changes occurring with age can result in alterations of xenobiotic disposition, such that the toxicity of xenobiotics may be altered in older individuals. The realization of these physiological changes has already led to more individualized (and thus more effective) dosing regimens of therapeutic agents for elderly people. Exposure to environmental agents, however, may occur under less controlled conditions and with more serious consequences. Although research on the effects of environmental toxicants in aged subjects is far from complete, it is reasonable to suggest that at present, aged persons are likely to be more susceptible to the deleterious effects of xenobiotics (National Research Council, 1987).

There is a need for further study of the effects on elderly persons of exposure to environmental toxicants. Although we know how some of the changes in physiological functions that occur with age can affect drug and xenobiotic disposition, we know less about how these changes affect the disposition of specific compounds, and the implications for toxicity in elderly individuals.

References

Anisimov, V. 1983. Carcinogenesis and aging. *Advances in Cancer Research* 40:365–424.

Anisimov, V. N. 1987. *Carcinogenesis and Aging* (Vol. 2). Boco Raton, FL: CRC Press.

Baird, M. B., and Birnbaum, L. S. 1979. Increased production of mutagenic metabolites of carcinogens by tissues from senescent rats. *Cancer Research* 39:4752–4755.

Banks, Y. B., Brewster, D. W., and Birnbaum, L. S. 1990. Age-related changes in dermal absorption of 2,3,7,8-tetrachlorodibenzo-p-dioxin and 2,3,4,7,8-pentachlorodibenzofuran. *Fundamental and Applied Toxicology* 15:163–173.

Baranovsky, A., and Myers, M. H. 1986. Cancer incidence and survival in patients 65 years of age and older. *Cancer Journal for Clinicians* 36:26–41.

Baron, J., Burke, J. P., Guengerich, F. P., Jakoby, W. B., and Voigt, J. M. 1988. Sites for xenobiotic activation and detoxication within the respiratory tract: Implications for chemically induced toxicity. *Toxicology and Applied Pharmacology* 93:493–505.

Beierschmitt, W. P. 1986. Age-related changes in renal metabolism of acetaminophen and their relationship to toxicity. Doctoral dissertation, University of Maryland at Baltimore.

Beierschmitt, W. P., Keenan, K. P., and Weiner, M. 1986. Age-related increased susceptibility of male Fischer 344 rats to acetaminophen nephrotoxicity. *Life Sciences* 39:2335–2342.

Beierschmitt, W. P., and Weiner, M. 1986. Age-related changes in renal metabolism of acetaminophen in male Fischer 344 rats. *Age* 9:7–13.

Bell, L. E., Hitt, B. A., and Mazze, R. I. 1975. The influence of age on the distribution, metabolism, and excretion of methoxyflurane in Fischer 344 rats: A possible relationship to nephrotoxicity. *Journal of Pharmacology and Experimental Therapeutics* 195:34–40.

Birnbaum, L. S. 1983. Distribution and excretion of 2,3,6,2,3',6'- and 2,4,5,2',4',5'-hexachlorobiphenyl in senescent rats. *Toxicology and Applied Pharmacology* 70:262–272.

Birnbaum, L. S. 1987. Age-related changes in carcinogen metabolism. *Journal of the American Geriatric Society* 35:51–60.

Birnbaum, L. S. 1988. Age-related changes in drug disposition. In Zenser, T. V., and Coe, R. M. (Eds.), New York, Springer-Verlag, pp. 125–138.

Birnbaum, L. S., and Baird, M. B. 1978. Induction of hepatic mixed function oxidases in senescent rodents: II. Effect of polychlorinated biophenyls. *Experimental Gerontology* 13:469–477.

Birnbaum, L. S., and Baird, M. B. 1979. Senescent changes in rodent hepatic epoxide metabolism. *Chemico-Biological Interactions* 26:245–256.

Borghoff, S. J., and Birnbaum, L. S. 1985. Age-related changes in glucuronidation and deglucuronidation in liver, small intestine, lung, and kidney of male Fischer-344 rats. *Drug Metabolism and Disposition* 13:62–67.

Borghoff, S. J., and Birnbaum, L. S. 1986. Age-related changes in the metabolism and excretion of allyl isothiocyanate. *Drug Metabolism and Disposition* 14:417–422.

Borghoff, S. J., Stefanski, S. A., and Birnbaum, L. S. 1988. The effect of age on the glucuronidation and toxicity of 4,4′-thiobis(6-t-butyl-m cresol). *Toxicology and Applied Pharmacology* 92:453–466.

Calabrese, E. J. 1986. *Age and Susceptibility to Toxic Substances*. New York, John Wiley and Sons.

Cameron, I. L., and Thrasher, J. D. 1976. Cell renewal and cell loss in the tissues of aging mammals. In Cutler, R. G. (Ed.), *Interdisciplinary Topics in Gerontology*. Basel, Karger, pp. 108–129.

Chadwick, R. W., and Copeland, M. F. 1985. Effects of age and obesity on the metabolism of lindane by black a/a, yellow A^{vy}/a, and pseudoagouti A^{vy}/a phenotypes of (ys × vy) F_1 hybrid mice. *Journal of Toxicology and Environmental Health* 16:771–796.

Cory-Slechta, D. A. 1988. Heightened vulnerability to lead during advanced age (abstract). *Toxicologist* 8:22.

Cotgreave, I. A., Moldeus, P., and Orrenius, S. 1988. Host biochemical defense mechanisms against prooxidants. *Annual Review of Pharmacology and Toxicology* 28:189–212.

Emanuel, N. M. 1976. Free radicals and the action of inhibitors of radical processes under pathological states and ageing in living organisms and in man. *Quarterly Review of Biophysics* 9:283–308.

Ganguly, R., Desai, U., and Khakoo, R. 1988. Lung defenses in aging: Responses to influenza vaccine and inflammatory stimuli. *Age* 11:15–18.

Ghanayem, B. I., Blair, P. C., Thompson, M. B., Maronpot, R. R., and Matthews, H. B. 1987. Effect of age on the toxicity and metabolism of ethylene glycol monobutyl ether (2-butoxyethanol) in rats. *Toxicology and Applied Pharmacology* 91:222–234.

Ghanayem, B. I., Sanders, J. M., Clark, A., Bailer, J., and Matthews, H. W. 1990. Effects of dose, age, inhibition of metabolism and elimination on the toxicokinetics of 2-butoxyethanol and its metabolites. *Journal of Pharmacology and Experimental Therapeutics* 253(1):136–143.

Gram, T. E. 1980. *Extrahepatic Metabolism of Drugs and Other Foreign Compounds*. New York, SP Medical and Scientific Books.

Gregus, Z., Stein, A. F., and Klaassen, C. D. 1987. Age-dependent biliary excretion of glutathione-related thiols in rats: Role of gamma-glutamyltransferase. *American Journal of Physiology* 253:686–692.

Hazelton, G. A., and Lang, C. A. 1985. Glutathione peroxidase and reductase activities in the aging mouse. *Mechanisms of Ageing and Development* 29:71–81.

Hebert, C. D., and Birnbaum, L. S. 1987. The influence of aging on intestinal absorption of TCDD in rats. *Toxicology Letters* 37:47–55.

Huckle, H. R., Tait, G. H., and Millburn, P. 1981. Species variations in the renal and hepatic conjugation of 3-phenoxybenzoic acid with glycine. *Xenobiotia* 11:635–644.

Imre, S., and Juhasz, E. 1987. The effect of oxidative stress on inbred mice of different ages. *Mechanisms of Ageing and Development* 38:259–266.

Ioannides, C., and Parke, D. V. 1987. The cytochromes P-448—a unique family of enzymes involved in chemical toxicity and carcinogenesis. *Biochemical Pharmacology* 36:4197–4207.

Kato, R., Vassanelli, P., Frontino, G., and Chiesara, E. 1964. Variation in the activity of liver microsomal drug-metabolizing enzymes in rats in relation to age. *Biochemical Pharmacology* 13:1037–1051.

Kim, J. C. S., and Kaminsky, L. S. 1988. 2,2,2-triflouroethanol toxicity in aged rats. *Toxicologic Pathology* 16:35–45.

Kimbrough, R. D. 1980. Environmental pollution of air, water, soil. In Kimbrough, R. D. (Ed.), *Halogenated Biphenyls, Terphenyls, Naphthalenes, Dibenzodioxins and Related Products.* Amsterdam, Elsevier/North-Holland, pp. 77–80.

Kyle, M. E., and Kocsis, J. J. 1985. The effect of age on salicylate-induced nephrotoxicity in male rats. *Toxicology and Applied Pharmacology* 81:337–347.

Langaniere, S., and Yu, B. P. 1987. Anti-lipoperoxidation action of food restriction. *Biochemical and Biophysical Research Communications* 45: 1185–1191.

Loi, C. M., and Vestal, R. E. 1988. Drug metabolism in the elderly. *Pharmacology and Therapeutics* 36:131–149.

Lubet, R. A., Lemaire, B. N., Avery, D., and Kouri, R. E. 1986. Induction of immunotoxicity in mice by polyhalogenated biphenyls. *Archives of Toxicology* 59:71–77.

Massie, H. R., Williams, T. R., and Aiello, V. R. 1985. Excess dietary aluminum increases drosophila's rate of aging. *Gerontology* 37:309–314.

Matthews, H. B., and Anderson, M. W. 1975. Effect of chlorination on the distribution and excretion of polychlorinated biphenyls. *Drug Metabolism and Disposition* 3:371–380.

Matthews, H. B., and Tuey, D. B. 1980. The effect of chlorine position on the distribution and excretion of four hexachlorobiphenyl isomers. *Toxicology and Applied Pharmacology* 53:377–388.

McMahon, T. F., Diliberto, J. J., and Birnbaum, L. S. 1989. Age-related changes in the disposition of benzyl acetate: A model compound for glycine conjugation. *Drug Metabolism and Disposition* 17:506–512.

McMahon, T. F., Beierschmitt, W. P., and Weiner, M. 1987. Changes in phase I and phase II biotransformation pathways with age in male Fischer 344 rat colon: Relationship to colon carcinogenesis. *Cancer Letters* 36:273–282.

McMartin, D. N., O'Connor, J. A., Fasco, M. J., and Kaminsky, L. S. 1980. Influence of aging and induction of rat liver and kidney microsomal mixed function oxidase systems. *Toxicology and Applied Pharmacology* 54: 411–419.

Miller, E. C., and Miller, J. A. 1981. Mechanisms of chemical carcinogenesis. *Cancer* 47:1055–1064.

Mukhtar, H., Athar, M., and Bickers, D. R. 1987. Cytochrome P-450 dependent metabolism of testosterone in rat skin. *Biochemical and Biophysical Research Communications* 145:749–753.

National Research Council. 1987. *Aging in Today's Environment*. Washington, DC, National Academy Press.

Newaz, S. N., Fang, W., and Strobel, H. W. 1983. Metabolism of the carcinogen, 1,2-dimethylhydrazine by isolated human colon microsomes and human colon tumor cells in culture. *Cancer* 52:794–798.

Nohl, H., Hegner, D., and Summer, K. H. 1979. Responses of mitochondrial superoxide dismutase, catalase and glutathione peroxidase activities to aging. *Mechanisms of Ageing and Development* 11:145–151.

Paigen, B., Holmes, P. A., Morrow, A., and Mitchell, D. 1986. Effect of 3-methylcholanthrene on atherosclerosis in two congenic strains of mice with different susceptibilities to methylcholanthrene-induced tumors. *Cancer Research* 46:3321–3324.

Preussmann, R., and Wiessler, M. 1987. The enigma of the organ specificity of carcinogenic nitrosamines. *Trends in Pharmacological Sciences* 8:185–189.

Rabovsky, J., Marion, K. J., Groseclose, R. D., Lewis, T. R., and Peterson, M. 1984. Low dose chronic inhalation of diesel exhaust and/or coal dust by rats: effect of age and exposure on lung and liver cytochrome P-450. *Xenobiotica* 14:595–598.

Radojicic, R., Spasic, M., Milic, B., Saicic, Z., and Petrovic, V. M. 1987. Age-related differences in the effect of diethyldithiocarbamate and cycloheximide on the liver copper, zinc containing superoxide dismutase in the rat. *Iugolslavica Physiologica et Pharmacologica Acta* 23:227–233.

Richter, E., Zwickenpflug, W., and Wiessler, M. 1988. Intestinal first-pass metabolism of nitrosamines. 2. Metabolism of N-nitrosodibutylamine in isolated perfused rat small intestinal segments. *Carcinogenesis* 9:499–506.

Rikans, L. E., and Kosanke, S. D. 1984. Effect of aging on liver glutathione levels and hepatocellular injury from carbon tetrachloride, allyl alcohol, or galactosamine. *Drug and Chemical Toxicology* 7:595–604.

Rikans, L. E., and Moore, D. R. 1987. Effect of age and sex on allyl alcohol hepatotoxicity in rats: Role of liver alcohol and aldehyde dehydrogenase activities. *Journal of Pharmacology and Experimental Therapeutics* 243: 20–26.

Rikans, L. E., and Moore, D. R. 1988. Aqueous-phase antioxidant concentrations in tissues of aging rats. *FASEB Journal* 2:A1730.

Robertson, I. G. C., and Birnbaum, L. S. 1982. Age-related changes in mutagen activation by rat tissues. *Chemico-Biological Interactions* 38:243–252.

Schmucker, D. L. 1985. Aging and drug disposition: An update. *Pharmacological Reviews* 37:133–148.

Schumann, A. M., Fox, T. R., and Watanabe, P. G. 1982. A comparison of the fate of inhaled methyl chloroform (1,1,1-trichloroethane) following single or repeated exposure in rats and mice. *Fundamental and Applied Toxicology* 2:27–32.

Sipes, I. G., and Gandolfi, A. J. 1986. Biotransformation of toxicants. In Klaassen, C. D., Amdur, M. O., and Doull, J. (Eds.), *Toxicology: The Basic Science of Poisons*. New York, Macmillan, pp. 64–98.

Sorokin, S. P. 1970. The cells of the lung. In Nettesheim, P., Hanna, M. G., Jr., and Deatherage, J. W. (Eds.), *Morphology of Experimental Respiratory Carcinogenesis*. Oak Ridge, TN: U.S. Atomic Energy Commission.

Spearman, M. E., and Liebman, K. C. 1983. Hepatic and pulmonary cytosolic metabolism of epoxides: Effects of aging on conjugation with glutathione. *Life Sciences* 33:2615–2625.

Spearman, M. E., and Liebman, K. C. 1984a. Effects of aging on hepatic and pulmonary glutathione-S-transferase activities in male and female Fischer 344 rats. *Biochemical Pharmacology* 33:1309–1313.

Spearman, M. E., and Liebman, K. C. 1984b. Aging selectively alters glutathione-S-transferase isozyme concentrations in liver and lung cytosol. *Drug Metabolism and Disposition* 12:661–671.

Stenbeck, F., Weisburger, J. H., and Williams, G. M. 1988. Effect of lifetime administration of dimethylaminoethanol on longevity, aging changes, and cryptogenic neoplasms in C3H mice. *Mechanisms of Ageing and Development* 42:129–138.

Stern, K., Hinds, E. G., and Askonas, B. P. 1945. Aging and detoxication. *American Journal of Psychiatry* 102:325–329.

Stiles, J., and Tyler, W. S. 1988. Age-related morphometric differences in responses of rat lungs to ozone. *Toxicology and Applied Pharmacology* 92:274–285.

Stohs, S. J., and Lawson, T. 1986. The role of glutathione and its metabolism in aging. In Kitani, K. (Ed.), *Liver and Aging*. Amsterdam, Elsevier, pp. 59–70.

Storm, J. E., Stewart, R. F., and Bronaugh, R. L. 1988. Interstrain and species differences in xenobiotic metabolizing capacity in skin: Evidence of enhanced activity in SENCAR mice (abstract). *Toxicologist* 8:126.

Sun, J., and Strobel, H. W. 1986. Aging affects the drug metabolism systems of rat liver, kidney, colon, and lung in a differential fashion. *Experimental Gerontology* 21:523–534.

Sun, J., Lau, P. O., and Strobel, H. W. 1986. Aging modifies the expression of hepatic microsomal cytochrome P-450 after pre-treatment of rats with β-naphthoflavone or phenobarbital. *Experimental Gerontology* 21:65–73.

Weiner, M., McMahon, T., and Centra, M. 1988. Age-related changes in colonic glucuronidation of 4-methylumbelliferone (4-MU): Inhibition by methylazoxymethanol (MAM) (abstract). *Toxicologist* 8:184.

Williams, G. M., and Weisburger, J. H. 1986. Chemical carcinogens. In Klaassen, C. D., Amdur, M. O., and Doull, J. (Eds.), *Toxicology: The Basic Science of Poisons* (3rd ed.). New York, Macmillan, p. 132.

Wynne, H., Mutch, E., James, O. F. W., Rawlins, M. D., and Woodhouse, K. W. 1987. The effect of age on monooxygenase enzyme kinetics in rat liver microsomes. *Age and Ageing* 16:153–158.

Videla, L. A., Fernandez, V., and Valenzuela, A. 1987. Age-dependent changes in rat liver lipid peroxidation and glutathione content induced by acute ethanol ingestion. *Cell Biochemistry and Function* 5:273–280.

2

Free Radicals, Aging, and Toxicology

Andrew T. Canada, Ph.D.

Edward J. Calabrese, Ph.D.

Free radicals are defined as substances that contain one or more unpaired electrons. The tendency toward electron pairing accounts for the elevated reactivity of free radicals. Free radicals can achieve electron pairing and thus stability by dimerization or by donating or receiving an electron. This tendency to donate or take an electron has the consequence that in reacting with nonradicals, free radicals will generate other free radicals. This is the basis for self-propagating chain reactions that can be initiated by free radicals. Because of the length of the reaction chains, this leads to amplification of the consequences resulting from the introduction of the initiating free radicals.

As a result of their high reactivity, free radicals can inactivate enzymes (Kim et al., 1986), produce DNA damage (Brawn and Fridovich, 1985), and induce mutagenesis (Hsie et al., 1986). Although this chapter focuses specifically on those compounds and exposures that likely involve free radical toxicity, a number of compounds such as thiourea (Hollinger, Giri, and Budd, 1976) and bromobenzene (Mitchell et al., 1971) have an age-related toxicity component and may act through a free radical mechanism. However, data supporting a free radical mechanism for their toxicity are inadequate at this time.

The Effect of Age on Antioxidant Protection

Aging may be the result of accumulation of unrepaired damage due to the attack of free radicals on cellular components. Alternatively, aged mammals may be affected to a greater extent by free radical stress. In the latter case, one may propose an age-related reduction in intracellular antioxidant protection systems or a reduced capacity to repair damage imposed by free radicals. There is evidence to support this explanation. Among the antioxidant protective systems affected by age are catalase, superoxide dismutase (SOD), and glutathione (GSH).

Catalase

Imre, Toth, and Fachet (1984) studied the effects of low and high doses of hydrogen peroxide on catalase activity in mouse liver homogenates. With the high hydrogen peroxide dose, the 5-month-old mice had almost twice the liver catalase of 3-month-old mice. The high hydrogen peroxide dose also induced liver catalase activity in 3-, 5-, and 14-month-old mice; however, no induction was observed in 27-month-old animals (Imre and Juhasz, 1987).

It is well recognized that reduction in caloric intake increases the life span of rodents (Yu et al., 1982). Koizumi, Weindruch, and Walford (1987) measured both catalase activity and the amount of lipid peroxidation in liver homogenates from 12- versus 24-month-old mice on control (nonrestricted) or calorically restricted diets. The 24-month-old mice on the restricted diet had 40 percent more catalase activity and 43 percent less lipid peroxidation than 24-month-old mice on control diets.

Baird and Samis (1971) provided data suggesting that there may be an age dependence in the ability of mice to regenerate catalase. They first treated young (44 weeks), middle-aged (90 weeks), and old (140 weeks) mice with the catalase inhibitor, 3-amino-1,2,4-triazole (AT). Following the rate of recovery of the lost catalase activity, they found that young and middle-aged animals recovered the original catalase activity within 24 hr whereas old animals had no recovery during the same period (Figure 2.1). This study provided support for the hypothesis that old animals, although no more sensitive to an initial oxidant exposure, may be more sensitive to constant or repetitive exposures.

In rats, liver catalase was found to slowly increase during the first year of life by 1.5 to 3-fold (Ross, 1969). Then between the first and second years, the activity slowly decreased by approximately 10–20 percent.

Red blood cells (RBC) from young, middle-aged, and elderly people who were donating blood were measured for catalase activity. There was a 20 percent increase in catalase from RBC taken from young compared with the old age group (Jozwiak and Jasnowska, 1985). Despite this increase, RBC from the old donors underwent greater spontaneous lipid peroxidation than those from any other age group.

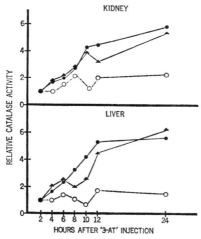

Figure 2.1. Recovery of catalase activity in C57BL/6J male mice following injection with 3-amino-1,2,4-triazole (3-AT). The activity was based on the number of units of catalase per micromolar DNA relative to the activity 2 hours after injection with 3-AT. *Source:* Reprinted with permission from Baird and Samis, 1971. Copyright 1971 by S. Karger AG.

Superoxide Dismutase

In mice, there does not appear to be any difference in hepatic SOD activity between animals ages 14 and 27 months (Imre and Juhasz, 1987). However, Reiss and Gershon (1976) did find that liver SOD-specific activity was lower in 32-month compared with 8-month animals. Similar to their results with catalase, Imre and Juhasz found that adult mice ages 3, 5, and 14 months responded to dietary hydrogen peroxide with an induction in liver SOD, whereas no effect occurred in aged (27 months) mice.

Thirty-month-old rats had lower SOD activity in liver homogenates than 8-month-old rats (Reiss and Gershon, 1976). They also reported that although there was no change in total brain catalase activity, catalytic activity per milligram of protein decreased, implying age-related protein damage. SOD activity also was measured in different sections of brains taken from 1- and 30-month-old rats (Vanella et al., 1982). Only in the cerebral cortex was a difference found, with a decrease observed in Cu,Zn SOD. In contrast, Mn SOD increased over the same period.

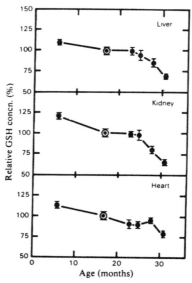

Figure 2.2. Concentrations of glutathione (GSH) in the liver, kidney, and heart during the life span of the mouse. *Source:* Reprinted with permission from Hazelton and Lang, 1980. Copyright 1980 by the Biochemical Society and Portland Press.

Glutathione

GSH is the major component of the GSH oxidation-reduction (redox) cycle, the intracellular antioxidant protective system against hydroperoxide-induced oxidant stress. A significant reduction of the intracellular GSH could reduce the ability to detoxify hydroperoxides and predispose the cell to oxidant stress injury. There is also evidence that this antioxidant activity decreases with age.

With mice, GSH concentrations show an age-related change in content in kidneys, intestinal mucosa, and RBC (Stohs et al., 1980). No age-related changes were found in the liver. GSH concentrations rose from young to middle-aged animals and then decreased in the old animals. Similar results were found by Hazelton and Lang (1980), who found an age-dependent decrease in GSH in the kidney, heart, and liver (Figure 2.2). This decrease was most noticeable in senescent animals, 28 months and older.

GSH concentrations in RBC taken from human blood donors of different ages showed a clear age-dependent relationship (Stohs et al., 1984). After a small increase in GSH from young to middle-aged donors, there was a substantial GSH decrease in RBC from elderly donors.

Age-Related Free Radical Toxicity

A number of xenobiotics and radiation have been shown, either directly or indirectly, to exert their toxicity through production of free radical intermediates or activated oxygen species. For many of the exposures, an age relationship for these toxic effects has been reported, with aged animals appearing to be the most sensitive and neonatal animals the least. These compounds/exposures are discussed below on an individual basis.

Acetaminophen

In addition to being a readily available over-the-counter drug, acetaminophen (AAP) is one of the more common compounds ingested with suicidal intent. The most significant toxicity associated with a suicidal ingestion is hepatic necrosis (Davidson and Eastham, 1966; Prescott et al., 1976). Shortly after the first report of the hepatic necrosis, there was evidence that it was free radical related. Liver GSH was found to decrease by more than 80 percent following massive AAP doses (Potter et al., 1974). If GSH was administered prior to AAP exposure, the amount of liver damage was significantly reduced (Malnoe et al., 1975; Mitchell et al., 1974).

Animals on diets deficient in the antioxidant vitamin E were found to experience a greater degree of hepatic damage than those on vitamin E supplemented diets (Walker et al., 1974). This provided additional evidence for oxidant stress's being the source of the liver damage.

On the basis of these and similar data, the mechanism of action for AAP liver toxicity was proposed to be the depletion of GSH by a free radical metabolite that, upon reduction of GSH to 20 percent of normal, would covalently bind to DNA and produce cell injury (Gillette, 1981). An alternate hypothesis was proposed by Rosen et al. (1983), who found that oxidation of AAP by cytochrome P-450 resulted in a free radical signal detected by electron spin resonance (ESR). They hypothesized that the radical resulted from a one-electron oxidation of AAP, which, when combined with dioxygen, produced superoxide and other oxyradical species. AAP toxicity was markedly reduced by the addition of desferoxamine to hepatocytes before exposure to AAP (Gerson et al., 1985; Kyle et al., 1987). The success of this iron chelator suggests that the toxic oxygen species is the hydroxyl radical, formed as a result of a Fenton reaction.

AAP was reported to be less toxic to neonatal than to adult mice

(Hart and Timbrell, 1979). Following a dose of 350 mg/kg of body weight, virtually all of the adult mice died, whereas all of the neonates survived. Moreover, the adult animals had a much greater loss of GSH than did the neonatal animals. In a similar study, adult (age not stated) mice were four times more sensitive to the lethality of AAP than neonates and rats showed increasing lethality from 7- to 14-day-old animals with little change thereafter (Mancini, Sonawane, and Yaffe, 1980).

In addition to the hepatic toxicity of AAP, nephrotoxicity may also be a consequence of an overdose (Brown, 1968; Kleinman, Breitenfield, and Roth, 1980). As with the liver, AAP was found to be metabolized in situ to a toxic metabolite that also produced a depletion of kidney GSH (McMurtry, Snodgrass, and Mitchell, 1978).

Age has been reported to be a determinant of the extent of AAP-induced kidney damage. Beierschmitt, Keenan, and Weiner (1986) studied the effects of three different AAP doses on the kidneys of young (2.5 months), middle-aged (13 months), and aged (23 months) rats. No kidney lesions were observed in young animals with any dose. Both middle-aged and aged rats given the two higher doses experienced an increase in blood urea nitrogen and decrease in urine osmolality (Figure 2.3). With the intermediate dose, acute tubular necrosis (ATN) was more prominent in aged compared with middle-aged animals, whereas at the highest dose ATN was present in both of the older age groups.

Bleomycin

Bleomycin is an antineoplastic drug that can produce pulmonary toxicity. The hypothesis that this toxicity is due to a free radical mechanism is supported by a number of studies. Among these were the findings that the toxicity of bleomycin to isolated human sarcoma cells was oxygen dependent (Yamauchi et al., 1987) and that hyperoxia potentiated the pulmonary toxicity (Tryka, Godleski, and Brain, 1984). In the latter study, the mortality following both intratracheal bleomycin and hyperoxia was 70 percent compared with 15 percent in bleomycin-only controls. Bleomycin-induced DNA damage was found to depend on the presence of both oxygen and elemental iron (Mahmutoglu, Scheulen, and Kappus, 1987). Both bleomycin-induced lipid peroxidation in the lung and the subsequent increase in collagen content were reduced by pretreating hamsters with desferoxamine (Chandler et al., 1988). These studies taken collectively suggest that the toxic oxygen species involved in bleomycin pulmonary toxicity is the hydroxyl radical.

There is some evidence that age may be a determinant of the extent

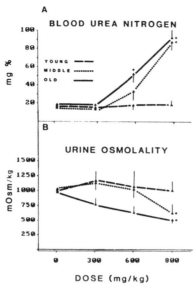

Figure 2.3. The effect of in vivo acetaminophen on blood urea nitrogen and urine osmolality from young, middle-aged, and old male Fischer 344 rats. Determinations were made 24 hours after dosing. Data are shown as means ± SEM. *Source:* Reprinted with permission from Beierschmitt et al., 1986. Copyright 1986 by Pergamon Press.
* Significantly different ($p < .05$) from corresponding controls.

of bleomycin toxicity. The amount of bleomycin-induced DNA damage was greater and the extent of DNA repair was less in 20-month-old compared with 3-month-old rats (Kennah, Coetzee, and Ove, 1985).

Adriamycin

Like bleomycin, adriamycin is an antineoplastic drug that is hypothesized to exert its toxicity, primarily cardiac, through a free radical mechanism. The generation of a free radical has been confirmed by the identification of an NADPH-dependent hydroxyl radical through ESR (Komiyama, Kikuchi, and Sugiura, 1982; Thornalley and Dodd, 1985). The presence of an iron-dependent adriamycin radical was also reported by Zweier (1985). In vivo confirmation of an oxidant stress mechanism for adriamycin cardiotoxicity was based on the finding that the combination of vitamins A and E reduced posttreatment electrocardiogram changes and hydroperoxide-initiated chemiluminescence (Milei et al., 1986). Microscopically, hearts from animals that received the vitamins had fewer damaged fibers than control animals. Additional evidence for a free radical mechanism of adriamycin toxicity is the ability of various oxyradical scavengers to suppress adriamycin-induced lipid peroxidation (Mimnaugh, Trush, and Gram, 1986).

Adriamycin toxicity was compared in young (1 month) and adult (6 months) rats (Weinberg and Singal, 1987). After the same milligram/kilogram of body weight dose, the adult animals appeared to be more adversely affected than the young rats. Many of the adult animals developed ascites, an effect not seen in young animals. In addition, 30 percent of the adult animals died from adriamycin toxicity compared with 17 percent of the young. Cardiac morphology showed less damage in hearts from young animals than from old. Lipid peroxidation in hearts of adult animals increased twofold over controls whereas no change occurred in the hearts of young rats.

Although there are conflicting data in humans, Von Hoff et al. (1979) reported that the probability of developing heart failure after adriamycin treatment correlated with increasing age of the patient. Those over age 70 had the highest incidence of cardiotoxicity. Contrary results showing no age–adriamycin toxicity correlation have been reported by Praga et al. (1979).

Gentamicin

Gentamicin is an antibiotic used for Gram-negative infections that can also produce nephrotoxicity. There is recent evidence that the nephrotoxicity side effect is a result of a free radical mechanism. Renal cortical mitochondria incubated with gentamicin showed an increased production of hydrogen peroxide (Walker and Shah, 1987). The same investigators showed the in vivo nephrotoxicity of gentamicin could be reduced if animals were pretreated with either a hydroxyl radical scavenger or an iron chelator (Walker and Shah, 1988). Both compounds that affected hydroxyl radical formation decreased histological evidence of toxicity as well as reducing the gentamicin-induced increase in blood urea nitrogen.

Although there is evidence of an age-related difference in gentamicin toxicity between neonates and adult humans, there are no studies conclusively showing that nephrotoxicity is more frequent in elderly humans than in other age groups. However, there are animal data to support this hypothesis. Old rats, defined as 260 g or larger, given the same milligram/kilogram dose, experienced greater nephrotoxicity than did young (90 g) rats (Marre et al., 1980). Nephrotoxicity was evaluated by the appearance of tubular cells and malic dehydrogenase in the urine (Figure 2.4). Another study (McMartin and Engel, 1982) evaluated gentamicin toxicity in young (7 months) and old (26 months) rats given similar milligram/kilogram doses. The authors reported that

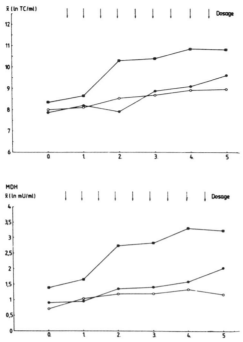

Figure 2.4. Tubular cell excretion (top) and malic dehydrogenase (MDH) activity (bottom) plotted against the number of days after gentamicin dose. Line with solid squares indicates 260-g rats; line with solid circles indicates 210-g rats; line with open circles indicates 90-g rats. *Source:* Reprinted with permission from Marre et al. Copyright 1980 Springer-Verlag.

the amount of microscopic renal tubular damage was dose related and, at each dose investigated, was greater in the old than in the young.

Cephaloridine

Cephaloridine is one of a group of cephalosporin antibiotics. Although the majority of the cephalosporins are relatively nontoxic, cephaloridine is nephrotoxic. Because of this unique toxicity, there is an interest in understanding the mechanism for its nephrotoxicity. Recently, the possibility that oxyradicals are responsible for the kidney damage has been studied. Cephaloridine was found to induce a significant decrease in kidney GSH as well as an increase in diene conjugation products, a measure of lipid peroxidation (Kuo et al., 1983). Cephaloridine also produced a significant time- and dose-related increase in malondialde-

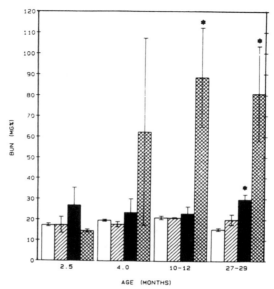

AGE (MONTHS)

Figure 2.5. Blood urea nitrogen (BUN) in rats of different ages 24 hr after a single intraperitoneal dose of cephaloridine. Values represent means ± SEM. Open bar indicates control; diagonal-filled bar indicates 500 mg/kg; solid bar indicates 1,000 mg/kg; x-filled bar indicates 2,000 mg/kg. *Source:* Reprinted from Goldstein et al., 1986. Copyright 1986 Elsevier Scientific Publishers.
* Statistically significant ($p < .05$) difference from age-matched control.

hyde (MDA) production (Cojocel, Hannemann, and Baumann, 1985). This increase could be inhibited by the antioxidants vitamin E and N,N′-diphenyl-p-phenylene-diamine, by the combination of SOD plus catalase, and by the hydroxyl radical scavenger mannitol (Cojocel et al., 1985).

An in vivo study showed an age-related difference in cephaloridine nephrotoxicity (Goldstein, Pasino, and Hook, 1986). Comparing rats 2.5, 4, 11, and 28 months old, they found an age-related increase in relative kidney weight (presumably reflecting edema) and blood urea nitrogen. Isolated cortical slices from the same animal groups showed an age-related decrease in accumulation of the organic anion p-amino-hippurate and tetraethylammonium (Figure 2.5).

Ethyl Alcohol

Ethyl alcohol (ethanol) has been reported to be another compound that may exert part of or all of its acute and chronic toxicity by a free radical mechanism. Both acute and chronic ethanol ingestion produces an increase in hepatic MDA and conjugated diene production, both indirect measures of lipid peroxidation (MacDonald, 1973; Shaw, Rubin, and Lieber, 1983). Shaw, Rubin, and Lieber also reported that patients with alcoholic liver disease had reduced GSH levels compared with nonalcoholic controls also with liver disease. Another measure of lipid peroxidation, pentane exhalation, was also increased after acute ethanol ingestion in rats (Litov et al., 1978).

Animal age was found to be a factor in a number of measured variables following acute ethanol ingestion. Adult (12 months) rats were found to be more susceptible to acute ethanol poisoning than young rats (Wiberg, Trenholm, and Coldwell, 1970). Another study reported that 37-week-old rats had a greater increase in liver thiobarbituric acid reacting substances (MDA being the major component) than 13-week-old rats after acute ethanol ingestion (Videla, Fernandez, and Valenzuela, 1987). Rats (53 weeks old) experienced a greater decrease in liver GSH and increase in GSSG than the other age groups. These observations suggest that given a similar ethanol exposure, the older age group lost the ability to detoxify ethanol-produced lipid peroxides compared with the younger age groups.

Allyl Alcohol and Acrolein

Allyl alcohol is metabolized in the liver by alcohol dehydrogenase to acrolein, a toxic metabolite and industrial chemical that is hepatotoxic (Ohno, Jones, and Ormstad, 1985). In addition to these two compounds being used as synthetic intermediates in the chemical industry, acrolein is one of the metabolites of the antineoplastic drug, cyclophosphamide. Acrolein is a strong electrophile which requires GSH for metabolism to a less toxic compound. Following the oral administration of acrolein to mice, virtually complete depletion of hepatic GSH was observed (Jaeschke, Kleinwaechter, and Wendel, 1987; Zitting and Heinonen, 1980). Simultaneously with the GSH loss there was a large increase in ethane exhalation, an indication of increased lipid peroxidation (Jaeschke, Kleinwaechter, and Wendel, 1987). Suggesting an oxyradical mechanism, Jaeschke, Kleinwaechter, and Wendel found that desferoxamine prevented both the increase in pentane exhalation and the cell damage. Ohno et al. (1985) found that increasing the intracellular GSH level in isolated renal epithelial cells decreased the toxicity of allyl alcohol.

Rikans (1984) evaluated the effect of age (rats ages 4, 14, and 24 months) on the hepatotoxicity of allyl alcohol. Judged both on the severity of hepatocellular necrosis and the release of alanine aminotransferase and aspartate aminotransferase, older rats experienced

Table 2.1. Aging Modification of Cytotoxic Injury

| | Serum enzyme activity (Sigma-Frankel units/ml) | | |
| | Alanine aminotransferase | Aspartate aminotransferase | Hepatocellular necrosis |
Treatment/age			
Control			
Young	57 ± 3^a	309 ± 17^a	0
Middle aged	65 ± 4^a	308 ± 19^a	0
Old	62 ± 4^a	240 ± 20^b	0
Allyl alcohol			
Young	200 ± 50^b	620 ± 130^c	0
Middle aged	$2,200 \pm 500^c$	$3,600 \pm 1,200^d$	$+1$
Old	$5,000 \pm 1,500^c$	$5,000 \pm 1,300^d$	$+2$
D-Galactosamine			
Young	$11,700 \pm 2,800^{d,e}$	$16,800 \pm 3,500^{e,f}$	$+2$
Middle aged	$11,300 \pm 900^e$	$16,100 \pm 1,900^f$	$+2$
Old	$6,600 \pm 1,800^{c,d}$	$7,700 \pm 2,000^{d,e}$	$+1$
Bromobenzene			
Young	$6,000 \pm 1,500^c$	$7,100 \pm 2,300^d$	$+2$
Middle aged	$6,400 \pm 1,400^c$	$7,100 \pm 1,600^d$	$+2$
Old	$4,300 \pm 1,300^c$	$4,600 \pm 1,500^d$	$+2$

Note: Values for enzyme activity are means and standard errors for six or more rats. Means with unlike superscripts vertically are significantly different at $p < .05$. Necrosis values are median score for each group. Median values coincided with means. From "Influence of Aging on the Susceptibility of Rats to Hepatotoxic Injury," by L. E. Rikans, 1984, *Toxicology and Applied Pharmacology, 73*, p. 245. Copyright 1984 by Academic Press. Adapted by permission.

much more damage than did the young (Table 2.1). Using hepatocytes isolated from rats ages 5, 15, and 26 months, Rikans and Hornbrook (1986) reported an age-related difference in toxicity following incubation with allyl alcohol. As measured by trypan blue exclusion and lactic acid dehydrogenase, hepatocytes from the old rats showed damage not only earlier but also at lower allyl alcohol doses. The mechanism for the age-related sensitivity appears to be increased metabolism to allyl alcohol in old compared with young animals (Rikans and Moore, 1987). This increased metabolism occurred because the old rats were found to have approximately 50 percent more alcohol dehydrogenase in the liver than the young animals.

Carbon Tetrachloride

Carbon tetrachloride (CCl_4) was a widely used industrial solvent until it was identified as a hepatotoxin. The formation of a free radical metabolite was suggested when GSH was found to protect rat liver microsomes against CCl_4 damage, which was also found to be oxygen-dependent (Burk, Patel, and Lane, 1983). Incubation of liver slices with CCL_4 resulted in a significant increase in thiobarbituric-acid-reacting (TBAR) substances, indicating lipid peroxidation (Fraga, Leibovitz, and Tappel, 1987). A free radical mechanism was further suggested when it was found that desferoxamine not only suppressed CCl_4-induced lipid peroxidation but also reduced hepatotoxicity (Younes and Siegers, 1985). As with other studies, the oxygen dependence of the toxicity coupled with the ability of desferoxamine to reduce CCl_4 toxicity suggest the hydroxyl radical as the mediator of toxicity.

CCl_4 is a hepatocarcinogen in animal models. There is evidence that xenobiotic-related carcinogenicity is a result of free-radical-induced DNA damage. Reuber and Glover (1967) investigated the carcinogenicity of subcutaneous CCl_4 in rats 4–52 weeks old. Whereas no hyperplasia occurred in the young animals, older rats developed hyperplastic nodules with occasional nodules identified as carcinoma.

Ozone

Ozone is an air pollutant that is a common component of air pollution in heavily populated and industrial areas. As would be expected, the primary target of ozone toxicity is the lung. Although there is no conclusive evidence that ozone toxicity is a result of free radicals, there is considerable evidence to suggest active oxygen species as the cause of the pulmonary damage. This evidence includes the depletion of intracellular antioxidant protection systems by acute ozone exposure (DeLucia et al., 1972); the ability of antioxidants, particularly vitamin E, to mitigate the pulmonary damage (Chow and Tappel, 1973); and the formation of MDA in the lung after exposure to ozone, indicating lipid peroxidation (Chow and Tappel, 1973).

A number of studies have shown an age-related difference in susceptibility to ozone toxicity. Comparing 1-year-old with 1-month old rats, Mustafa et al. (1985) reported that after 3 days of ozone exposure the 1-year-old animals displayed increased lung:body weight ratio whereas no increase was observed in the young (1 month old) rats. These data implied pulmonary fluid accumulation (edema) in the 1-year-old animals, whereas no edema was observed in the young animals. The 1-year-old animals also showed an induction of components of the GSH redox system, whereas none occurred in the young. Ozone-induced pulmonary edema and tolerance were investigated in rats 3–33 weeks old (Nambu and Yokoyama, 1981). After exposure to 2 ppm for 3 hr, the young animals showed resistance to a further

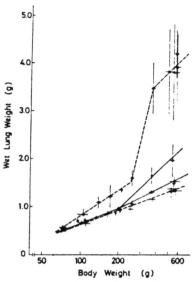

Figure 2.6. The relationship between lung weight and body weight of rats exposed to ozone. Data are shown as means ± SEM. Top line represents 5.6 ppm for 3 hr; next line represents 2 ppm for 3 hr; next line represents 2 ppm for 3 hr followed by reexposure at the same concentration; bottom line represents a nonexposed control. *Source:* Reprinted from Nambu and Yokoyama, 1981. Copyright 1981.

exposure at 5.6 ppm but the old animals were able to develop only partial resistance. When exposed to 5.6 ppm acutely, the lung wet weight of the old animals increased significantly over that of non-exposed controls whereas virtually no change occurred in the young and middle-aged animals.

The loss of intracellular reducing equivalents, particularly NADPH, may be an important step preceding cell injury and death. Rats (5 and 25 months old) were exposed to 1.5 ppm of ozone for 8 hr and then were assessed for lung NADPH and NADP (Montgomery, Raska-Emery, and Balis, 1987). The young animals experienced a 45 percent loss of pulmonary NADPH and the old animals, a 73 percent loss; the difference was statistically significant.

Nitrogen Dioxide

Nitrogen dioxide (NO_2), like ozone, is a common constituent of industrial pollution. The evidence that NO_2 produces its toxicity through a free radical mechanism is also circumstantial. NO_2 exposure in rats produced a dose-related increase of ethane exhalation indicating increased lipid peroxidation (Sagai et al., 1981, 1983). An increase in pentane exhalation also was detected in NO_2- exposed vitamin E- and selenium-deficient rats (Dillard, Sagai, and Tappel, 1980). An increase in another indicator of lipid peroxidation, TBAR, was found in rats exposed to NO_2 (Cavanagh and Morris, 1987; Sagai, Ichinose, and Kubota, 1984). Another study found an increase in TBAR in lung microsomes from vitamin E-deficient rats exposed to NO_2 (Sevanian, Hacker, and Elsayed, 1982).

As observed with ozone, there appears to be an age-related sensitivity to the pulmonary toxicity of NO_2. In a study comparing the toxicity of NO_2 in 6- and 20-month-old mice, there was more histopathological damage in the lungs of the old than of the young mice (Bils and Romanovsky, 1967). In another study, male rats ages 1 to 25 months were exposed to NO_2 for up to 15 days and evaluated on both histopathological changes and survival (Cabral-Anderson, Evans, and Freeman, 1977). The 1- and 3-month-old rats tolerated exposures up to 17 ppm with no mortality whereas significant mortality occurred in the older animals beginning with 11-month-old rats. There was more pulmonary damage and less repair at Day 2 in the older animals compared with the young. Rats ages 9, 18, and 27 months were exposed to low, medium, and high concentrations of NO_2 (Sagai et al., 1983). The two lowest doses of NO_2 produced an increase in ethane exhalation that showed a clear age-related response (Figure 2.7). No age-related increase was observed at the highest exposure. Sagai et al. had no explanation for the disappearance of the age-related effect at the highest dose.

Ultraviolet Light

The evidence that ultraviolet light can produce intracellular free radicals is limited. One study showed that lipid peroxidation products could be detected in the skin of neonatal rats exposed to ultraviolet radiation (Meffert, Diezel, and Sonnichsen, 1976). Pathak and Stratton (1968), using ESR, found that pigmented human skin, guinea pig hair, and melanosomes irradiated with wavelengths greater than 320 nm yielded a stronger ESR signal than before irradiation.

The occurrence of unscheduled DNA synthesis is used as an index of DNA repair within cells. Plesko and Richardson (1984) isolated hepatocytes from rats ages 6–32 months and irradiated them at 254 nm. There was a clear age-related difference in the ability to initiate DNA repair. Repair was the most rapid in 14- and 20-month-old animals, whereas virtually no repair was observed in cells from the 32-

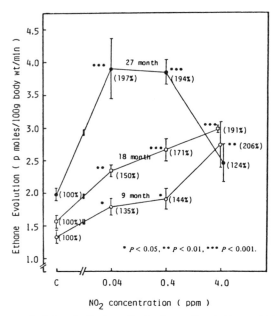

Figure 2.7. Ethane exhalation in the breath of rats continuously exposed to nitrogen dioxide for 9, 18, and 27 months. Data are shown as means ± SEM. Asterisks represent the statistically significant difference from control value. *Source:* Reprinted with permission from Sagai et al., 1983. Copyright 1984 Academic Press.

month-old animals. Kennah, Coetzee, and Ove (1985), using a different exposure dose, found that hepatocytes from 20-month-old rats had significantly less unscheduled DNA synthesis (repair) than 3-month-old rats.

Radiation

Radiation is recognized as exerting its toxicity through the formation of intracellular radicals, primarily hydroxyl (Dertinger and Jung, 1970; Huttermann, Kohnlein, and Teoule, 1978). The evidence that the hydroxyl radical is involved in radiation toxicity is further confirmed by the ability of various hydroxyl scavengers to mitigate radiation-induced hemolysis in RBC (Miller and Raleigh, 1983), increase the survival of Chinese hamster ovary cells (Chapman et al., 1979), and decrease single-strand DNA breaks following radiation (Repine et al., 1981).

There appears to be clear evidence of an age-related sensitivity to both the acute toxicity of radiation and radiation-induced carcinogenicity. In animals, Storer (1965) determined the LD_{50} (in rads) of mice of various ages. Radiation resistance slowly increased with age until the animals were 240 days old, whereupon the resistance slowly decreased over the ensuing 580 days. Then the LD_{50} decreased rapidly until for 960-day-old animals, it was 33 percent lower than in the 240-day-old animals. In another study the mean lethal radiation dose in 630-day-old mice was only 25 percent that of 315-day-old mice, showing a precipitous increase in radiation sensitivity in the aged animals (Spalding and Trujillo, 1962).

In humans, a study of Japanese atomic bomb survivors revealed that the rate of leukemia was highest in those who were younger than 10 and older than 50 at the time of exposure (Finch, 1979).

Ischemia–Reperfusion Injury

The tissue damage that occurs following ischemia of an organ has been proposed to comprise both an ischemic and a reperfusion component. The reperfusion component has been hypothesized to be a result of production of oxyradicals either within the ischemic tissue (McCord and Roy, 1982) or by activated neutrophil-mediated damage to capillary endothelial cells (Grisham and Granger, 1988). The evidence that oxyradicals are involved in this type of injury is primarily circumstantial. The injury following ischemia and reperfusion of the cat intestine was reduced if the animals were pretreated with SOD (Granger, Rutili, and McCord, 1981). This pioneering investigation was followed by many others implicating oxyradicals as the source of reperfusion injury in virtually every major organ in the body (Ambrosio et al., 1986; Atalla et al., 1985; Baker, Corry, and Autor, 1985; Flamm et al., 1978).

Few studies have investigated the effect of age on ischemia–reperfusion injury. One of these compared the effects of kidney ischemia with reperfusion in rats 3 and 37 months old (Miura et al., 1987). Using both biochemical and histopathological measurements, the authors found that the old rats experienced much greater damage than the young. Although there was a transient increase in blood urea nitrogen and serum creatinine in the young animals, these measurements of kidney function were markedly elevated in the old rats (Figure 2.8). The old rats also showed more histological damage and less restoration of tubular architecture than the young.

Discussion

Although aged humans are exposed to drugs and environmental toxins as frequently or more so than infants, the number of studies in either

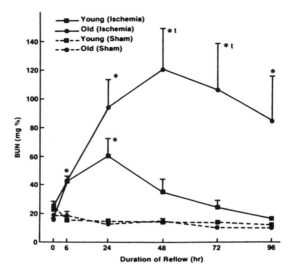

Figure 2.8. The effect of ischemia on the concentration of blood urea nitrogen (BUN). Data are shown as means ± SEM. Asterisk denotes statistically significant ($p < .05$) difference compared with age-matched controls; t indicates significant ($p < .05$) difference compared with young rats. *Source:* Reprinted with permission from Miura et al., 1987. Copyright 1987 Academic Press.

animals or humans that have focused specifically on age as a risk factor for toxicity is limited. Age-related toxicity studies in humans have a common problem in the inability to control for all the factors that could affect outcome. Another problem is determining how much of an age-related toxic effect comes from the coexistence of diseases seen more frequently in elderly persons rather than an age-related sensitivity of old cells to free radical damage. However, the outcome is still the same, that is, an apparent age-related sensitivity to free radical toxicity.

This lack of controlled studies exists despite a growing body of evidence that age, even in the absence of underlying disease, may well be a significant risk factor in determining the extent of toxic damage or repair following free radical stress. As more xenobiotic toxicity is attributed to free radical reactions, the aspect of animal age will take on increasing importance, particularly in the area of drug toxicology because elderly humans are likely to receive many more drugs than any other age group. A hypothesis that a xenobiotic may exert its toxicity through a free-radical-mediated process should prompt investigations into the variable of age on toxicity, particularly if the compound is to be used in the treatment of disease(s) associated with the aging process.

We would like to express our appreciation to Dr. Irwin Fridovich for his contribution to this chapter.

References

Ambrosio, G., Becker, L. C., Hutchins, G. M., Weisman, H. F., and Weisfeldt, M. L. 1986. Reduction in experimental infarct size by recombinant human superoxide dismutase: Insights into the pathophysiology of reperfusion injury. *Circulation* 74:1424–1433.

Atalla, S. L., Toledo-Pereyra, L. H., MacKenzie, G. H., and Cederna, J. P. 1985. Influence of oxygen-derived free radical scavengers on ischemic livers. *Transplantation* 40:584–590.

Baird, M. B., and Samis, H. V., Jr. 1971. Regulation of catalase activity in mice of different ages. *Gerontologia* 17:105–115.

Baker, G. L., Corry, R. J., and Autor, A. P. 1985. Oxygen-free radical induced damage in kidneys subjected to warm ischemia and reperfusion. *Annals of Surgery* 202:628–641.

Beierschmitt, W. P., Keenan, K. P., and Weiner, M. 1986. Age-related increased susceptibility of male Fisher 344 rats to acetaminophen nephrotoxicity. *Life Sciences* 39:2335–2342.

Bils, R. F., and Romanovsky, J. C. 1967. Ultrastructural alterations in alveolar tissue of mice. II. Synthetic photochemical smog. *Archives of Environmental Health* 14:844–858.

Brawn, M. K., and Fridovich, I. 1985. Increased superoxide radical production evokes inducible DNA repair in *Escherichia coli*. *Journal of Biological Chemistry* 260:922–925.

Brown, R. A. G. 1968. Hepatic and renal damage with paracetamol overdosage. *Journal of Clinical Pathology* 21:793.

Burk, R. F., Patel, K., and Lane, J. M. 1983. Reduced glutathione protection against rat liver microsomal injury by carbon tetrachloride. *Biochemical Journal* 215:441–445.

Cabral-Anderson L. J., Evans, M. J., and Freeman, G. 1977. Effects of NO_2 on the lungs of aging rats. I. Morphology. *Experimental and Molecular Pathology* 27:353–365.

Cavanagh, D. G., and Morris, J. B. 1987. Mucous protection and airway peroxidation following nitrogen dioxide exposure in the rat. *Journal of Toxicology and Environmental Health* 22:313–328.

Chandler, D. B., Butler, T. W., Briggs, D. D., III, Grizzle, W. E., Barton, J. C., and Fulmer, J. D. 1988. Modulation of the development of bleomycin-induced fibrosis by deferoxamine. *Toxicology and Applied Pharmacology* 92:358–367.

Chapman, J. D., Doern, S. D., Reuvers, A. P., Gillespie, C. J., Chatterjee,

A., Blakely, E. A., Smith, K. C., and Tobias, C. A. 1979. Radioprotection by DMSO of mammalian cells exposed to X-rays and to heavy charged-particle beams. *Radiation and Environmental Biophysics* 16:29–41.

Chow, C. K., and Tappel, A. L. 1973. Activities of pentose shunt and glycolytic enzymes in lungs of ozone-exposed rats. *Archives of Environmental Health* 26:205–208.

Cojocel, C., Hannemann, J., and Baumann, K. 1985. Cephaloridine-induced lipid peroxidation initiated by reactive oxygen species as a possible mechanism of cephaloridine nephrotoxicity. *Biochimica et Biophysica Acta* 834: 402–410.

Cojocel, C., Laeschke, K. H., Inselmann, G., and Baumann, K. 1985. Inhibition of cephaloridine-induced lipid peroxidation. *Toxicology* 35:295–305.

Davidson, D. G. D., and Eastham, W. N. 1966. Acute liver necrosis following overdose of paracetamol. *British Medical Journal* 2:497–499.

DeLucia, A. J., Hoque, P. M., Mustafa, M. G., and Cross, C. E. 1972. Ozone interaction with rodent lung: Effect on sulfhydryls and sulfhydryl-containing enzyme activities. *Journal of Laboratory and Clinical Medicine* 80:559–566.

Dertinger, H., and Jung, H. 1970. *Molecular Radiation Biology.* New York, Springer-Verlag.

Dillard, C. J., Sagai, M., and Tappel, A. L. 1980. Respiratory pentane: A measure of in vivo lipid peroxidation applied to rats fed diets varying in polyunsaturated fats, vitamin E, and selenium and exposed to nitrogen dioxide. *Toxicology Letters* 6:251–256.

Finch, S. C. 1979. The study of atomic bomb survivors in Japan. *American Journal of Medicine* 66:899–901.

Flamm, E. S., Demopoulos, H. B., Seligman, M. L., Poser, R. G., and Ransohoff, J. 1978. Free radicals in cerebral ischemia. *Stroke* 9:445–447.

Fraga, C. G., Leibovitz, B. E., and Tappel, A. L. 1987. Halogenated compounds as inducers of lipid peroxidation in tissue slices. *Free Radical Biology and Medicine* 3:119–123.

Gerson, R. J., Casini, A., Gilfor, D., Serroni, A., and Farber, J. L. 1985. Oxygen-mediated cell injury in the killing of cultured hepatocytes by acetaminophen. *Biochemical and Biophysical Research Communications* 126:1129–1137.

Gillette, J. R. 1981. An integrated approach to the study of chemically reactive metabolites of acetaminophen. *Archives of Internal Medicine* 141:375–379.

Goldstein, R. S., Pasino, D. A., and Hook, J. B. 1986. Cephaloridine nephrotoxicity in aging male Fischer-344 rats. *Toxicology* 38:43–53.

Granger, D. N., Rutili, G., and McCord, J. M. 1981. Superoxide radicals in feline intestinal ischemia. *Gastroenterology* 81:22–29.

Grisham, M. B., and Granger, D. N. 1988. Neutrophil-mediated mucosal injury. Role of reactive oxygen metabolites. *Digestive Diseases and Sciences* 33(3 Suppl.): 6S–15S.

Hart, J. G., and J. A. Timbrell, J. A. 1979. The effect of age on paracetamol hepatotoxicity in mice. *Biochemical Pharmacology* 28:3015–3017.

Hazelton, G. A., and Lang, C. A. 1980. Glutathione contents of tissues in the aging mouse. *Biochemical Journal* 188:25–30.

Hollinger, M. A., Giri, S. N., and Budd, E. 1976. A pharmacodynamic study of [14C]thiourea toxicity in mature, immature, tolerant, and nontolerant rats. *Toxicology and Applied Pharmacology* 37:545–556.

Hsie, A. W., Recio, L., Katz, D. S., Lee, C. Q., Wagner, M., and Schenley, R. L. 1986. Evidence for reactive oxygen species inducing mutations in mammalian cells. *Proceedings of the National Academy of Sciences* (USA) 83:9616–9620.

Huttermann, J., Kohnlein, W., and Teoule, R. 1978. *Effects of Ionizing Radiation on DNA*. Berlin, Springer-Verlag.

Imre, S., and Juhasz, E. 1987. The effect of oxidative stress on inbred mice of different ages. *Mechanisms of Ageing and Development* 38:259–266.

Imre, S., Toth, F., and Fachet, J. 1984. Superoxide dismutase, catalase and lipid peroxidation in liver of young mice of different ages. *Mechanisms of Ageing and Development* 28:297–304.

Jaeschke, H., Kleinwaechter, C., and Wendel, A. 1987. The role of acrolein in allyl alcohol-induced lipid peroxidation and liver cell damage in mice. *Biochemical Pharmacology* 36:51–57.

Jozwiak, Z., and Jasnowska, B. 1985. Changes in oxygen-metabolizing enzymes and lipid peroxidation in human erythrocytes as a function of age of donor. *Mechanisms of Ageing and Development* 32:77–83.

Kennah, H. E., II, Coetzee, M. L., and Ove, P. 1985. A comparison of DNA repair synthesis in primary hepatocytes from old and young rats. *Mechanisms of Ageing and Development* 29:283–298.

Kim, H., Minard, P., Legoy, M., and Thomas, D. 1986. Inactivation of 3-α-hydroxysteroid dehydrogenase by superoxide radicals. *Biochemical Journal* 233:493–497.

Kleinman, J. G., Breitenfield, R. V., and Roth, D. A. 1980. Acute renal failure associated with acetaminophen ingestion: Report of a case and review of the literature. *Clinical Nephrology* 14:201–205.

Koizumi, A., Weindruch, R., and Walford, R. L. 1987. Influences of dietary restriction and age on liver enzyme activities and lipid peroxidation in mice. *Journal of Nutrition* 117:361–367.

Komiyama, T., Kikuchi, T., and Sugiura, Y. 1982. Generation of hydroxyl radical by anticancer quinone drugs, carbazilquinone, mitomycin c, aclacinomycin A and adriamycin, in the presence of NADPH-cytochrome P-450 reductase. *Biochemical Pharmacology* 31:3651–3656.

Kuo, C., Maita, K., Sleight, S. D., and Hook, J. B. 1983. Lipid peroxidation: A possible mechanism of cephaloridine-induced nephrotoxicity. *Toxicology and Applied Pharmacology* 67:78–88.

Kyle, M. E., Miccadei, S., Nakae, D., and Farber, J. L. 1987. Superoxide dismutase and catalase protect cultured hepatocytes from the cytotoxicity of acetaminophen. *Biochemical and Biophysical Research Communications* 149:889–896.

Litov, R. E., Irving, D. H., Downey, J. E., and Tappel, A. L. 1978. Lipid peroxidation: A mechanism involved in acute ethanol toxicity as demonstrated by in vivo pentane production in the rat. *Lipids* 13:305–307.

MacDonald, C. M. 1973. The effects of ethanol on hepatic lipid peroxidation and on the activities of glutathione reductase and peroxidase. *FEBS Letters* 35:227–230.

Mahmutoglu, I., Scheulen, M. E., and Kappus, H. 1987. Oxygen radical formation and DNA damage due to enzymatic reduction of bleomycin-Fe (III). *Archives of Toxicology* 60:150–153.

Malnoë, A., Louis, A., Benedetti, M. S., Schneider, M., Smith, R. L., Kreber, L., and Lam, R. 1975. Effect of liposomal entrapment on the protective action of glutathione against paracetamol-induced liver necrosis. *Biochemical Society Transactions* 3:730–732.

Mancini, R. E., Sonawane, B. R., and Yaffe, S. J. 1980. Developmental susceptibility to acetaminophen toxicity. *Research Communications in Chemical Pathology and Pharmacology* 27:603–606.

Marre, R., Tarara, N., Louton, T., and Sack, K. 1980. Age-dependent nephrotoxicity and the pharmacokinetics of gentamicin in rats. *European Journal of Pediatrics* 133:25–29.

McCord, J. M., and Roy, R. S. 1982. The pathophysiology of superoxide: Roles in inflammation and ischemia. *Canadian Journal of Physiology and Pharmacology* 60:1346–1352.

McMartin, D. N., and Engel, S. G. 1982. Effect of aging on gentamicin nephrotoxicity and pharmacokinetics in rats. *Research Communications in Chemical Pathology and Pharmacology* 38:193–207.

McMurtry, R. J., Snodgrass, W. R., and Mitchell, J. R. 1978. Renal necrosis, glutathione depletion, and covalent binding after acetaminophen. *Toxicology and Applied Pharmacology* 46:87–100.

Meffert, H., Diezel, W., and Sonnichsen, N. 1976. Stable lipid peroxidation products in human skin: Detection, ultraviolet light-induced increase, pathogenic importance. *Experientia* 32:1397–1398.

Milei, J., Boveris, A., Llesuy, S., Molina, H. A., Storino, R., Ortega, D., and Milei, S. E. 1986. Amelioration of adriamycin-induced cardiotoxicity in rabbits by prenylamine and vitamins A and E. *American Heart Journal* 111:95–102.

Miller, G. G., and Raleigh, J. A. 1983. Action of some hydroxyl radical scavengers on radiation-induced haemolysis. *International Journal of Radiation Biology and Related Studies in Physics, Chemistry and Medicine* 43:411–419.

Mimnaugh, E. G., Trush, M. A., and Gram, T. E. 1986. A possible role for membrane lipid peroxidation in anthracycline nephrotoxicity. *Biochemical Pharmacology* 35:4327–4335.

Mitchell, J. R., Reid, W. D., Christie, B., Moskowitz, J., Krishna, G., and Brodie, B. B. 1971. Bromobenzene-induced hepatic necrosis: Species differences and protection by SKF 525-A. *Research Communications in Chemical Pathology and Pharmacology* 2:877–888.

Mitchell, J. R., Thorgeirsson, S. S., Potter, W. Z., Jollow, D. J., and Keiser, H. 1974. Acetaminophen-induced hepatic injury: Protective role of glutathione in man and rationale for therapy. *Clinical Pharmacology and Therapeutics* 16:676–684.

Miura, K., Goldstein, R. S., Morgan, D. G., Pasino, D. A., Hewitt, W. R., and Hook, J. B. 1987. Age-related differences in susceptibility to renal ischemia in rats. *Toxicology and Applied Pharmacology* 87:284–296.

Montgomery, M. R., Raska-Emery, P., and Balis, J. U. 1987. Age-related difference in pulmonary response to ozone. *Biochimica et Biophysica Acta* 890:271–274.

Mustafa, M. G., Elsayed, N. M., Ospital, J. J., and Hacker, A. D. 1985. Influence of age on the biochemical response of rat lung to ozone exposure. *Toxicology and Industrial Health* 1:29–41.

Nambu, Z., and Yokoyama, E. 1981. The effect of age on the ozone-induced pulmonary edema and tolerance in rats. *Japanese Journal of Industrial Health* 23:146–149.

Ohno, Y., Jones, T. W., and Ormstad, K. 1985. Allyl alcohol toxicity in isolated renal epithelial cells: Protective effects of low molecular weight thiols. *Chemico-Biologic Interactions* 52:289–299.

Ohno, Y., Ormstad, K., Ross, D., and Orrenius, S. 1985. Mechanism of allyl alcohol toxicity and protective effects of low molecular-weight thiols studied with isolated rat hepatocytes. *Toxicology and Applied Pharmacology* 78:169–179.

Pathak, M. A., and Stratton, K. 1968. Free radicals in human skin before and after exposure to light. *Archives of Biochemistry and Biophysics* 123:468–476.

Plesko, M. M., and Richardson, A. 1984. Age-related changes in unscheduled DNA synthesis by rat hepatocytes. *Biochemical and Biophysical Research Communications* 118:730–735.

Potter, W. Z., Thorgeirsson, S. S., Jollow, D. J., and Mitchell, J. R. 1974. Acetaminophen-induced hepatic necrosis-V. Correlation of hepatic necrosis, covalent binding and glutathione depletion in hamsters. *Pharmacology* 12:129–143.

Praga, C., Beretta, G., Vigo, P. L., Lenaz, G. R., Pollini, C., Bonadonna, G., Canetta, R., Castellani, R., Villa, E., Gallagher, C. G., von Melchner, H., Hayat, M., Ribaud, P., DeWasch, G., Mattsson, W., Heinz, R., Waldner, R., Kolaric, K., Buehner, R., Bokkel-Huyninck, W., Perevodchikova, N. I., Manziuk, L. A., Senn, H. J., and Mayr, A. C. 1979. Adriamycin cardiotoxicity: A survey of 1273 patients. *Cancer Treatment Reports* 63:827–834.

Prescott, L. F., Park, J., Sutherland, G. R., Smith, I. J., and Proudfoot, A. T. 1976. Cysteamine, methionine, and penicillamine in the treatment of paracetamol poisoning. *Lancet* 2:109–113.

Reiss, U., and Gershon, D. 1976. Comparison of cytoplasmic superoxide dismutase in liver, heart and brain of aging rats and mice. *Biochemical and Biophysical Research Communications* 73:255–262.

Repine, J. E., Pfenninger, O. W., Talmage, D. W., Berger, E. M., and Pettijohn, D. E. 1981. Dimethyl sulfoxide prevents DNA nicking mediated by ionizing radiation or iron/hydrogen peroxide-generated hydroxyl radical. *Proceedings of the National Academy of Sciences (USA)* 78:1001–1003.

Reuber, M. D., and Glover, E. L. 1967. Hyperplastic and early neoplastic lesions of the liver in Buffalo strain rats of various ages given subcutaneous carbon tetrachloride. *Journal of the National Cancer Institute* 38:891–899.

Rikans, L. E. 1984. Influence of aging on the susceptibility of rats to hepatotoxic injury. *Toxicology and Applied Pharmacology* 73:243–249.

Rikans, L. E., and Hornbrook, K. R. 1986. Isolated hepatocytes as a model for aging effects on hepatotoxicity: Studies with allyl alcohol. *Toxicology and Applied Pharmacology* 84:634–639.

Rikans, L. E., and Moore, D. R. 1987. Effect of age and sex on allyl alcohol hepatotoxicity in rats: Role of liver alcohol and aldehyde dehydrogenase activities. *Journal of Pharmacology and Experimental Therapeutics* 243: 20–26.

Rosen, G. M., Singletary, W. V., Jr., Rauckman, E. J., and Killenberg, P. G. 1983. Acetaminophen hepatotoxicity. An alternate mechanism. *Biochemical Pharmacology* 32:2053–2059.

Ross, M. H. 1969. Aging, nutrition and hepatic enzyme activity patterns in the rat. *Journal of Nutrition* 97:565–601.

Sagai, M., Ichinose, T., Kobayashi, T., and Kubota, K. 1983. Changes of lipid peroxidation and antioxidative protective systems in rat lungs upon life span exposure to low levels of nitrogen dioxide. *Developments in Toxicology and Environmental Science* 11:483–486.

Sagai, M., Ichinose, T., and Kubota, K. 1984. Studies on the biochemical effects of nitrogen dioxide. IV. Relation between the change of lipid peroxidation and the antioxidative protective system in rat lungs upon life span exposure to low levels of NO_2. *Toxicology and Applied Pharmacology* 73:444–456.

Sagai, M., Ichinose, T., Oda, H., and Kubota, K. 1981. Studies on biochemical effects of nitrogen dioxide: I. Lipid peroxidation as measured by ethane exhalation of rats exposed to nitrogen dioxide. *Lipids* 16:64–67.

Sevanian, A., Hacker, A. D., and Elsayed, N. 1982. Influence of vitamin E and nitrogen dioxide on lipid peroxidation in rat lung and liver microsomes. *Lipids* 17:269–277.

Shaw, S., Rubin, K. P., and Lieber, C. S. 1983. Depressed hepatic glutathione and increased diene conjugates in alcoholic liver disease. Evidence of lipid peroxidation. *Digestive Diseases and Sciences* 28:585–589.

Spalding, J. F., and Trujillo, T. T. 1962. Radiosensitivity of mice as a function of age. *Radiation Research* 16:125–129.

Stohs, S. J., El-Rashidy, F. H., Lawson, T., Kobayashi, R. H., Wulf, B. G., and Potter, J. F. 1984. Changes in glutathione and glutathione metabolizing enzymes in human erythrocytes and lymphocytes as a function of age of donor. *Age* 7:3–7.

Stohs, S. J., Hassing, J. M., Al-Turk, W. A., and Masoud, A. N. 1980. Glutathione levels in hepatic and extrahepatic tissues of mice as a function of age. *Age* 3:11–14.

Storer, J. B. 1965. Radiation resistance with age in normal and irradiated populations of mice. *Radiation Research* 25:435–459.

Thornalley, P. J., and Dodd, N. J. F. 1985. Free radical production from normal and adriamycin-treated rat cardiac sarcosomes. *Biochemical Pharmacology* 34:669–674.

Tryka, A. F., Godleski, J. J., and Brain, J. D. 1984. Differences in effects of immediate and delayed hyperoxia exposure on bleomycin-induced pulmonary injury. *Cancer Treatment Reports* 68:759–764.

Vanella, A., Geremia, E., D'Urso, G., Tiriolo, P., DiSilvestro, I., Grimaldi, R., and Pinturo, R. 1982. Superoxide dismutase activities in aging rat brain. *Gerontology* 28:108–113.

Videla, L. A., Fernandez, V., and Valenzuela, A. 1987. Age-dependent changes in rat liver lipid peroxidation and glutathione content induced by acute ethanol ingestion. *Cell Biochemistry and Function* 5:273–280.

Von Hoff, D. D., Layard, M. W., Basa, P., Davis, H. L., Jr., Von Hoff, A. L., Rozencweig, M., and Muggia, F. M. 1979. Risk factors for doxorubicin-induced congestive heart failure. *Annals of Internal Medicine* 91:710–717.

Walker, B. E., Kelleher, J., Dixon, M. F., and Losowsky, M. S. 1974. Vitamin E protection of the liver from paracetamol in the rat. *Clinical Science and Molecular Medicine* 47:449–459.

Walker, P. D., and Shah, S. V. 1987. Gentamicin enhanced production of hydrogen peroxide by renal cortical mitochondria. *American Journal of Physiology* 253:C495–C499.

Walker, P. D., and Shah, S. V. 1988. Evidence suggesting a role for hydroxyl radical in gentamicin-induced acute renal failure in rats. *Journal of Clinical Investigations* 81:334–341.

Weinberg, L. E., and Singal, P. K. 1987. Refractory heart failure and age-related differences in adriamycin-induced myocardial changes in rats. *Canadian Journal of Physiology and Pharmacology* 65:1957–1965.

Wiberg, G. S., Trenholm, H. L., and Coldwell, B. B. 1970. Increased ethanol toxicity in old rats: Changes in LD_{50}, in vivo and in vitro metabolism, and liver alcohol dehydrogenase activity. *Toxicology and Applied Pharmacology* 16:718–727.

Yamauchi, T., Raffin, T. A., Yang, P., and Sikic, B. I. 1987. Differential protective effects of varying degrees of hypoxia on the cytotoxicities of etoposide and bleomycin. *Cancer Chemotherapy and Pharmacology* 19:282–286.

Younes, M., and Siegers, C. 1985. The role of iron in the paracetamol- and CCl_4-induced lipid peroxidation and hepatotoxicity. *Chemico-Biologic Interactions* 55:327–334.

Yu, B. P., Masoro, E. J., Murata, I., Bertrand, H. A., and Lynd, F. T. 1982. Life span study of SPF Fischer 344 male rats fed ad libitum or restricted diets. Longevity, growth, lean body mass and disease. *Journal of Gerontology* 37:130–141.

Zitting, A., and Heinonen, T. 1980. Decrease of reduced glutathione in isolated rat hepatocytes caused by acrolein, acrylonitrile, and the thermal degradation products of styrene copolymers. *Toxicology* 17:333–341.

Zweier, J. L. 1985. Iron-mediated formation of an oxidized adriamycin free radical. *Biochimica et Biophysica Acta* 839:209–213.

3

Molecular Aspects of Aging
and Carcinogenesis

S. Spence McCachren, M.D.
Jeffrey Crawford, M.D.
Harvey Jay Cohen, M.D.

Cancer is a major cause of morbidity and mortality in the aged population. In the United States more than 50 percent of cancers occur in the 11 percent of the population over age 65. Review of data from the National Cancer Institute's Surveillance, Epidemiology, and End Results (SEER) Program reveals that the absolute age-specific incidence of and mortality from cancer rise as a function of age (Mathe and Reizenstein, 1985; Young et al., 1981). These data refute earlier reports, based on comparison of cancer mortality with total population mortality, that cancer mortality decreases with age (Brody, 1983). In fact, the SEER program reported that the 5-year survival for most types of cancer decreases with advancing age. The increased ratio of cancer mortality to cancer incidence suggests that cancer is more lethal in elderly people than in young people (Ries, Pollack, and Young, 1983). Clearly, the belief that elderly people tend more "to die with cancer than of cancer" is no longer tenable (Fries, 1980).

To understand the increased incidence of neoplasia in elderly persons, one must understand the basic mechanisms of carcinogenesis and how the involved metabolic pathways are altered with age. It has been estimated that most tumors arise from exposure to exogenous factors that may be avoidable (Doll and Peto, 1981; Horton, 1983; National Research Council, 1988). Lung cancer is an instructive example. Tobacco smoking is estimated to cause 30–40 percent of all cancer deaths in the United States (Loeb et al., 1984). The SEER program showed an apparent decrease in lung cancer incidence in older age groups (U.S. Department of Health and Human Services, 1985), but this was best explained by a reduced prevalence of smoking in these groups. Data from the Lung Cancer Early Detection Project were available for annual cancer incidence in men over age 45 with reference to smoking status (Melamed et al., 1984). When the annual age-specific cancer incidence for the population at highest risk (smokers) is corrected lung cancer risk increases dramatically with age. Although these data demonstrate in smokers a higher incidence of lung cancer with increasing age, age itself has not been shown to be a risk factor independent of prolonged smoking (Loeb et al., 1984). These data do suggest that the aged population may deal with external carcinogenic insults differently than the younger population. The known reduction in risk of lung cancer after cessation of smoking suggests that the steps in development of cancer may be partially reversible. If these steps can be identified, then a rational plan for reduction in cancer risk by avoidance of carcinogenic toxicants and perhaps preventive use of "anticarcinogens" may become practical.

The theories attempting to explain the increased incidence of cancer with aging may be grouped into several categories: (1) increased duration of exposure to carcinogenic agents, (2) decreased ability to accurately repair DNA damage induced by carcinogens, (3) increased susceptibility of aged cells to carcinogenic insults, and (4) decreased host defenses against cancer. In this chapter, we briefly review the mechanisms in the multistep development of cancer and the role of oncogenes in this process. The effects of carcinogens in elderly persons, particularly in metabolism, free radical generation, and DNA repair are then discussed. Finally, we attempt to determine if a rational approach to cancer prevention is suggested by the data.

The Nature of Cancer Development

Much of our understanding of carcinogenesis has arisen from the use of animal models and chemical carcinogens (Farber, 1981). A multistep model has been developed that also fits with the observed development of cancer in humans (Farber, 1984). The detailed mechanisms at each step of the model are slowly being elucidated, with the role of oncogenes and growth factors being major targets of research.

The development of a cancer proceeds in steps from initiation, through promotion, and eventually progression from a premalignant group of cells to a frankly malignant lesion (Farber, 1984). Initiation, the first step, involves the introduction of an irreversible lesion into the genomic DNA of a stem cell. Such a change may result from exposure to chemicals, physical agents, and viruses, or from endogenous errors in DNA replication. All but the last may be controlled to some extent by reducing exposure to external agents. It is estimated that a spontaneous somatic mutation occurs in 1 in 10^6 cell divisions. Such lesions may be potentially carcinogenic, and, with approximately 10^{16} cell divisions occurring in a human lifetime, the number of such mutations may be high at advanced age (Ebbesen, 1984). The accumulation of these spontaneous somatic mutations has been invoked by some to explain the increased incidence of cancer with age (Cairns, 1983). Given that the time required for a single cellular mutation to progress to a clinically apparent tumor may require 10–30 percent of an organism's life span, this is consistent with the experimental data on cancer incidence.

It is not clear whether initiated cells can be recognized phenotypically. Such a phenotype would be characterized by loss of some features of normal cellular differentiation but without the development of an abnormal proliferative stage. Possible examples of initiated lesions include epithelial dysplasia (carcinoma in-situ) and preleukemia (Scott and Wille, 1984). Because initiation involves introduction of lesions in genomic DNA, the accuracy and integrity of DNA repair mechanisms are vital in protection from carcinogens. Some compounds behave as carcinogens only when activated metabolically, so an understanding of the metabolism of toxicants is relevant to our discussion. Changes in DNA repair and toxicant metabolism have been documented with age and are discussed below.

The second step in carcinogenesis is promotion, the initial proliferative phase. Many substances function as promoters, including polyunsaturated fatty acids, phenobarbital, hormones, and phorbol diesters. These have the common property of inducing mitogenesis in the initiated cell. These substances will not induce transformation without prior initiation, although compounds do exist that can function as both initiators and promoters (Newbold, Overell, and Connell, 1982). Promotion can occur immediately after initiation or may be delayed. It is dose dependent and is most effective with constant or repetitive stimuli rather than a single exposure. Most important, promotion may be reversible. An example is the regression of pulmonary epithelial dysplasia after cessation of smoking (Loeb et al., 1984).

The final step of carcinogenesis, progression, may be divided into three stages: transformation, clonal progression, and metastasis. Transformation involves the conversion of a premalignant hyperplastic group of cells to frankly malignant cells. An example may be the progression of an adenomatous polyp to adenocarcinoma. The clinical recognition of this stage usually depends on recognition of invasiveness of the abnormal cells into surrounding tissues. The genetic events associated with progression are not clear. Activated *ras* oncogenes are frequently found in colon adenocarcinomas (Bos et al., 1987). Recent investigations reveal that they may also be found in adenomatous polyps and thus may be a marker of initiation and promotion, rather than of the final transformation to frank neoplasia (Forrester et al., 1987). Cancer cells are also frequently characterized by genomic instability. This is most easily recognized by the abnormal karyotypes of many tumors, which may change over time (Yunis, 1983). One result of this instability is the development of clones of cancer cells with varying degrees of invasiveness, growth rate, drug resistance, and so forth. Thus, as tumors grow, they consist of a heterogeneous population of cancer cells (Heppner, 1984; Schnipper, 1985). The major clinical significance of this heterogeneity is that treatment will usually select for the growth of a clone of resistant cells. Another consequence is the occasional emergence of a clone of cells with a markedly increased growth rate or invasiveness. One example may be the transformation of a slow-growing chronic granulocytic leukemia to a rapidly growing acute leukemia, "blast crisis." Thus, as is familiar to clinicians, the behavior of a given tumor in a patient may vary dramatically over time. This may reflect in part a variation in tumor cell surface antigens and escape from host immunological surveillance. The final component of tumor progression is metastasis. The propensity of a tumor to metastasize (spread to distant sites in the body) may vary over time, in part because of clonal selection but also because of variations in host defense mechanisms.

It is now generally accepted that the initial step in the development of cancer is a genomic mutation. This suspicion originally arose from the observation of well-defined karyotypic abnormalities associated with some cancers, such as chronic myelocytic leukemia (Yunis, 1983). Further evidence for the importance of genomic mutation was provided by Bruce Ames and co-workers (McCann and Ames, 1976). They showed that the mutagenic potential of many chemicals was positively correlated with carcinogenic activity. Their system used prokaryotic mutagenesis, but culture systems for mammalian cells were soon adapted to allow evaluation of mutagenic and transforming activity of exogenous agents.

With these systems it was conclusively shown that chemicals could transform cells in vitro, as could certain viruses and radiation. It still was unproven that the cellular transformation was purely the result of a genetic mutation. The development of DNA transfection into cells by coprecipitation with calcium phosphate by Graham and van der Eb (1973) allowed this hypothesis to be tested. The transformed phenotype could be transferred from cell to cell by DNA transfection, and, furthermore, specific gene sequences could be cloned that were responsible for this transformation (Shih et al., 1979). Such sequences could be found in cancer cells or tumor viruses and were termed onco-genes.

The discovery soon followed that normal cells contained DNA se-quences closely related to these oncogenes, termed *protooncogenes* (Stehelin et al., 1976). The surprising finding that tumor-associated *ras* oncogenes differed from the normal cellular *ras* proto-oncogene by only a single base mutation demonstrated conclusively that a minor change in a gene could lead to a major change in genetic regulation of the cell and ultimately neoplastic transformation (Parada et al., 1982; Tabin et al., 1982). Changes such as this point mutation are frequently the result of chemical and physical mutagens and carcinogens. This supports concepts to identify and then limit exposure to these stimuli and also highlights the role DNA repair mechanisms may play in pro-tection from cancer.

A single mutation or expression of a single oncogene is usually insufficient to cause transformation in normal cell lines and, presum-ably, in vivo. Neither *myc* nor *ras* oncogene transfection alone will transform rat embryo fibroblasts, but together they efficiently trans-form the cells (Land, Parada, and Weinberg, 1983). This apparent re-quirement for the activation or expression of more than one oncogene is consistent with the multistep model of carcinogenesis advanced ear-lier. Further evidence for the multistep nature of cancer development and for tissue specificity was obtained by Leder and associates using a transgenic mouse model (Stewart, Pattengale, and Leder, 1984). A transgenic strain of mice was made whose cells contained the *myc* oncogene under the control of a mouse mammary tumor virus pro-moter. This strain of mice had a higher incidence of mammary carci-noma than the wild-type strain, but both malignant and normal mam-mary epithelial cells overexpressed the foreign *myc* gene, implying that a subsequent event was required for tumor development. There is now evidence in human systems for the involvement of several oncogenes in the malignant phenotype: HL-60 human promyelocytic leukemia cells contain *myc* and *ras* oncogenes, and both *myc* and *neu* oncogenes have been implicated in breast carcinomas (Collins et al., 1987; Slamon et al., 1987).

Thus far, evidence of activated oncogenes has been found in only a minority of human tumor DNAs. Recently anti-oncogenes have been postulated. When mutated, these may be recognized as "cancer sus-ceptibility" genes, such as is now known to be important in retinoblas-toma. In general, one would expect a mutation to more easily interfere with the action of a gene than to activate it. Therefore, the inactivation of anti-oncogenes may be of major importance in the development of cancer. Evidence that this is the case has been obtained in colorectal carcinoma and in small cell lung cancer, in addition to retinoblastoma (Friend et al., 1986; Naylor et al., 1987; Solomon, Voss, and Hall, 1978).

The evidence accumulated to date implicates DNA mutation as the fundamental lesion leading to the development of cancer. We have briefly reviewed the multistep nature of carcinogenesis and have shown how current research on the function of oncogenes supports this model. The role of growth factors in development of cancer shall not be reviewed here other than to state that many oncogenes are involved in systems of signal transduction and therefore may lead to alterations in response to growth factors when mutated.

The increasing incidence of cancer with age suggests that as a person ages he or she may have a greater susceptibility to one or more steps of cancer development. The discussion of this topic is broken down into the following sections: (1) The ability of the aged organism to detoxify (or to activate) carcinogens metabolically is one area of change. (2) The containment of damage induced by carcinogens (directly or indirectly, as by free radicals) is the next step that may change with age. (3) Subsequently, DNA repair mechanisms become of major importance. (4) The genomic stability and characteristics of aging organisms also may alter. (5) Data regarding changes in tumor promotion with aging are largely limited to evaluation of changes in metabolism of tumor promoters. (6) Finally, damage containment by the immune system may be affected. Age-related declines in immune function as well as effects of environmental toxicants on immune function shall be considered. An approach to cancer prevention in elderly individuals based on the multistep model of carcinogenesis and the metabolic pathways involved shall be addressed.

Changes in Metabolism of Carcinogens with Age

Many cancers appear to be the result of exposure to environmental carcinogens. Central to the cancer–aging relationship is whether age is merely permissive in the development of neoplasia through the accumulation and potential expression of carcinogenic cellular events, or whether the altered physiology of the aged person contributes directly to accelerate the steps of carcinogenesis. It is well known that elderly people respond differently to drugs than do young people (Geokas and Haverback, 1969; Ouslander, 1981). These changes result from altered absorption, distribution, metabolism, and excretion. Decrements in function of the liver and kidney, regional alteration in blood flow, and change in body composition are all involved in the elderly person's response to drugs. Responses to environmental toxicants, including carcinogens, as a function of age are less well studied.

The metabolism of environmental carcinogens involves two main steps. The first step, functionalization, results in increased polarity of compounds via oxidation, reduction, or hydrolysis (Williams, 1959). This is accomplished mainly by the mixed function oxidase system, a series of enzymes associated with the endoplasmic reticulum membrane and found at highest levels in the liver and kidney. From molecular oxygen, one atom of oxygen is transferred to substrate and one to water. Electrons are transferred from NADPH to cytochrome P-450 via NADPH-dependent cytochrome P-450 reductase. Lipid also has a necessary role in the process, and changes in lipid components of the system will alter overall activity. The next step of carcinogen metabolism is conjugation of the polar compound with an endogenous acceptor such as glucuronic acid, glutathione, sulfate, or other groups (Williams, 1959). A single polar metabolite may be conjugated to a variety of ligands depending on the supply of potential acceptor molecules and the tissue studied. Most of the studies on carcinogen metabolism at advanced age have used rodent models. Limited primate studies have been performed. Comparison of the studies is difficult because of differences in analytical techniques used, controls, animal strains, and definitions of advanced age. A common problem is that important changes in metabolic function with age may be of small amplitude and therefore difficult to detect. Also, if the major changes are in reaction kinetics, studies using saturating doses of carcinogens may not reveal significant changes with age.

Lipid is an integral part of the mixed function oxidase system. A decrease in the ratio of phospholipid to lipid in hepatic microsomes from older rats has been reported (Birnbaum and Baird, 1978b; Grinna, 1977). In mice, however, Birnbaum (1980) noted no change in the ratio with age. There is, though, a decrease in the phosphatidyl choline in mouse hepatic microsomes and an increase in the relative amount of cholesterol in mouse and rat microsomal membranes with aging (Birnbaum, 1980; Hawcroft, Jones, and Martin, 1982). It is unclear if functional differences in the mixed function oxidase system result from these changes in lipid composition.

Several groups have reported a decrease in activity of NADPH-dependent cytochrome P-450 reductase with aging (Kato, Takanaka, and Onoda, 1970; Rikans and Notley, 1984; Schmucker and Wang, 1980). In one strain of rat the reduced activity was felt to be due to lowered substrate affinity resulting from posttranslational modifications (Schmucker and Wang, 1983). These results were contradicted by one group who found no changes related to age in either mice or rats (Birnbaum, 1980; Birnbaum and Baird, 1978a, 1978b). Some of the contradictions may be explained by use of different strains of animals and different ages for the study. No consistent change across all species has yet been described.

The level of total liver microsomal cytochrome P-450 activity does not appear to change with age in rats (Abraham, Levere, and Freedman, 1985; Kao and Hudson, 1980; Schmucker and Wang, 1980). Peggins, Shipley, and Weiner (1984) reported no change in P-450 level with age in miniature swine. In hamsters, however, both sexes were reported to develop increases in P-450 as they aged (Brrt, Hruza, and Baker, 1983). The cytochrome P-450 system comprises a number of species of molecules, and Fujita et al. (1985) suggested that only specific forms change with age but the total P-450 level remains constant. In particular, they found a loss with age of those forms specific only to males, suggesting sex differences may be important during aging. In nonhuman primates the situation is less well studied. No change in total phospholipids has been noted in the mixed function oxidase system in monkeys (Maloney et al., 1986). There is little change with age in the total cytochrome P-450 level or reductase activity. This is also true in the primate *Macaca nemestrina,* even though there is an age-related increase in phospholipid and cholesterol in hepatic microsomes of this species (Sutter et al., 1985). Thus, the data suggest little overall change in cytochrome P-450 levels or reductase activity with aging. Some isozymes of the mixed function oxidase system may change with age, but the significance of this change for carcinogen activation or inactivation remains uncertain.

The cytochrome P-450 system can be induced by a variety of agents, including phenobarbital and polycyclic aromatic hydrocarbons. The effects of aging on induction of the system may be inducer specific, as well as species and strain specific. For instance, phenobarbital has been reported to induce hepatic mixed function oxidases equally in young and aged mice and rats (Kato, Takanaka, and Onoda, 1970; Rikans and Notley, 1984). Birnbaum and Baird (1978b), however, showed increased induction in senescent rats by a mixture of polychlorinated biphenyls. Kato and Takanaka (1968a) showed that there was a decrease in a specific P-450 peptide after phenobarbital induction in senescent rats. Thus, studies measuring overall levels or activities of enzyme systems with aging may lack the sensitivity required to detect potentially significant changes in single components or isozymes. The changes may also vary between tissues. In rat kidneys, cytochrome P-450 and reductase activities have been shown to decrease with age, and their induction is also impaired (McMartin et al., 1980).

To illustrate the problems in interpreting studies with different substrates, tissues, and species it is useful to consider the metabolism of a procarcinogen whose metabolism has been well studied, benzo(a)-pyrene (BP). The metabolism of BP yields diols and epoxides, the carcinogenic products. Free radicals are involved in some of the damage to macromolecules caused by BP (Rabovsky et al., 1984) and shall be reviewed later. Birnbaum reported a greater than 40 percent decrease in BP oxidation by the hepatic mixed function oxidase system in senescent rats, but inducibility by 3-methylcholanthrene was still effective (Birnbaum and Baird, 1978a). In mice, however, there was an apparent threefold increase in BP oxidation with age, but poor inducibility with 3-methylcholanthrene (Birnbaum, 1980). Thus, effects of age vary with species studied. Rabovsky et al. (1984) showed a large increase in BP oxidation with age in rat lung tissue, an important result because most exposure to BP is by inhalation. Yet in female monkeys no changes have yet been reported with age (Sutter et al., 1985).

A more direct means of testing effects of age-related changes in the mixed function oxidase system on carcinogen metabolism is to use the metabolic products in the Ames mutagen assay (Ames, 1979; Ames, Magaw, and Gold, 1987; McCann and Ames, 1976). Using this method Baird and Birnbaum (1979) found that liver homogenates from senescent rats and mice produced more mutations from BP than did homogenates from young animals. The mutagenicity of aflatoxin B_1 decreased with aging, demonstrating the substrate specificity of the effect (Jayaraj and Richardson, 1981). Homogenates from other tissues also alter the activation of procarcinogens with age. Kidney homogenates from aged mice and rats produced lower mutagen levels from aflatoxin B_1 and 2-aminofluorene than did homogenates from young animals (Sutter et al., 1982). Other studies confirm the substrate-, tissue-, species-, and strain-specific effects of age on metabolism (Baird and Birnbaum, 1979; Guttenplan and Blenakov, 1981).

Phenobarbital is a tumor promoter in rat liver (Schate-Hermann, 1985). Its metabolism has been reported to decrease in liver from aged rats and induction of its metabolic system has also been seen to decline with age (Kapetanovic, Sweeny, and Rapoport, 1982; Kato and Takanaka, 1968b). The net result is an increase in phenobarbital half-life in old animals and possibly an increased risk of tumor promotion from phenobarbital. If confirmed for other tumor promoters, such results could explain part of the increased incidence of tumors with aging. Such a promotion effect might be enhanced because phenobarbital may induce systems of activation for other procarcinogens to mutagenic compounds. Currently, the data are contradictory on effects of age on promotion. In one mouse model system, for instance, using a phorbol ester promoter and DMBA initiator, there was no change in initiation with age, but a decrease in promoter activity (Robertson and Birnbaum, 1982).

The literature dealing with conjugation of metabolites is just as contradictory and confusing as that on the mixed function oxidase system. Glucuronidation is a major pathway to conjugation for a variety of compounds. There are at least three different glucuronyl transferase systems, which vary in substrate specificity and inducibility. The glucuronyl transferase induced by polycyclic hydrocarbons also conjugates thyroid hormones and does not seem to change in liver during adulthood, but it may decline in kidney (Borghoff and Birnbaum, 1985). The glucuronyl transferase system responsible for conjugating bilirubin, however, has been reported to decline with aging (Borghoff and Birnbaum, 1985, 1986). Because glucuronidation is often looked at as a detoxification mechanism, declines in activity may be important in increasing effectiveness of carcinogens. Complicating the picture is a reported increase in glucuronidase activity with age (Borghoff and Birnbaum, 1985; Schmucker and Wang, 1979). The studies on conjugation to sulfate and glutathione also are complicated by the existence of multiple enzymes with overlapping activities, and varying reported changes with age depending on substrate, tissue, and species studied (Fujita et al., 1985a, 1985b; Kosta et al., 1981; Spearman and Liebmen, 1984).

In summary, numerous studies have examined the effects of aging on metabolic activation and inactivation of environmental carcinogens in a variety of animal models. No fundamental change has been noted across all species and tissues studied. In many cases, although total activity of an enzyme system remains unchanged with aging, there may be a biologically significant shift in the balance of isozymes involved that would not have been detected in older studies. With more sophisticated analytical techniques it is likely that important changes with age in the metabolism of environmental toxicants will be more thoroughly defined. These may well be tissue and species specific. Also, though age may increase the risk of mutagenesis or tumor promotion from some compounds, it may reduce the risk from others. The data thus far suggest that the elderly do respond differently to a variety of carcinogenic compounds, whether ingested (aflatoxins and N-nitroso compounds), inhaled (benzo(a)pyrene, polycyclic hydrocarbons, and tars), or contacted topically (alkyl halides and polycyclic hydrocarbons).

Genetic Stability, DNA Damage, and DNA Repair in Aging

All normal mammalian cells contain proto-oncogenes, DNA sequences that upon activation or altered expression give a cell a malignant phenotype. As previously discussed, environmental carcinogens can give rise to mutation and subsequent malignancy. Whether aging itself predisposes to malignancy without the action of exogenous carcinogens is under investigation. There is evidence for changes in gene regulation with aging. Nakamura and Hart (1987) found no change in expression of several oncogenes in fresh human fibroblasts from donors ages 0–70 years. Little change was observed during subsequent culture. Srivastava et al. (1985) observed, however, that during the limited replicative life span of human diploid fibroblasts in vitro there was up to a fourfold amplification of the c-Ha-*ras*-1 proto-oncogene and a corresponding increase in its mRNA and protein product.

The frequency and significance of such gene amplification with age are under investigation. If such overexpression were to occur in a population of cell in vitro it could predispose to transformation by mutation of a cooperating oncogene (Land, Parada, and Weinberg, 1983). There is also evidence that c-*myc* transcript levels increase in the liver of aging mice (Matocha et al., 1987). The expression of c-*src* or c-*sis* was not increased. No differences were seen with age in brain cells. The elevation in c-*myc* transcript levels did not correlate with the age-related polyploidy commonly seen in hepatocyte nuclei (Abraham, Levere, and Freedman, 1985; Kao and Hudson, 1980). One hypothesis to explain the increase in hepatic growth is that hormones involved in hepatic growth such as insulin, glucagon, and epidermal growth factor may be elevated in aging (Leffert et al., 1982). Another is that the increase in c-*myc* may be due to an age-related loss of normal regulatory mechanisms.

Gene expression is regulated at the levels of transcription initiation, transcript processing, and transcript degradation. Transcript initiation may be regulated by local DNA supercoiling and methylation, among other mechanisms. In mice the methylation of c-*myc* changed during aging (Ono et al., 1986). Methylation of *myc* was decreased in spleen, increased in liver, and unchanged in brain from aged mice. No changes in methylation were noted in actin and dihydrofolate reductase, suggesting the alterations were limited to the oncogene. Changes have also been seen in methylation of H-*ras* and c-*src*. The functional significance of methylation changes with aging are not clear but similar changes in methylation of genes are often seen in cancer cells (Mays-Hoppes, 1985; Riggs and Jones, 1983). In old mice, T-cell proliferative responses to mitogenic lectins are decreased. This is accompanied by a decline in levels of c-*myc* expression. Yet c-*myc* transcription rate and degradation are unchanged, suggesting that an age-related alteration in posttranscriptional processing is present (Buckler et al., 1988). Thus, there is evidence for changes in gene regulation with aging, and it is against this background that the effects of carcinogens must be viewed.

The data indicating that DNA mutations are responsible for cancer have been reviewed. Interactions with agents from the environment or endogenous to the cell may lead to the induction of mutation, which must be heritable to cause malignancy. The types of damage caused by chemical and physical agents, the repair systems that protect the cells from such damage, and the effect of aging on these processes shall be discussed. Among the most common types of lesions are noncoding lesions, typified by ultraviolet radiation-induced pyrimidine dimers, but also caused by aflatoxin B_1, benzo(a)pyrene, and 2-acetylamino-fluorene, among many other agents (Friedberg, 1985; Schendel, 1981). Strand breaks are induced by ionizing radiation, radiomimetic drugs, and free radicals (Friedberg, 1985; Schendel, 1981). Cross-links arise from psoralens, nitrogen mustard derivatives, and mitomycin D (Friedberg, 1985; Schendel, 1981). Altered bases may result from incorporation of base analogues (2-aminopurine or 5-bromouracil), thermal or chemical deamination of adenine, 3-alkylation of adenine, or hydroxylamine. Miscoding alkylation damage results from alkylnitrosoureas or nitrosodialkylamines and, via O6-alkylation of guanine, may alter base pairing followed by base transition (Friedberg, 1985; Schendel, 1981). We shall review the characteristics during aging of repair of DNA damage due to ultraviolet irradiation and related drugs, repair of strand breaks, and alkylation of bases.

DNA damage from a number of insults may increase with age. Price, Modak, and Makinodan (1971) showed that DNA strand breaks increased with age in mice. Total body X-irradiation of young mice replicated these changes. Using alkaline sucrose nucleoid sedimentation, Wheeler and Lett (1974) found an age-related increase in DNA strand breaks in beagles, but DNA repair capability was not noted to be impaired. In a preliminary study Burns, Sargent, and Albert (1981) exposed rat epidermis to 1,220-rad electron beam irradiation at various ages, finding similar amounts of damage induced at all ages, but that the rate of repair decreased fivefold with aging.

Repair of DNA damage due to ultraviolet irradiation, and mutagens such as benzo(a)pyrene and aflatoxin B_1, is referred to as *excision repair* and proceeds in several steps (Friedberg, 1985). A lesion is recognized and repair is initiated by incision of the DNA strand nearby, either directly or after glycosylation. An exonuclease excises the altered base and nearby nucleotides. The excised area is resynthesized by DNA polymerase using the unaltered opposite strand as a template. Finally, ligase seals the gap. This excision repair can be measured by several techniques: (1) repair replication, (2) bromodeoxyuridine photolysis, and (3) measurement of unscheduled DNA synthesis. The last method is generally the simplest and the most often used. The repair of strand breaks, or postreplicative repair, consists of recombination between sister chromatids or de novo synthesis. Repair of these lesions is usually rapid. Alkaline sucrose gradient sedimentation is the method commonly used to measure strand breaks, although alkaline elution may also be used. Alkylation of DNA is typical of damage caused by N-nitroso compounds. Tumor induction by these compounds correlates with O6-alkylation of guanine or O4-alkylation of thymine. Repair of other alkylation damage is accomplished by excision repair, but these two lesions are also repaired by transfer of the methyl (or ethyl) group to cysteine in a methyltransferase protein. No reparative synthesis is required.

Numerous studies have evaluated the efficacy of DNA repair mechanisms in relation to age. Care must be taken in interpreting the results of these studies because several groups have reported that DNA excision repair may decrease markedly in some cells maintained in culture when compared with the corresponding in vivo situation. This has been noted for mouse embryo fibroblasts and rat epithelium (Peleg, Raz, and Ben-Ishai, 1977; Vijg et al., 1985; Vijg, Mullaart, and Roza, 1985). These changes may only be apparent with specific insults rather than generalized phenomena.

Ishikawa and Sakurai (1986) studied ultraviolet-induced unscheduled DNA synthesis (UDS) in mouse skin in intact animals. Low doses of ultraviolet light or 4-hydroxyaminoquinoline-1-oxide gave the same increase in UDS in 2- and 18-month-old mice. At high doses of ultraviolet light the old mice had a much lower increase in UDS than young mice, suggesting a possible decline in DNA repair mechanisms with age. This result is confounded by the fact that high-dose ultraviolet light may inactivate enzymes by interaction with cysteine. Because protein turnover is decreased with age it is possible that damaged enzymes are not replaced quickly. In subsequent studies in rat hepatocytes, a postmitotic cell, treatment with ultraviolet irradiation in moderate doses and with N-hydroxyacetylaminofluorene or N-nitroso-N-methylurea (NMU) resulted in similar increases in UDS in young and old animals (Sawada and Ishikawa, 1988). DNA repair systems appeared preserved up to doses that would prove lethal for both young and old cells. Interestingly, the capacity for replicative DNA synthesis was markedly reduced in the cells from old rats. This may have a partial protective effect on hepatic carcinogenesis, because cell proliferation plays an important role in chemical carcinogenesis. For instance, hepatocyte regeneration induced by partial hepatectomy enhances both initiation and promotion of tumors (Craddock and Frei, 1974).

Evidence is accumulating for reduced excision repair with aging in humans. Patients older than age 60 are at greater risk of developing nonmelanoma skin cancer than those younger than 60, given the same amount of sun exposure (Vitaliano and Urbach, 1980). Smith (1978) noted an accumulation of DNA damage with age. Lambert, Ringbord, and Swanbeck (1976) and Sbano (1978) describe a decrease in UDS in skin fibroblasts and lymphocytes from patients with extensive photoaged skin. The number of epidermal melanocytes has also been noted to decrease with age (Gilchrest, Blog, and Zabo, 1979). This may therefore lead to increased ultraviolet sensitivity. The skin's immune function may also decrease with age (Epstein, 1983). Both processes may predispose to cancer formation. The number of cell generations in vitro of keratinocytes from chronically sun-exposed skin is reduced compared with that of nonexposed skin from the same donor (Gilchrest, 1979). This is similar to the effect of aging on cultured cells and provides support that in some ways photodamage results in premature aging of skin (Schneider and Mitsui, 1976; Smith and Lincoln, 1984; Stanulis-Praeger, 1987). Exceptions have been noted. Liu, Parsons, and Hanawalt (1982) found no change in ultraviolet-induced UDS in keratinocytes with age. Similarly, no change in UDS with age was noted in isolated human kidney cells after ultraviolet irradiation (Nette et al., 1983). Nette et al. (1984) found an overall decrease with age in ultraviolet-induced UDS in the epidermis of women. Lambert, Ringbord, and Skoog (1979) found a decrease with aging in UDS in response to ultraviolet irradiation in isolated peripheral blood leukocytes of 58 donors ages 13 to 94 years. Kutlaca, Seshadri, and Morley (1982) reported that lymphocytes of older individuals were more sensitive to X rays, and this was confirmed by Licastro et al. (1982) in gamma-irradiated human lymphocytes.

Changes in DNA repair may vary between species and tissues. Ultraviolet-induced UDS in rat retina does not change with age, whereas a dramatic decline is noted in hepatocytes of the same species (Ishikawa, Takayama, and Kitagawa, 1978; Richardson, Birchenall-Sparks, and Plesko, 1984). In hepatocytes in vitro ultraviolet-induced UDS peaks at 14 months, and declines thereafter, being undetectable at 32 months (Richardson, Birchenall-Sparks, and Plesko, 1984). Mouse fibroblasts also apparently lose their excision repair capacity as the donor ages (Kempf et al., 1984). In contrast, in hamster brain, lung, kidney, and liver there is no change in ultraviolet-induced UDS with age (Gensler, 1981a, 1981b).

Damage due to chemicals is also frequently repaired via the excision repair mechanism operative in ultraviolet-induced damage. In rat retinal cells 4-nitroquinoline-1-oxide, N-nitrosoethylnitrosourea, or methyl methane-sulfonic acid all induced UDS, but no age-related differences were seen (Ishikawa, Takayama, and Kitagawa, 1978). This agrees with the data for ultraviolet irradiation in the same tissue. Human peripheral blood lymphocytes had an increased sensitivity to damage by N-acetoxy-2-acetylaminofluorene. Induction of UDS decreased with age and plateaued at age 60 years (Pero and Norden, 1981).

Changes in DNA repair mechanisms with age depend on the agent studied as well as the tissue. This is elegantly shown in the work of Niedermuller (1982). He administered intraperitoneally NMU, N-nitrosodimethylamine (DMNA), or methyl methanesulfonate (MMS) to male rats. UDS in response to NMU decreased with age in skin, lung, brain, heart, spleen, and gonads. DMNA-induced UDS declined with age in kidney, duodenum, lung, liver, spleen, and gonads. MMS-induced UDS was reduced with aging in heart, liver, lung, and gonads. This suggests that some tissues may become more sensitive to the carcinogenic actions of a chemical than others during normal aging. For example, the hepatocarcinogen DMNA induced less UDS in the liver of aged rats.

Other methods of analysis support the evidence from UDS that there may be a decrease in DNA repair capability with age. Using an alkaline elution technique, Fort and Cerutti (1981) showed that N-ethylnitrosourea (NEU)-induced damage in cultured fibroblasts from young animals was more effectively excised than in cells from old animals. Using alkaline sucrose gradient sedimentation as a measure of DNA repair, Kanagalingam and Balis (1975) studied rat intestinal mucosa. Rats were treated with the carcinogen 1,2-dimethylhydrazine and noncarcinogens (nitrogen mustard and MMS) for intestinal mucosa. The carcinogen induced a high level of repair in the intestinal epithelium of young rats, but the induction in old rats was slower and less pronounced.

Alkylation damage of DNA may be reversed by the excision repair mechanism, but, as described earlier, O6-alkylguanine and O4-alkylthymine may be repaired by methyltransferases. These particular miscoding lesions correlate with the carcinogenic effect of alkylating agents (Montesano, 1981). O6-methylguanine disturbs normal base pairing and leads to misreading of information during replication and transcription. These lesions also alter helical structure, potentially altering DNA folding into higher order structures (Mehta and Ludlum, 1976). Changes in helical structure may affect nucleoid sedimentation and render repair estimates by this method questionable. Alkylation damage can also cause DNA strand breaks from DNA depurination after excision of adducts such as 7-methylguanine or 3-methyladenine (Lipetz, Galsky, and Stephens, 1982).

DNA repair ability of cells for O6-alkylguanine and O4-alkylthymine residues can be measured by quantitating the number of lesions in DNA after alkylating damage or by measuring methyltransferase activity directly in cell extracts. The activity of O6-methyl(ethyl)guanine:DNA alkyltransferase has been measured in various species and tissues. There is wide interindividual variation in activity, but no consistent change with age has been documented (Craddock, Henderson, and Gash, 1984). In humans no change in enzyme activity with age has been noted in lymphocytes, liver, and gastrointestinal tract (Myrnes, Giercksky, and Krokan, 1983; (Pegg et al., 1982; Waldstein et al., 1982). In one study there was evidence for greater inducibility of the enzyme with age in some species (Margison, 1985).

In rats treated with a known intestinal carcinogen, N-methyl(acetoxymethyl)nitrosamine, O6-methylguanine persisted for a longer time in aged animals (Likhachev et al., 1983). Surprisingly, repair of this lesion was less efficient in the livers of young animals, while no differences were noted in the lungs. The authors also examined this agent's effect on DNA structure in peripheral blood mononuclear cells by nucleoid sedimentation. The results suggested either more damage or less efficient repair in older animals. Likhachev, Anisimov, and Ovsyannikov treated rats with a single dose of ^{14}C-N-nitrosodiethylamine and measured the levels of ethylated purines in hepatic and renal DNA (Anisimov, 1987). Alkylguanine residues persisted at higher levels in the kidneys and livers from old rats than from younger animals.

In general, cells that are rapidly proliferating seem more sensitive to carcinogenesis. For instance, partially hepatectomized rats develop liver tumors when treated with NMU, but sham-operated animals developed no tumors (Craddock and Frei, 1974). In a similar experiment, ionizing radiation induced tumors in animals after partial hepatectomy or heminephrectomy (Alexandrov, 1982). Induction of proliferation of intestinal epithelium by placement of a suture enhanced tumor development at the suture site in response to dimethylhydrazine (Pozharisski, 1975). In older animals, there is a general decrease in cellular proliferation, although focal hyperplasias do occur. Therefore, from this line of reasoning, older animals could be somewhat protected from carcinogenic insults. However, this would appear to be outweighed by the defects in DNA repair that develop with cellular aging. Impairment of host mechanisms for limiting tumor growth may also contribute to accelerated carcinogenesis in the aged.

Free Radicals, Aging, and Cancer

Many of the reactions by which xenobiotics affect DNA and protein proceed through the generation of free radicals, and this has been shown for a number of carcinogens. Toxins that are themselves free radicals or contain free radicals include NO, NO_2, soot, tar, and tobacco smoke (Church and Pryor, 1985; Kerr, Calvert, and Demerjian, 1976; Pryor, Jerauchi, and Davis, 1976). Polluted air and cigarette smoke contain high levels of these components. These radicals are capable of oxidizing polyunsaturated fatty acids and other compounds in vivo (Pryor and Lightsey, 1981). At low levels of NO_2 hydrogen ions can be abstracted from olefins, producing nitrous acid as a by-product (Pryor and Lightsey, 1981). This can in turn react with amines, forming the highly carcinogenic nitrosamines. Semiquinones in tobacco smoke are also capable of generating superoxide and eventually hydroxyl radicals (Cosgrove et al., 1985). Cigarette tar has been shown to induce in a dose-dependent manner single-strand breaks in DNA (Borish et al., 1985). This can be inhibited by superoxide dismutase, catalase, and hydroxyl radical scavengers. Strand breaks induced by cigarette tar block subsequent DNA replication (Henner, Grunberg, and Haseltine, 1983). Similar lesions, with 3′-phosphate and 3′-phosphate-glycolate esters, are induced by ionizing radiation (Henner, Grunberg, and Haseltine, 1983; Nilsson and Magnusson, 1982). DNA ligase, like DNA polymerase, has a 3′-OH recognition site and is unable to accurately join some lesions induced by cigarette tar or radiation. The impaired DNA repair mechanisms in the elderly patient may exacerbate the damage as a result of these free-radical-generating agents.

Ozone, although not a radical itself, is very reactive, and is capable of causing free radical formation in a variety of target compounds (Menzel, 1976). Free-radical-mediated reactions are responsible for part of the pathology caused by breathing ozone at the levels found in smog (Menzel, 1976). Although ozone itself does not gain access to DNA in vivo, free radical cascades can lead to damage to DNA and to enzymes, including those involved in DNA repair.

Polycyclic aromatic compounds are common environmental contaminants. Benzo(a)pyrene has already been discussed. Its activation to carcinogens can involve an epoxidation system that results in diols, but it may also be metabolized by a single electron transfer system, involving free radicals, to yield primarily phenols and quinones (Marnett and Reed, 1979; Morgenstern et al., 1981). We have already discussed changes in benzo(a)pyrene metabolism with age. Other compounds that undergo autoxidation to form superoxide and/or hydrogen peroxide (e.g., dopa) may show similar changes in metabolism with age.

Other toxicants may interrupt cellular electron flow and, via single electron transfer reactions, form radicals. Among these agents are alkyl halides (carbon tetrachloride and chloroform), nitrofuran drugs, bleomycin, paraquat, and nitroaromatic compounds (Autor, 1977; Recknagel, Glenda and Hruszkewycz, 1977; Horwitz, Sausville, and Peisach, 1979).

The final source of free radicals is endogenous production (Cerutti, 1985; McCord and Fridovich, 1977). Hydrogen peroxide and superoxide are produced during normal cellular metabolism. Both of these compounds are capable of yielding free radicals by metal-catalyzed production of hydroxyl radicals. Superoxide may also yield free radicals by reaction with lipid hydroperoxides. During phagocytosis high levels of reactive oxygen species are produced and may be a prominent source of free radicals (Babior, 1978).

Are free radicals important in aging and carcinogenesis? Antioxidants, such as vitamin E, may extend the mean life span of primitive organisms, and other antioxidants have been shown to lengthen the mean life span of mice (Harman, 1968, 1982; Sohal, 1981). In general, animals with higher metabolic rates have shorter mean life spans. Production of free radicals correlates with metabolic rate (Tolmasoff, Ona, and Cutler, 1980). Some of these free radicals may then produce pathological damage. Sohal (1981) showed that by reducing respiratory (and metabolic) rate in houseflies, the maximum life span is increased. Fluorescent age pigment also developed to a much less extent in these flies. Increases in life span by as much as 260 percent were noted. This effect has also been seen in studies of caloric restriction and temperature reduction.

Organisms have developed many defense mechanisms against damage from reactive oxygen species. Among these defenses are superoxide dismutase, catalase, glutathione peroxidase, tocopherols, beta-carotene, and uric acid (Ames, 1983; Ames et al., 1981). In spite of these protective mechanisms the reactive oxygen species can persist long enough to damage molecules in the cell. Antioxidants inhibit the production of tumors induced by many carcinogens in several species and organs. This protective effect of antioxidants against chemical carcinogenesis is well established (Ts'o, Caspary, and Lorentzen, 1977). It therefore seems that the production of tumors by many chemicals involves free radical mechanisms.

Oxidative damage to DNA can be estimated by urinary excretion of thymine glycol and thymidine glycol. Measurements in patients from 24 to 84 years of age suggest that the rate of oxidative DNA damage in humans does not significantly change with age (Ames and Saul, 1986). Other forms of DNA damage, including strand breaks and altered repair of such lesions in elderly persons, have been described. Abnormal methylation of DNA, resulting in altered transcription and altered methylation of some oncogenes with aging, may be the potential result of oxidative DNA damage (Denda et al., 1985; Saul, Gee, and Ames, 1987). (Evidence for altered methylation of some oncogenes with aging has already been presented.)

Free radicals may also contribute to carcinogenesis in elderly people by alterations of immune function. Some antioxidants have been shown to enhance immune responsiveness of cells from aged patients (Fidelus and Tsan, 1987). Increased mean life span and increased immune function have been described in mice in response to antioxidants.

In summary, free radicals are involved in the induction of tumors by many environmental toxicants. The background rate of free-radical-induced damage may be constant during aging, but there is evidence of accumulated damage with age in cellular macromolecules (collagen, elastin, DNA, and aging pigment) (Harman, 1986). The finding in animals that antioxidants can reduce cancer incidence and prolong mean life span suggests that similar intervention should further be studied in humans. Finally, free radical damage may contribute to the immune deficiency of aging. Reduced exposure to radical-generating toxicants and dietary changes designed to reduce free radical generation are reasonable in attempts to prolong active life and reduce cancer incidence.

Immune Function, Tumor Surveillance, and Aging

Defects in immune function are a common feature of aging in humans (Weksler, 1982; Weksler and Siskind, 1984). They are reviewed elsewhere in this book in detail. More than one-half of people over 60 years of age have evidence for impaired delayed cutaneous hypersensitivity (Schwab, Staiano-Coico, and Weksler, 1983). This is illustrative of the general impairment of T-cell-dependent functions. By the age of 15 involution of the thymus is well progressed (Boyde, 1932). With increasing age there is a continuing decline in production of thymic hormones and subsequent impairment of T-cell maturation (Lewis et al., 1978; Schwab, Staiano-Coico, and Weksler, 1983). An imbalance in helper and suppressor functions may partially explain the emergence of the monoclonal immunoglobulins and autoimmune syndromes with age (Hallgren et al., 1973; Rodl et al., 1980). Several investigators have demonstrated a decrease in lymphocyte chromosomal stability during aging (Staiano-Coico et al., 1983). This is partially manifested as a wide variation in cellular DNA content in human peripheral blood mononuclear cells in elderly people (Staiano-Coico et al., 1982). T cells from old animals have impaired ability to proliferate in culture, produce less interleukin-2 (IL-2) and have fewer IL-2 receptors (Gillis et al., 1981; Hefton et al., 1980; Nagel et al., 1988). The aging of the immune system may well increase susceptibility to cancer. Evidence for this comes from two observations: (1) Patients with primary immunodeficiencies have an increased risk of tumor development. (2) Similarly, patients on immunosuppressant therapy have an increased risk of tumor development.

Numerous metabolic changes occur with age. Studies suggest that alterations in normal metabolism may interfere with immune function. In mice caloric restriction caused a dramatic increase in lectin-stimulated mitogenesis, a result most marked in the oldest animals (Weindruch et al., 1979). Production of IL-2 was also enhanced in these animals (Richardson and Cheung, 1982). Low density and very low density lipoprotein inhibit lymphocyte mitogenesis in vitro and inhibit macrophage killing of tumor cells (Justement et al., 1984; Waddell, Tauton, and Twomey, 1978). They also decrease marrow stem cell proliferation (Zucker et al., 1979). Response of T cells to concanavalin A can be impaired by cholesterol (Alderson and Green, 1975). In patients with breast cancer and elevated lipids, normalization of serum lipid profiles with drugs improved measures of cell-mediated immunity (Revskoy et al., 1985). Whether these metabolic changes cause or merely accompany immune suppression is not clear. It does seem that metabolic abnormalities, such as those frequently seen in elderly individuals may be associated with immunodepression and that their correction may be beneficial.

If immunosenescence is a significant factor in the development of cancer in elderly people, one might expect an increased rate of growth of transplanted tumors in old animals. The data are contradictory. This may be due in part to variations in rate of decline of immune function with age in different strains of animals, but histological tumor type may play a role in growth rate. In general, squamous cell tumors and some adenocarcinomas and fibrosarcomas grow more rapidly in older animals, although the numbers are small and exceptions have been found. Hematological neoplasm growth does not seem to vary with age (Flood et al., 1981; Goldin et al., 1955; Teller et al., 1964; Thompson, 1976). Anisimov, (1987) has extensively reviewed the studies on this subject.

In summary, the evidence suggests that immunosenescence may increase risk of tumor development in old age. Tumors may more easily escape immune surveillance. There is evidence that dietary and metabolic manipulations may partially improve the immune defects of aging. Similarly, antioxidants have been shown to improve lymphocyte function. The use of immunostimulators such as thymosin alpha-1 and interleukins may be of use in the future. However, definitive recommendations for use of immunostimulatory agents await formal clinical trials.

Summary

During aging there is a continuing increase in the risk of developing cancer. According to current knowledge, the majority of human cancers arise from exposure to environmental toxicants and hence may be preventable. The metabolism of many toxicants varies with age so that the carcinogenic potential of specific compounds may be either higher or lower in elderly persons. Currently, it is difficult to generalize about toxicant metabolism. Free radical mechanisms are involved in the carcinogenicity of many of these toxicants. This would suggest that antioxidant therapy may have protective effects on cancer development. Evidence for this in humans is not yet available, although the beneficial effect is clear in mice. There is a demonstrable accumulation with aging of free-radical-damaged macromolecules: Changes have been noted in collagen, elastin, and DNA, among others. Age-related pigment is also a product of free-radical-mediated reactions. Such accumulated damage may impair cellular functioning, and the DNA damage may increase the risk of cellular transformation.

Carcinogenesis has been shown to result from DNA damage. We have reviewed the general means by which carcinogens, both physical and chemical, may alter DNA. There is accumulating evidence that DNA damage induced by a variety of agents may not be repaired as efficiently in elderly as in young people. Data have been reviewed for decreased genetic stability in aging, as evidenced by variations of DNA content in human peripheral blood mononuclear cells, polyploidy of hepatocytes, and altered expression of oncogenes. The latter may be accompanied by alterations in DNA methylation. This decreased DNA repair ability and lack of genomic stability suggest that elderly persons are certainly at higher risk for potentially carcinogenic genetic damage (both initiation and promotion). Tumors initiated earlier in life may be more efficiently promoted in old age.

Finally, the mechanisms of tumor surveillance are diminished in elderly people. The immunodysregulation of old age is accompanied by an increased susceptibility to infections, monoclonal immunoglobulin disorders, autoimmune syndromes, and possibly cancer. With the ongoing elucidation of immune regulatory mechanisms and the purification of the involved hormones/growth factors, potential means of enhancing immune surveillance in elderly people may be available. The significance of the alterations in immune function with age has been questioned by Siskind (1987), but most investigators believe they are potentially harmful. Many of the immune changes are accompanied by metabolic alterations, and correction of abnormalities in lipid metabolism and restriction of caloric intake have been associated with improved immune function in some species. Whether this may result in improved tumor surveillance remains to be seen.

The major risk factors for human cancer in the United States are tobacco; dietary imbalances; and ingestion of carcinogens, hormones, radiation (predominately ultraviolet-induced skin cancer and radon-related pulmonary tumors), and viruses. Avoidable factors include tobacco, ultraviolet light, and radon. Avoidance of excess fat and calories in the diet also is likely to be of benefit in reducing cancer incidence, in addition to the benefit of reducing morbidity due to obesity and atherosclerosis. The animal evidence for increased cancer morbidity related to excess calorie and fat intake is compelling.

Although the elderly person is at increased risk of cancer development, prevention should start earlier in life. The American Cancer Society recommendations for reducing risks of cancer are the most reasonable guidelines at present. In the near future we may expect advances in the areas of toxicant metabolism, prevention of free radical damage, enhancement of DNA repair or prevention of damage, and enhancement of immune tumor control. The American Cancer Society recommendations are as follows:

1. Avoid obesity.

2. Reduce total fat intake.

3. Increase dietary fiber, as by use of whole-grain cereals and vegetables.

4. Include foods rich in vitamins A and C in daily diet.

5. Include cruciferous vegetables (cabbage, broccoli, brussels sprouts, and cauliflower) in the diet.

6. Be moderate in consumption of alcohol.

7. Be moderate in consumption of salt-cured, smoked, and nitrite-cured foods.

To these we would add the testing of home and work environments for radon, and use of chemical- and pesticide-free food and water to the extent practical. The rapid growth of our knowledge of the mechanisms involved in aging and carcinogenesis should continue, and it is hoped that advances in cancer prevention and amelioration of age-related pathology will soon follow.

References

Abraham, N. G., Levere, R. D., and Freedman, M. L. 1985. Effect of age on rat liver heme and drug metabolism. *Experimental Gerontology* 20: 277–284.

Alderson, J. C. E., and Green, C. 1975. Enrichment of lymphocytes with cholesterol and its effects on lymphocyte activation. *FEBS Letters* 52:208–211.

Alexandrov, S. N. 1982. Late radiation pathology of mammals. In Graffi, A., Magdon, E., Matthes, T., and Tanneberger, S. (Eds.), *Fortschritte der Onkologie* (Band 6). Berlin, Academic-Verlag, pp. 203–234.

Ames, B. N. 1979. Identifying environmental chemicals causing mutation and cancer. *Science* 204:587–593.

Ames, B. N. 1983. Dietary carcinogens and anticarcinogens: Oxygen radicals and degenerative diseases. *Science* 221:1256–1264.

Ames, B. N., Cathcart, R., Schwiers, E., and Hochstein, P. 1981. Uric acid provides an antioxidant defense in humans against oxidant- and radical-caused aging and cancer: A hypothesis. *Proceedings of the National Academy of Sciences (USA)* 78:6848–6862.

Ames, B. N., Magaw, R., and Gold, L. S. 1987. Ranking possible carcinogenic hazards. *Science* 236:271–280.

Ames, B. N., and Saul, R. L. 1988. Cancer, aging, and oxidative DNA damage. In Iversen, O. H. (Ed.), *Theories of Carcinogenesis*. New York, Hemisphere, pp. 203–220.

Anisimov, V. N. 1987. *Carcinogenesis and Aging*. Boca Raton, FL: CRC Press.

Autor, A. P. 1977. *Biochemical Mechanisms of Paraquat Toxicity*. New York, Academic Press.

Babior, B. A. 1978. Oxygen-dependent microbial killing by phagocytes. *New England Journal of Medicine* 298:721–725.

Baird, M. B., and Birnbaum, L. S. 1979. Increased production of mutagenic metabolites of carcinogens by tissues from senescent rodents. *Cancer Research* 39:4752–4755.

Birnbaum, L. S. 1980. Altered hepatic drug metabolism in senescent mice. *Experimental Gerontology* 15:259–267.

Birnbaum, L. S., and Baird, M. B. 1978a. Induction of hepatic mixed function oxidase in senescent rodents. *Experimental Gerontology* 13:299–303.

Birnbaum, L. S., and Baird, M. B. 1978b. Induction of hepatic mixed function oxidase in senescent rodents. II. Effect of polychlorinated biphenyls. *Experimental Gerontology* 13:469–477.

Borghoff, S. J,. and Birnbaum, L. S. 1985. Age-related changes in glucuronidation and deglucuronidation in liver, small intestine, lung, and kidney of male Fischer rats. *Drug Metabolism and Disposition* 13:62–67.

Borghoff, S. J., and Birnbaum, L. S. 1986. Alterations in glucuronidation with age in vivo and in vitro using 4,4'-thiobis(6-t-butyl-m-cresol) as a model compound. *The Toxicologist* 6:147–150.

Borish, E. T., Cosgrove, J. P., Church, D. F., Deutsch, W. A., and Pryor, W. A. 1985. Cigarette tar causes single stranded breaks in DNA. *Biochemical and Biophysical Research Communications* 133:780–786.

Bos, J. L., Fearon, E. R., Hamilton, S. R., Verlaan-de Vries, M., van Boom, J. H., van der Eb, A. J., and Vogelstein, B. 1987. Prevalence of *ras* gene mutations in human colorectal cancers. *Nature* 327:293–297.

Boyde, E. 1932. The weight of the thymus gland in health and disease. *American Journal of Diseases of Children* 43:1162–1214.

Brody, J. A. 1983. Limited importance of cancer and of competing-risk theories in aging. *Journal of Clinical and Experimental Gerontology* 5:141–154.

Brrt, D. F., Hruza, D. S., and Baker, P. Y. 1983. Effects of dietary protein level on hepatic mixed function oxidase systems during aging in two generations Syrian hamsters. *Toxicology and Applied Pharmacology* 68:77–86.

Buckler, A. J., Vie, H., Sonenshein, G. E., and Miller, R. A. 1988. Defective T lymphocytes in old mice. Diminished production of nature c-*myc* RNA after mitogen exposure not attributable to alterations in transcription or RNA stability. *Journal of Immunology* 140:2441–2446.

Burns, F. J., Sargent, E. V., and Albert, R. E. 1981. Carcinogenicity and DNA break repair as a function of age in irradiated rat skin. *Proceedings of the American Association of Cancer Research* 22:910.

Cairns, J. 1983. Aging and the natural history of cancer. In Yancile, R., Carbone, P. P., Patterson, W. B., Steel, K., and Terry, W. D. (Eds.), *Perspectives on Prevention and Treatment of Cancer in the Elderly*. New York, Raven Press, pp. 19–24.

Cerutti, P. A. 1985. Prooxidant states and tumor promotion. *Science* 227:375–381.

Church, D. F., and Pryor, W. A. 1985. Free radical chemistry of cigarette smoke and its toxicological implications. *Environmental Health and Perspectives* 64:111–126.

Collins, S. J. 1987. The HL-60 promyelocytic leukemia cell line: Proliferation, differentiation, and cellular oncogene expression. *Blood* 70:1233–1244.

Cosgrove, J. P., Borish, E. T., Church, D. F., and Pryor, W. A. 1985. The metal-mediated formation of hydroxyl radical by aqueous extracts of cigarette tar. *Biochemical and Biophysical Research Communications* 132:390–396.

Craddock, V. M., and Frei, J. V. 1974. Induction of liver cell adenomata in the rat by a single treatment with N-methyl-N-nitrosourea given at various times after partial hepatectomy. *British Journal of Cancer* 30:503–509.

Craddock, V. M., Henderson, A. R., and Gash, S. 1984. Repair and replication of DNA in rat brain and liver during fetal and post-natal development in relation to nitroso-alkylurea induced carcinogenesis. *Journal of Cancer Research and Clinical Oncology* 108:30–35.

Denda, A., Rao, P. M., Rajelakshmi, S., and Sarma, D. S. R. 1985. 5-azacytidine potentiates initiation induced by carcinogens in rat liver. *Carcinogenesis* 6:145–146.

Doll, R., and Peto, R. 1981. The causes of cancer: Quantitative estimates of avoidable risks of cancer in the United States today. *Journal of the National Cancer Institute* 66:1195–1305.

Ebbesen, P. 1984. Cancer and normal aging. *Mechanisms of Aging and Development* 25:269–283.

Epstein, J. H. 1983. Photocarcinogenesis, skin cancer, and aging. *Journal of the American Academy of Dermatology* 9:487–502.

Farber, E. 1981. Chemical carcinogenesis. *New England Journal of Medicine* 305:1379–1389.

Farber, E. 1984. The multistep nature of cancer development. *Cancer Research* 44:4217–4223.

Fidelus, R. K., and Tsan, M. F. 1987. Glutathione and lymphocyte activation: A function of aging and autoimmune disease. *Immunology* 61:503–508.

Flood, P. M., Urban, J. L., Kripke, M. L., and Schreiber, H. 1981. Loss of tumor-specific and idiotype specific immunity with age. *Journal of Experimental Medicine* 154:245–290.

Forrester, K., Almuguerac, C., Han, K., Grizzle, W. E., and Perucho, M. 1987. Detection of high incidence of K-*ras* oncogenes during human colon tumorigenesis. *Nature* 327:298–303.

Fort, F. L., and Cerutti, P. A. 1981. Altered DNA repair in fibroblasts from aged rats. *Gerontology* 27:306–312.

Friedberg, E. C. 1985. *DNA Repair.* New York, W. H. Freeman.

Friend, S., Bernards, R., Rogelj, S., Weinborg, R. A., Rapaport, J. M., Albert, D. M., and Dryja, T. P. 1986. A human DNA segment with properties of the gene that predisposes to retinoblastoma and osteosarcoma. *Nature* 323:643–646.

Fries, J. F. 1980. Aging, natural death, and the compression of morbidity. *New England Journal of Medicine* 303:130–135.

Fujita, S., Kitagawa, H., Chiba, M., Suzuki, T., Okata, M., and Kitani, K. 1985a. Age and sex associated differences in the relative abundance of multiple species of cytochrome P450 in rat liver microsomes. A separation by HPLC of hepatic microsomal cytochrome P450 species. *Biochemical Pharmacology* 34:1861–1864.

Fujita, S., Kitagawa, H., Ishizawa, H., Suzuki, T., and Kitani, K. 1985b. Age associated alterations in hepatic glutathione-S-transferase activities. *Biochemical Pharmacology* 34:3891–3894.

Gensler, H. L. 1981a. The effect of hamster age on uv-induced unscheduled DNA synthesis in freshly isolated lung and kidney cells. *Experimental Gerontology* 16:59–68.

Gensler, H. L. 1981b. Low level of UV induced unscheduled DNA syntheses in post-mitotic brain cells of hamsters: Possible relevance to aging. *Experimental Gerontology* 16:199–207.

Geokas, M. C., and Haverback, B. J. 1969. The aging gastrointestinal tract. *American Journal Surgery* 117:881–892.

Gilchrest, B. A. 1979. Relationship between actinic damage and chronological aging in keratinocyte cultures of human skin. *Journal of Investigative Dermatology* 72:219–223.

Gilchrest, B. A., Blog, F. B., and Zabo, G. 1979. Effects of aging and chronic sun exposure on melanocytes in human skin. *Journal of Investigative Dermatology* 73:141–143.

Gillis, S., Kozak, R. W., Durante, M., and Weksler, M. E. 1981. Immunological studies of aging. Decreased production of and response to T-cell growth factor by T lymphocytes from aged humans. *Journal of Clinical Investigations* 67:937–942.

Goldin, A., Vendetti, J. M., Humphreys, S. R., Sennis, D., and Mantel, N. 1955. Factors influencing the specificity of action of an antileukemic agent (aminopterin): Host age and weight. *Journal of the National Cancer Institute* 16:709–721.

Graham, F. L., and van der Eb, A. J. 1973. A new technique for the assay of infectivity of human adenovirus 5 DNA. *Virology* 52:456–467.

Grinna, L. 1977. Age related changes in the lipids of the microsomal and mitochondrial membranes of rat liver and kidney. *Mechanisms of Ageing and Development* 6:197–205.

Guttenplan, J. B., and Blenakov, E. G. 1981. Activation of procarcinogens by liver homogenates isolated from female mice at different ages: Lack of significant differences. *Mechanisms of Ageing and Development* 16:29–36.

Hallgren, H. M., Buckley, C. E., Gilbertsen, V. A., and Yunis, E. J. 1973. Lymphocyte phytohemagglutinin responsiveness, immunoglobulins and autoantibodies in aging humans. *Journal of Immunology* 111:1101–107.

Harman, D. 1968. Free radical theory of aging: Effort of free radical inhibitors on the mortality rate of male LAF mice. *Journal of Gerontology* 23:476–482.

Harman, D. 1982. The free radical theory of aging. In Pryor, W. A. (Ed.), *Free Radicals in Biology*. New York, Academic Press, pp. 255–271.

Harman, D. 1986. Free radical theory of aging: Role of free radicals in the origination and evolution of life, aging, and disease processes. In Johnson, J. E., Walford, R., Harman, D., and Miguel, J. (Eds.), *Free Radicals, Aging, and Degenerative Diseases*. New York, Alan R. Liss, pp. 3–49.

Hawcroft, D., Jones, T., and Martin, P. 1982. Studies on age-related changes in cytochrome P450, cytochrome B5, and mixed function oxidase activity in mouse liver microsomes in relation to their phospholipid composition. *Archives of Gerontology and Geriatrics* 1:55–74.

Hefton, J. M., Darlinton, G., Casazza, B. A., and Weksler, M. E. 1980. Immunologic studies of aging. V. Impaired proliferation of PHA responsive human lymphocytes in culture. *Journal of Immunology* 125:1007–1010.

Henner, W. D., Grunberg, S. M., and Haseltine, W. A. 1983. Enzyme action at 3' termini of ionizing radiation-induced DNA strand breaks. *Journal of Biological Chemistry* 258:15198–15205.

Heppner, G. H. 1984. Tumor heterogeneity. *Cancer Research* 44:2259–2265.

Horton, J. 1983. On the avoidance and prevention of cancer. *Clinical Cancer Briefs* July:3–16.

Horwitz, S. B., Sausville, E. A., and Peisach, J. 1979. A role for iron in the degradation of DNA by bleomycin. In Hecht, S. M. (Ed.), *Bleomycin*. New York, Springer-Verlag, pp. 170–183.

Ishikawa, T., and Sakurai, J. 1986. In vivo studies on age dependency of DNA repair with age in mouse skin. *Cancer Research* 46:1344–1348.

Ishikawa, T., Takayama, S., and Kitagawa, T. 1978. DNA repair synthesis in rat retinal ganglion cells treated with chemical carcinogens or ultraviolet light in vitro with special reference to aging and repair level. *Journal of the National Cancer Institute* 61:1101–1105.

Jayaraj, A., and Richardson, A. 1981. Metabolic activation of aflatoxin B1 by liver tissue from male Fischer F344 rats of different ages. *Mechanisms of Ageing and Development* 17:163–171.

Justement, L. B., Patel, S. T., Newman, H. A., and Zwilling, B. S. 1984. Inhibition of macrophage-mediated tumor cell destruction by oxidized lipoproteins. *Journal of the National Cancer Institute* 43:469–474.

Kanagalingam, K., and Balis, M. E. 1975. In vivo repair of rat intestinal DNA damage by alkylating agents. *Cancer* 36:2364–2372.

Kao, J., and Hudson, P. 1980. Induction of the hepatic cytochrome P.450 dependent mono oxygenase system in young and geriatric rats. *Biochemical Pharmacology* 29:1191–1194.

Kapetanovic, I. M., Sweeny, D. J., and Rapoport, S. I. 1982. Phenobarbital pharmacokinetics in rat as a function of age. *Drug Metabolism and Disposition* 10:586–589.

Kato, R., and Takanaka, A. 1968a. Effect of phenobarbital on election transport system, oxidation, and reduction of drugs in liver microsomes of rats of different ages. *Journal of Biochemistry* 63:406–408.

Kato, R., and Takanaka, A. 1968b. Metabolism of drugs in old rats. II. Metabolism in vivo and effects of drugs on old rats. *Japanese Journal of Pharmacology* 18:389–406.

Kato, R., Takanaka, A., and Onoda, K. T. 1970. Studies on age differences in mice for the activity of drug-metabolizing enzymes of liver microsomes. *Japanese Journal of Pharmacology* 20:572–576.

Kempf, C., Schmitt, M., Dance, J. M., and Kempf, J. 1984. Correlation of DNA repair synthesis with aging in mice evidenced by quantitative autoradiography. *Mechanisms of Ageing and Development* 26:183–194.

Kerr, J. A., Calvert, J. G., and Demerjian, K. L. 1976. Free radical reactions in the production of photochemical smog. In Pryor, W. A. (Ed.), *Free Radicals in Biology*. New York, Academic Press, pp. 159–178.

Kutlaca, R., Seshadri, R., and Morley, A. A. 1982. Effect of age on sensitivity of human lymphocytes to radiation. *Mechanisms of Ageing and Development* 19:97–101.

Kosta, H. I., Halsenia, J., Scholtens, E., Knippers, M., and Mulder, G. J. 1981. Dose dependent shifts in sulfation and glucuronidation of phenolic compounds in the rat in vivo and in isolated hepatocytes. *Biochemical Pharmacology* 30:2569–2575.

Lambert, B., Ringbord, U., and Swanbeck, G. 1976. Ultraviolet induced DNA repair synthesis in lymphocytes from patients with extensive actinic keratoses. *Journal of Investigative Dermatology* 67:594–598.

Lambert, B., Ringbord, U., and Skoog, L. 1979. Age-related decrease of ultraviolet light induced DNA repair synthesis in human peripheral leukocytes. *Cancer Research* 39:2792–2795.

Land, H., Parada, L. F., and Weinberg, R. A. 1983. Tumorigenic conversion of primary embryo fibroblasts requires at least two cooperating oncogenes. *Nature* 304:596–602.

Leffert, H. L., Koch, K. S., Moran, T., and Rabalcava, B. 1982. Hormonal control of rat liver regeneration. *Gastroenterology* 76:1470–1482.

Lewis, V. M., Twomey, J. J., Bealmear, P., Goldstein, G., and Good, R. A. 1978. Age, thymic involution, and circulating thymic hormone activity. *Journal of Clinical Endocrinology and Metabolism* 48:145–150.

Licastro, F., Francheshii, C., Chiricolo, M., Battelli, M. G., Tabacchi, P., Cenci, M., Barboni, F., and Pallenzona, D. 1982. DNA repair after gamma irradiation and superoxide dismutase activity from subjects of far advanced age. *Carcinogenesis* 3:45–50.

Likhachev, A. J., Ohsima, H., Anisimov, W. N., Ovsyannikov, A. I., Revskoy, S. Y., Keefer, L. K., and Reist, E. J. 1983. Carcinogenesis and aging. II. Modifying effect of aging on metabolism of methly (acetoxymethyl) nitrosamine and its interaction with DNA of various tissues in rats. *Carcinogenesis* 4:967–971.

Lipetz, P. D., Galsky, A. G., and Stephens, R. E. 1982. Relation of DNA tertiary and quaternary structure to carcinogenic processes. *Advances in Cancer Research* 36:165–210.

Liu, S. C. C., Parsons, C. S., and Hanawalt, P. C. 1982. DNA repair response in human epidermal keratinocytes from donors of different age. *Journal of Investigative Dermatology* 79:330–335.Loeb, L. A., Ernster, V. L., Warner, K. E. 1984. Smoking and lung cancer. *Cancer Research* 44:5940–5958.

Loeb, L. A., Ernster, V. L., Warner, K. E., et al. 1984. Smoking and lung cancer. *Cancer Research* 44:5940–5958.

Maloney, A. G., Schmucker, D. L., Vessey, D. A., and Wang, R. K. 1986. The efforts of aging on the hepatic mixed function oxidase system of male and female monkeys. *Hepatology* 6:282–287.

Margison, G. P. 1985. The effect of age on the metabolism of chemical carcinogens and inducibility of O^6-methyl transferase. *IARC Scientific Publications (Lyon)* 58:225–229.

Marnett, L. J., and Reed, G. A. 1979. Peroxidatic oxidation of benzo(a)pyrene and prostaglandin biosynthesis. *Biochemistry* 18:2923–2929.

Mathe, G., Reizenstein, P. 1985. Aging and human cancer. In Mathe, G., and Reizenstein, P. (Eds.), *Pathophysiological Aspects of Cancer Epidemiology*. Elmsford, NY, Pergamon Press, pp. 195–210.

Matocha, M. F., Cosgrove, J. W., Atuck, J. R., and Rapoport, S. I. 1987. Selective elevation of c-*myc* transcript levels in the liver of the aging Fischer-344 rat. *Biochemica et Biophysica Research Communications* 147:1–7.

Mays-Hoppes, L. L. 1985. DNA methylation: A possible correlation between aging and cancer. In Sohal, R. S., Birnbaum, L. S., and Cutler, R. G. (Eds.), *Molecular Biology of Aging: Gene Stability and Gene Expression*. New York, Raven Press, pp. 49–66.

McCann, J., and Ames, B. N. 1976. Detection of carcinogens as mutagens in the salmonella/microsome test: Assay of 300 chemicals. Discussion. *Proceedings of the National Academy of Sciences (USA)* 73:950–954.

McCord, J. M., and Fridovich, I. 1977. Superoxide dismutases: A history. In Michelson, A., McCord, J. M., and Fridovich, I. (Eds.), *Superoxide and Superoxide Dismutases.* New York, Academic Press, pp. 1–11.

McMartin, D. N., O'Conner, J. A., Fasco, M. J., and Kaminsky, L. S. 1980. Influence of aging and induction on rat liver and kidney microsomal mixed function oxidase systems. *Toxicology and Applied Pharmacology* 54: 411–419.

Mehta, J., and Ludlum, D. B. 1976. Synthesis and properties of poly(O^6-ethylguanylic acid) and poly(O^6-methylguanylic acid). *Biochemistry* 15: 4329–4333.

Melamed, M. R., Flehinger, B. J., Zaman, M. B., Heelar, R. T., Perchick, W. A., and Martin, N. 1984. Screening for lung cancer: Result of the Memorial Sloan-Kettering study in New York. *Chest* 86:44–53.

Menzel, D. B. 1976. The role of free radicals in the toxicity of air pollutants (nitrogen oxides and ozone). In Pryor, W. A. (Ed.), *Free Radicals in Biology* (Vol. 2). New York, Academic Press, pp. 181–202.

Montesano, R. 1981. Alkylation of DNA and tissue specificity in nitrosamine carcinogenesis. *Journal of Supramolecular Structure and Cellular Biochemistry* 17:259–266.

Morgenstern, R. J., Depierre, J. W., Lind, C., Guthenbert, C., Mannervik, B., and Ernster, L. 1981. Benzo(a)pyrene quinones can be generated by lipid peroxidation and are conjugated with glutathione by glutathione S-transferase B from rat liver. *Biochemical and Biophysical Research Communications* 99:682–688.

Myrnes, B., Giercksky, K. E., and Krokan, H. 1983. Interindividual variation in the activity of O^6-methylguanine-DNA methyltransferase and uracil-DNA glycosylase in human organs. *Carcinogenesis* 4:1565–1571.

Nagel, J. E., Chopra, R. K., Chrest, F. J., McCoy, M. T., Schneider, E. L., Holbrook, N. J., and Adler, W. H. 1988. Decreased proliferation, interluekin 2 synthesis, and interleukin 2 receptor expression are accompanied by decreased mRNA expression in phytohemagglutinin-stimulated cells from elderly donors. *Journal of Clinical Investigation* 81:1096–1102.

Nakamura, K. D., and Hart, R. W. 1987. Comparison of proto oncogene expression in seven primate fibroblast cultures. *Mechanisms of Ageing and Development* 39:177–187.

National Research Council Committee on the Biological Effects of Nonionizing Radiations. 1988. *Health Risks of Radon and Other Internally Deposited Alpha-Emitters.* Washington, DC, National Academy Press.

Naylor, S. L., Johnson, B. E., Minna, J. D., and Sakaguchi, A. Y. 1987. Loss of heterozygosity of chromosome 3p markers in small cell lung carcinoma. *Nature* 329:451–453.

Nette, E. G., Sun, Y. K., Xi, Y. P., and King, D. W. 1983. Correlation between aging and DNA repair syntheses in human epidermal and renal cells obtained at surgery. *Federation Proceedings* 42:750.

Nette, E. G., Xi, Y. P., Sun, Y. K., Andrews, A. D., and King, D. W. 1984. A correlation between aging and DNA repair in human epidermal cells. *Mechanisms of Ageing and Development* 24:283–292.

Newbold, R. F., Overell, R. W., and Connell, J. R. 1982. Induction of immortality is an early event in malignant transformation of mammalian cells by carcinogens. *Nature* 299:633–635.

Niedermuller, H. 1982. Age related dependency of DNA repair in rats after DNA damage by carcinogens. *Mechanisms of Ageing and Development* 19:259–271.

Nilsson, S. V., and Magnusson, G. 1982. Sealing of gaps in duplex DNA by T4 DNA ligase. *Nucleic Acids Research* 10:1425–1437.

Ono, T., Tawa, R., Shinya, K., Hirose, S., and Okada, S. 1986. Methylation of the c-*myc* gene changes during the aging process of mice. *Biochemical and Biophysical Research Communications* 139:1299–1304.

Ouslander, J. G. 1981. Drug therapy in the elderly. *American Journal of Surgery* 117:881–892.

Parada, L. F., Tabin, C. J., Shih, C., and Weinberg, R. A. 1982. Human EJ bladder carcinoma oncogene is homologue of Harvey sarcoma virus *ras* gene. *Nature* 297:474–478.

Pegg, A. E., Roberfroid, M., von Bahr, C., Foote, R. S., Mitra, S., Bresil, H., Likhachev, A., and Montesano, R. 1982. Removal of O^6-methylguanine from DNA by human liver fraction. *Proceedings of the National Academy of Sciences (USA)* 79:5162–5165.

Peggins, J. O., Shipley, L. A., and Weiner, M. 1984. Characteristics of age-related changes in hepatic drug metabolism in miniature swine. *Drug Metabolism and Disposition* 12:379–381.

Peleg, L., Raz, E., and Ben-Ishai, R. 1977. Changing capacity for DNA excision repair in mouse embryonic cells in vitro. *Experimental Cell Research* 104:301–307.

Pero, R. W., and Norden, A. 1981. Mutagen sensitivity in peripheral lymphocytes as a risk indicator. *Environmental Research* 24:409–424.

Pozharisski, K. M. 1985. The significance of nonspecific injury for colon carcinogenesis in rats. *Cancer Research* 35:3824–3830.

Price, G. B., Modak, S. P., and Makinodan, T. 1971. Age associated changes in the DNA of mouse tissue. *Science* 171:917–920.

Pryor, W. A., Jerauchi, K., and Davis, W. H. 1976. Electron spin resonance study of cigarette smoke by the use of spin trapped techniques. *Environmental Health Perspectives* 16:161–175.

Pryor, W. A., and Lightsey, J. W. 1981. Mechanisms of nitrogen dioxide reactions: Initiation of lipid peroxidation and the production of nitrous acid. *Science* 214:435–437.

Rabovsky, J., Marion, K. J., Groseclose, R. D., Lewis, T. R., and Petersen, M. 1984. Low dose chronic inhalation of diesel exhaust and/or coal dust by rats: Effects of age and exposure on lung and liver cytochrome P450. *Xenobiotica* 14:595–598.

Recknagel, R. O., Glenda, E. A., and Hruszkewycz, A. M. 1977. Chemical mechanisms in carbon tetrachloride toxicity. In Pryor, W. A. (Ed.), *Free Radicals in Biology* (Vol. 3). New York, Academic Press, pp. 97–132.

Revskoy, S. Y., Poroshina, T. E., Kovaleva, I. G., Bernstein, L. M., Ostrou-
mova, M. N., and Dilman, V. M. 1985. Age-dependent metabolic immunodepression and cancer. IARC *Scientific Publications* (Lyon) 58:253–260.

Richardson, A., Birchenall-Sparks, M. C., and Plesko, M. M. 1984. Age-
related changes in translation and transcription in isolated hepatocytes. In
Bezooijen, C. F. A. (Ed.), *Pharmacological, Morphological and Physiological Aspects of Liver Aging*. Rijswijk, the Netherlands, Eurage, pp. 3–12.

Richardson, A., and Cheung, H. T. 1982. The relationship between age-related
changes in gene expression, protein turnover, and the responsiveness of an
organism to stimuli. *Life Sciences* 31:605–614.

Ries, L. G., Pollack, E. S., and Young, J. L. 1983. Cancer patient survival:
Surveillance, epidemiology, and end results program, 1973–1979. *Journal of
the National Cancer Institute* 70:693–707.

Riggs, A. D., and Jones, P. A. 1983. 5-Methylcytosine, gene regulation, and
cancer. *Advances in Cancer Research* 40:1–30.

Rikans, L. E., and Notley, B. A. 1984. Effect of methyltestosterone administration on microsomal drug metabolism in aging rats. *Mechanisms of Ageing
and Development* 25:335–341.

Robertson, I. G. C., and Birnbaum, L. S. 1982. Age related changes in mutagen activation by rat tissues. *Chemico-Biologic Interactions* 38:243–252.

Rodl, J., DeGlopper, E., VandenBerg, P., and Van Zweiten, M. J. 1980. Idio-
pathic paraproteinemia. III. Increased frequency of paraproteinemia in the
thymectomized aging C57BL/KaLwRij and CBA/BrARij mice. *Journal of
Immunology* 125:31–35.

Saul, R. L., Gee, P., and Ames, B. N. 1987. Free radicals, DNA damage, and
aging. In Warner, H. R. (Ed.), *Modern Biological Theories of Aging*. New
York, Raven Press, pp. 113–130.

Sawada, N., and Ishikawa, T. 1988. Reduction of potential for replicative
but not unscheduled DNA synthesis in hepatocytes isolated from aged as
compared to young rats. *Cancer Research* 48:1618–1622.

Sbano, E. 1978. DNA repair after UV irradiation in skin fibroblasts from
patients with actinic keratoses. *Archives of Dermatological Research*
262:55–61.

Schate-Hermann, R. 1985. Tumor promotion in the liver. *Archives of Toxicology* 57:147–158.

Schendel, P. F. 1981. Inducible repair systems and their implications for toxicology. *CRC Critical Reviews of Toxicology* 8:311–330.

Schmucker, D. L., and Wang, R. K. 1979. Rat liver lysosomal enzymes: Effects of aging and phenobarbital. *Age and Ageing* 2:93–96.

Schmucker, D. L., and Wang, R. K. 1980. Age-related changes in liver drug-
metabolizing enzymes. *Experimental Gerontology* 15:321–329.

Schmucker, D. L., and Wang, R. K. 1983. Age dependent alterations in rat
liver microsome NADPH-cytochrome C(P450) reductase: A qualitative and
quantitative analysis. *Mechanisms of Ageing and Development* 21:137–156.

Schneider, E. L., and Mitsui, Y. 1976. The relationship between in vitro cellular aging and in vivo human age. *Proceedings of the National Academy of
Sciences (USA)* 73:3584–3588.

Schnipper, L. E. 1985. Clinical implications of tumor-cell heterogeneity. *New England Journal of Medicine* 314:1423–1431.

Schwab, R., Staiano-Coico, L., and Weksler, M. E. 1983. Immunological studies in aging: IX. Quantitative differences in T lymphocyte subsets in young and old individuals. *Diagnostic Immunology* 1:195–198.

Scott, R. E., and Wille, J. J. 1984. Mechanisms for the initiation and promotion of carcinogenesis: A review and a new concept. *Mayo Clinic Proceedings* 59:107–117.

Shih, C., Shilo, B., Goldfarb, M., Dannenberg, A., and Weinberg, R. A. 1979. Passage of phenotypes of chemically transformed cells via transfection of DNA and chromatin. *Proceedings of the National Academy of Sciences (USA)* 76:5714–5718.

Siskind, G. W. 1987. Aging and the immune system. In Warner, H. R., Butler, R. N., Sprott, R. L., and Schneider, E. L. (Eds.), *Modern Biological Theories of Aging*. New York, Raven Press, pp. 235–242.

Slamon, D. J., Clark, G. M., Wong, S. G., Levin, W. J., Ullrich, A., and McGuire, W. L. 1987. Human breast cancer: Correlation of relapse and survival with amplification of the HER-2/*neu* oncogene. *Science* 235:177–182.

Smith, J. R., and Lincoln, D. W. 1984. Aging of cells in culture. *International Review of Cytology* 89:151–177.

Smith, K. C. 1978. Aging carcinogenesis, and radiation biology. *Progress in Biochemical Pharmacology* 14:70–75.

Sohal, R. S. 1981. Metabolic rate, aging, and lipofuscin accumulation. In Sohal, R. S. (Ed.), *Age Pigments*. Amsterdam, Elsevier/North-Holland, pp. 303–311.

Solomon, E., Voss, R., and Hall, V. 1978. Chromosome 5 allele loss in human colorectal carcinomas. *Nature* 329:616–619.

Spearman, M. E., and Liebmen, K. C. 1984. Aging selectively alters glutathione-S tranferase isoenzyme concentrations in lung and liver cytosol. *Drug Metabolism and Disposition* 12:661–671.

Srivastava, A., Norris, J. S., Reis, R. J. S., and Goldstein, S. 1985. C-Ha-*ras*-1 protooncogene amplification and overexpression during the limited replicative life span of normal human fibroblasts. *Journal of Biological Chemistry* 260:6404–6409.

Staiano-Coico, L., Darzynkiewicz, Z., Melamed, M. K., and Weksler, M. E. 1982. Changes in DNA content of human blood mononuclear cells with senescence. *Cytometry* 3:79–83.

Staiano-Coico, L., Darzynkiewicz, Z., Melamed, M. K., and Weksler, M. E. 1983. Increased sensitivity of lymphocytes from people over age 65 to cell cycle arrest and chromosomal damage. *Science* 219:1335–1337.

Stanulis-Praeger, B. M. 1987. Cellular senescence revisited: A review. *Mechanisms of Ageing and Development* 38:1–48.

Stehelin, D., Varmus, H. E., Bishop, J. M., and Vogt, P. K. 1976. DNA related to the transforming gene(s) of avian sarcoma viruses is present in normal avian DNA. *Nature* 260:170–173.

Stewart, T. A., Pattengale, P. K., and Leder, P. 1984. Spontaneous mammary adenocarcinomas in transgenic mice that carry and express MTV/*myc* fusion genes. *Cell* 38:627–637.

Sutter, M. A., Chernesky, P., Jayaraj, A., and Richardson, A. 1982. Metabolic activation of chemical carcinogens by kidney from rats and mice of different ages. *Comparative Biochemistry and Physiology* 73C:435–438.

Sutter, M. A., Wood, W. G., Williamson, L. S., Strong, R., Pickham, K., and Richardson, A. 1985. Comparison of the hepatic mixed function mono oxygenase system of young, adult, and old nonhuman primates (*Macaca nemestrina*). *Biochemical Pharmacology* 34:2983–2987.

Tabin, D. H., Bradley, S. M., Bargmann, C. I., Weinberg, R. A., Papageorge, A. G., Scolnick, E. M., Dhar, R., Lowy, D. R., and Chang, E. H. 1982. Mechanism of activation of a human oncogene. *Nature* 300:143–149.

Teller, M. N., Stohr, G., Curlett, W., Kubisek, M. L., and Curtis, D. 1964. Aging and carcinogenesis. I. Immunity to tumor and skin grafts. *Journal of the National Cancer Institute* 33:649–656.

Thompson, S. C. 1976. Effect of age and sex on lung colony forming efficiency of injected mouse tumor cells. *British Journal of Cancer* 34:566–570.

Tolmasoff, J. M., Ona, T., and Cutler, R. G. 1980. Superoxide dismutase: Correlation with life-span and specific metabolic rate in primate species. *Proceedings of the National Academy of Sciences (USA)* 77:2777–2781.

Ts'o, O. P., Caspary, W. J., and Lorentzen, R. J. 1977. The involvement of free radicals in chemical carcinogenesis. In Pryor, W. A. (Ed.), *Free Radicals in Biology* (Vol. 3). New York, Academic Press, pp. 251–305.

U.S. Department of Health and Human Services. 1985. *The Health Consequences of Smoking: Cancer and Chronic Lung Disease in the Workplace. Report to the Surgeon General* (DHHS(PHS)85-50207). Rockville, MD, U.S. Department of Health and Human Services, Office on Smoking and Health.

Vijg, J., Mullaart, E., Lohman, P. H. M., and Knook, D. L. 1985. UV-induced unscheduled DNA synthesis in fibroblasts of aging inbred rats. *Mutation Research* 146:197–204.

Vijg, J., Mullaart, E., and Roza, L. 1986. Immunochemical detection of DNA in alkaline sucrose gradient fractions. *Journal of Immunologic Methods* 91:53–58.

Vitaliano, P. P., and Urbach, F. 1980. The relative importance of risk factors in nonmelanoma skin carcinoma. *Archives of Dermatology* 116:454–456.

Waddell, C. C., Tauton, O. D., and Twomey, J. J. 1978. Inhibition of lymphoproliferation by hyperlipoproteinemic plasma. *Journal of Clinical Investigation* 58:950–954.

Waldstein, E. A., Cao, E. H., Bender, M. A., and Setlow, R. B. 1982. Abilities of extracts of human lymphocytes to remove O^6-methylguanine from DNA. *Mutation Research* 95:405–416.

Weindruch, R. H., Kristie, J. A., Cheney, K. E., and Walford, R. L. 1979. Influence of controlled dietary restriction on immunologic function and aging. *Federation Proceedings* 38:2007–2016.

Weksler, M. E. 1982. Age-associated changes in the immune response. *Journal of the American Geriatric Society* 30:718–723.

Weksler, M. E., and Siskind, G. W. 1984. The cellular basis of immune senescence. *Monographs in Developmental Biology* 17:110–121.

Wheeler, K. T., and Lett, J. T. 1974. On the possibility that DNA repair is related to age in non-dividing cells. *Proceedings of the National Academy of Sciences (USA)* 71:1862–1865.

Williams, R. T. 1959. *Detoxification Mechanisms.* New York, John Wiley and Sons.

Young, S. L., Percy, C. L., Asire, A., Berg, J. W., Cusano, M. M., Gloeckler, L. A., Horn, J. W., Lourie, W. I., Pollack, E. S., and Shambaugh, E. M. 1981. Surveillance, epidemiology, and end results: Incidence and mortality data, 1973–1977. *National Cancer Institute Monographs* 57:1–188.

Yunis, J. J. 1983. The chromosomal basis of human neoplasia. *Science* 221:227–236.

Zucker, S., Michael, M. S., Lysik, R. M., Gluchsman, M. J., Reese, J., Rudin, A., and DiStefano, J. 1979. Lipoprotein inhibitor of bone marrow cells in tumor bearing rats. *Cell Tissues Kinetics* 12:393–404.

4

Environmental Influences
on Skin Aging
and Cutaneous Carcinogenesis

Gary S. Rogers, M.D.
Barbara A. Gilchrest, M.D.

The skin is the interface between organism and environment. Thus, the integument is an ideal organ for studying the effects of environmental agents on aging and on the formation of tumors. The skin is a large organ, diverse in appearance, easily manipulated, and readily sampled. Age- and toxicant-associated morphological alterations can be viewed and sampled with precision and alacrity. Environmental influences are widely theorized to contribute to aging of the organism. Perhaps the strongest data to support this hypothesis come from studies of cutaneous aging.

Aging of the skin is a function of chronological aging and environmental factors. The best studied of these factors is photoaging—changes in the structure and biological activity of skin due to habitual exposure to the sun. Only recently has photoaging been discriminated from "true" aging of the skin at the clinical, histological, and cellular levels (Gilchrest, 1987). Photoaging is estimated to account for more than 90% of age-associated cosmetic skin problems (Gilchrest, 1987). Clinically, photoaging, also known as *dermatoheliosis,* can be recognized by wrinkling, mottled pigmentation, coarseness, telangiectases, laxity, and atrophy of chronically sun-exposed skin. These cutaneous changes influence a person's self-esteem and society's perception of him or her (Dion, Berscheid, and Walster, 1972). The stigma attached to growing old is evidenced by the more than 12 billion dollars spent annually on cosmetics to camouflage the visible signs of aging (Weary, 1979). Epidemiological data indicate a causal role of photoaging in the development of skin cancer (Fears, Scotto, and Schneiderman, 1977).

Table 4.1. Benign Proliferative Growths Associated with Aging

Lesion	Cell or Tissue of Origin	Prevalence (%)
Lentigo senilis	Melanocyte	70.6
Seborrheic keratosis	Dermis, keratinocyte, melanocyte	61.2
Acrochordon	Dermis, keratinocyte, melanocyte	58.8
Cherry hemangioma	Capillaries	53.7
Sebaceous hyperplasia	Sebaceous glands	17.5

Note: Data are from a survey of 68 subjects, 50–91 years of age, with an average age of 74 years (Beauregard and Gilchrest, 1987).

Cutaneous neoplasia is one of the best documented interactions between aging of the organism and environmental toxicants. A variety of environmental factors, the most notable being ultraviolet (UV) light, have been shown to cause cancer of the skin in human subjects and animal models (Fears, Scotto, and Schneiderman, 1977; Kripke and Fisher, 1978). There is a wealth of recent information and new research efforts directed toward obtaining a better understanding of the interaction between aging and skin tumor development. This chapter reviews current concepts and new data pertaining to the influence of aging and the environment on cutaneous carcinogenesis.

The Formation of Cutaneous Tumors

Neoplasia and aging processes appear to be fundamentally intertwined. Benign and malignant tumors are prone to occur in every organ system with progressive aging. This is particularly true of the skin. One or more benign tumors is present on the skin of virtually all individuals over age 65 (Beauregard and Gilchrest, 1987). A representative list of the most common benign skin tumors associated with aging is shown in Table 4.1.

Skin cancer is the most common human malignancy. The number of skin malignancies reported each year is equal to that of all cancers from all anatomic sites combined (Gordon and Silverstone, 1976; Schottenfeld and Fraumeni, 1982; Scotto, et al., 1980). The incidence of cutaneous basal and squamous cell carcinoma increases dramatically with aging (Lin and Carter, 1986; National Cancer Institute, 1981; Scotto, Fears, and Fraumeni, 1983).

Is the skin therefore uniquely predisposed to neoplasia? Skin tumors are certainly easier to detect than a lesion developing in a visceral organ. Increased detection, however, cannot account for the overwhelming incidence of skin cancer. Cutaneous neoplasia is a function of the skin's exposure to the environment and decline in immunological homeostasis with aging (Johnson and Stern, 1979; Urbach, Rose, and Bonnem, 1972; Yunis and Lane, 1979). The skin is bombarded on a daily basis by environmental carcinogens. Although a plethora of chemical and physical factors are known to be carcinogenic in humans and experimental animals (Yuspa, 1983, 1986, 1987), the most significant of these carcinogens is electromagnetic radiation in the 290- to 320-nm spectrum, known as ultraviolet B (UVB) light. UV radiation with wavelengths shorter than 290 nm, also carcinogenic, is effectively filtered out by the earth's ozone layer. Thus, only a minute amount of this form of UV light reaches the earth's surface. UVB light is only partially filtered out by the atmosphere and presently constitutes approximately 0.5% of total terrestrial sunlight (Emmett, 1973; Epstein, 1970; Fitzpatrick and Sober, 1985). Depletion of the ozone layer with a corresponding increase in incident UV radiation is now the subject of intense interest. The release of chlorofluorocarbons, constituents of refrigerant gasses and aerosol propellants, into the earth's stratosphere is steadily and progressively depleting the ozone layer via a photocatalytic process (Beadle and Leach, 1982; Fears and Scotto, 1983; Rundel, 1983). However, substantial scientific uncertainty still exists whether emissions of these chemicals significantly threaten the stratospheric ozone layer and, if they do, to what extent the ozone depletion actually threatens human health (Pyle and Derwent, 1980; Sloss and Rose, 1985). A complicating factor is that greater than 20 years are necessary for chlorofluorocarbons to rise from the earth's surface to the upper levels of the atmosphere where the ozone layer is located (Rundel and Nachtway, 1983). Thus, today we are only measuring the cumulative effect of these chemicals released through the late 1960s.

What are the potential health implications of increased UV radiation? The quantitative impact of UV radiation on the incidence of basal and squamous cell skin cancer was determined in a 1977 study of 10 regions in the continental United States (Fears, Scotto, and Schneiderman, 1977). Statistical analysis of the data in dose–response models demonstrates an amplified effect of increased UV radiation on the number of cutaneous carcinomas. For each 1 percent increase in UVB, a 1.0–2.8 percent long-term increase in skin cancers is predicted (Fears, Scotto, and Schneiderman, 1977). It is important to note that the dose–response model for malignant melanoma (Scotto, Fears, and Gori, 1975) has not been determined. The calculation of projected incidence is extrapolated from indirect evidence and has been criticized as being too conservative (Green Alex and Hedinger, 1978; Scott and Straf, 1977). Dose-delivery factors, life-style, and local environmental factors are not considered. This estimate does not take into account

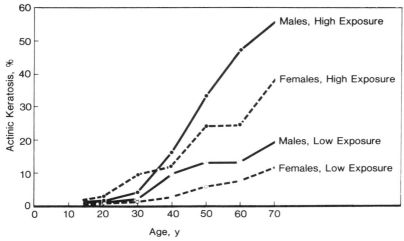

Figure 4.1. The prevalence rates of basal cell carcinoma per 100 white persons in the United States aged 65–74 years. Significance testing for no actinic damage versus severe damage. *Source:* Reprinted with permission from Engel et al. (1988) *Archives of Dermatology* 124:72–79. Copyright 1988 by the American Medical Association.

** $p < .01$.

the effect of an aging population that is already predisposed to skin cancer development. Increased amounts of UV radiation impinging on a growing population of individuals with photoaged skin (vide infra) may dramatically increase skin tumor formation.

UVB is known to have a dose-dependent effect on the incidence of squamous cell carcinoma development in both human subjects and animal models (de Gruijl and Van der Leun, 1979; Green Alex, 1978; Green Alex et al., 1976). The incidence of basal and squamous cell carcinoma increases proportionately with decreasing latitude (increasing insolation) of residence (Auerbach, 1982; Green Alex and Mo, 1974; Johnson and Stern, 1979). The prevalence of basal cell carcinoma is more than 10-fold higher in individuals over age 65 with evidence of severe actinic skin damage, compared with that in individuals of the same age without actinic damage (Figure 4.1) (Engel, Johnson, and Haynes, 1988).

Mechanisms of Cutaneous Carcinogenesis

What predisposes aging skin to the development of malignancies? Carcinoma development is theorized to be a multistage process involving at least three mechanistically distinct steps: initiation, promotion, and malignant conversion (Marks and Furstenberger, 1984; Scott and Maercklein, 1985; Ward et al., 1986; Yuspa, 1986). Initiation is the first change noted in the epidermal cell exposed to a carcinogen. There is experimental evidence that initiation is the result of deoxyribonucleic acid (DNA) damage resulting in a point-mutation-like genetic alteration. Initiated cells are not malignant, but may fail to respond to signals for terminal differentiation or halting of proliferation (Farber, 1984; Granstein and Sober, 1982; Hartley et al., 1985; Setlow, 1982). There is no clinical or histological alteration detectable in skin initiated by a carcinogen (Yuspa, 1986). However, the initiated cell and its progeny are irreversibly altered toward the capacity for tumor formation.

UVB light acting on a single-hit dose–response basis is a known initiator of epidermal cells (Green Alex, 1978; Hannan et al., 1984; Hennings and Yuspa, 1985; Rundel, 1983). This may occur through absorption of photons of specific energy by pyrimidine bases in DNA, resulting in cross-linking of immediately adjacent thymidine residues. These thymidine dimers are nontranslatable. Faulty excision repair of the dimer results in a point mutation. The mutation must be nonlethal and occur in a gene that affects proliferation or terminal differentiation (Yuspa, 1983, 1986, 1987). Activation of transforming genes, oncogenes, via a point mutation is currently an area of great research interest. In the mouse model, the c-*ras* oncogene is a target for initiating carcinogens (Androphy and Lowy, 1984; Balmain, 1985; Harper, Roop, and Yuspa, 1986; Ozato and Wakamatsu, 1983), and premalignant keratoses (papillomas) often contain mutated or amplified forms of the c-*ras* oncogene (Balmain et al., 1984).

DNA repair mechanisms are speculated to become progressively less efficient and less accurate with aging (Epstein, 1983; Setlow, 1982). In disease states such as xeroderma pigmentosum, DNA repair is known to be defective. This results in the development of skin cancers in sun-exposed areas at an early age. Thus, the statistical probability of tumor initiation increases with progressive aging, chronic sun exposure, and genetic predisposition.

Tumor promotion, the second stage of epidermal carcinogenesis, results in the selective clonal outgrowth of the initiated cell population. A premalignant clone of cells expanded from the initiated stem cell keratinocyte results in a clinically distinct cutaneous lesion in the mouse model (Ebbesen, 1985).

Actinic keratoses, precursors of squamous cell carcinoma, may represent such initiated clones of keratinocytes in human subjects. Clini-

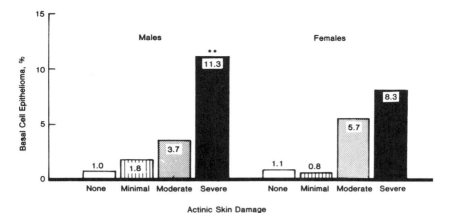

Figure 4.2. The prevalence rates of actinic keratoses per 100 white persons in the United States. The rates were plotted by age for each of the groups. *Source:* Reprinted with permission from Engel et al. (1988) *Archives of Dermatology* 124:72–79. Copyright 1988 by the American Medical Association.

cally, actinic keratoses increase in size and number with progressive aging (Hennings et al., 1985) and are found predominately in sun-exposed skin (Figure 4.2) (Graham and Helwig, 1966; Hennings and Yuspa, 1985). The clonality of actinic keratoses has not been determined. However, UVB-induced mouse papillomas, which histologically resemble actinic keratoses, have been shown to be monoclonal (Ebbesen, 1985; Hennings et al., 1985; Yuspa, 1987).

UVB light is a known promoter of initiated keratinocytes (Diamond, O'Brien, and Baird, 1980; Parkinson, 1985; Stenback and Arranto, 1985). A variety of nonmutagenic chemicals, such as anthralin and benzoyl peroxide may also act as tumor promoters (Argyris, 1985; Urbach, Forbes, and Davies, 1982; Yuspa, 1986). There is evidence that biochemical intermediates in melanin synthesis may act as tumor promoters. When pheomelanin is exposed to UV light, carcinogenic photoproducts are generated (Harsanyi et al., 1980). An autocarcinogenic mechanism has therefore been suggested for melanoma development.

Initiation and promotion are necessary but not sufficient steps for malignant conversion, and further cellular events are required for cancer development (Balmain, 1985; Balmain et al., 1984; Harper, Roop, and Yuspa, 1986). The exact mechanism is poorly understood, but there is experimental evidence in the mouse model that genetic damage is the *ras* oncogene is a central step in both initiation and malignant conversion in vivo (Harper, Roop, and Yuspa, 1986).

Immune Response to Tumorigenesis

A neoplasm must elude the host's immune defenses if it is to survive and grow. As the immunomodulatory role of the skin is increasingly well understood, age-associated and UV-induced changes in the dermis and epidermis are perceived as increasingly relevant to photocarcinogenesis (Burnett, 1971; Greenburg and Yunis, 1975; Kripke and Fisher, 1978). Specifically, age-associated decline in local and systemic immune status may act in a permissive manner toward furthering tumor growth and development.

The bone-marrow-derived epidermal Langerhans cell is the immune recognition cell of the skin (Thiers et al., 1984). There is a steady decline in the density of this dendritic cell population with progressive aging in human skin (Gilchrest, Murphy, and Soter, 1982; Thiers et al., 1984). Moreover, both acute and chronic UV light exposure has been repeatedly documented to decrease the number of epidermal Langerhans cells (Gilchrest, Murphy, and Soter, 1982; Thiers et al., 1984). Thus, there is presumed to be a progressive decrement in local immune surveillance with aging, especially in sun-exposed skin.

Systemic immune suppression, as seen in renal transplant recipients, is also associated with an increased propensity for skin cancer development (Lutzner, 1985). These individuals develop actinic keratoses and skin cancers, primarily squamous cell carcinoma, on sun-exposed skin at rates approximately five times those of age- and complexion-matched controls (Boyle et al., 1984; Lutzner, 1985). This phenomenon may also be explained in part by the reduction in density of Langerhans cells due to the immunosuppressive therapy, on the order of 30–63 percent compared with normal controls (Sontheimer et al., 1984). This reduction is particularly pronounced in sun-exposed skin (Sontheimer et al., 1984). The paucity of immune recognition cells in sun-exposed skin of these individuals is theorized to result in the excess of skin cancers. The alloantigen presenting capacity of Langerhans cells is also depressed in renal transplant recipients, again particularly in sun-exposed compared with sun-protected cutaneous Langerhans cells (Sontheimer et al., 1984).

These phenomena of diminished density and function of Langerhans cells are paralleled, to a lesser degree than in transplant recipients, with progressive aging. Thus, the combined effects of age and sun exposure on Langerhans cell function and density may facilitate tumor development.

Melanocytic Lesions

Melanocytes, derived from the neural crest, manufacture pigment to provide photoprotection for the skin. The melanocytic nevus (nevocellular nevus and nevus cell nevus) is a common yet unique neoplasm. In the stepwise progression from benignancy to malignancy, certain nevi are thought by some investigators to be the potential precursor of malignant melanoma (Clark et al., 1984).

We enter and leave life with few nevi. Melanocytic nevi are rare in infancy and childhood, increase in size and number during puberty and early adulthood, and involute during late adulthood (MacKie et al., 1985). The average adult has 15–40 acquired melanocytic nevi on his or her skin (Maize and Foster, 1979), and approximately 1–2 percent of Caucasians have a nevus present at birth (congenital moles) (Alper and Holmes, 1983). Thus, development of benign tumors of the melanocytic system is primarily a process of youth and middle age.

The relationship between normal melanocytes and nevus cells is poorly understood. Histologically, they are quite distinct, but cultured nevus cells strongly resemble cultured epidermal melanocytes in terms of growth rate and substrate responsiveness (Gilchrest et al., 1986). Whether local environmental factors transform melanocytes into nevus cells or their origins are intrinsically distinct is still the subject of speculation.

The risk of malignant conversion of these cells has yet to be determined. There are no data suggesting that the nevus cell represents an initiated cell phenotype. Melanocyte culture data indicate that transformation of epidermal malanocytes to melanoma entails at least two phenotypic changes, including escape from melanocyte growth factor responsiveness, probably through autocrine stimulation by such factors as basic fibroblast growth factor (Halaban and Alfano, 1984), and insensitivity to cyclic adenosine monophosphate modulation (Gordon et al., 1986).

Distinct age-associated changes in epidermal melanocytes and melanocytic nevi are apparent both in vivo and in vitro. The culture life span is shorter and mitotic rate slower in adult versus newborn melanocytes despite a similar ultrastructural appearance (Gilchrest et al., 1984). The significance of these phenomena for the several age-associated pigmentary alterations ranging from graying of hair to lentigines to decreased photoprotection remains to be determined. In human skin, melanocyte density decreases with age throughout adulthood (Gilchrest, Blog, and Szabo, 1979; Quevedo, Szabo, and Virks, 1969). There is a 6–20 percent decrease in 3,4-dihydroxyphenylalanine (dopa)-positive melanocytes with aging in all anatomic sites each decade after age 30 years (Quevedo, Szabo, and Virks, 1969). However, the density of dopa-positive cells is roughly twofold higher in chronically sun-exposed skin (Gilchrest, Blog, and Szabo, 1979). This accounts for the seemingly paradoxical hyperpigmentation of elderly sun-exposed skin despite declining melanocyte density. The basis of the stimulatory effect of sunlight on melanocyte proliferation is not known but may reflect the promoting effects of UV radiation (vide supra).

Nevi demonstrates characteristic aging changes as they progress from junctional (i.e., nevus cells limited to the dermal–epidermal [DE] junction), to compound (nevus cells above and below the DE junction), to intradermal tumors (Hu, 1979). The genesis of nevi appears at the DE junction where they exhibit proliferative and melanogenic activity (Nordlund, 1986). This activity is gradually lost with progressive descent into the dermis. Whether this represents aging, as felt by some investigators (e.g., Hu, 1979), or terminal differentiation is unknown. Similarly, nevus cells exhibit morphological changes with aging. They progress from small dendritic to large epithelioid cells in the upper dermis, to small lymphocytoid and finally spindle or neuroid forms in the deeper dermis. The neuroid type cells no longer contain pigment (Hu, 1979).

The association between melanocytic nevi and malignant melanoma is the subject of considerable controversy and is as yet poorly understood (Clark et al., 1984; Greene, 1985; Greene et al., 1985; Rhodes, 1984). On a statistical basis, roughly 20 percent of carefully analyzed melanomas show histologic evidence of a preexisting nevus in contiguity with the malignancy (Kopf, Rigel, and Friedman, 1982). Congenital nevi and dysplastic nevi (lesions with specific clinicopathological features) are thought by some investigators to be potential precursors of malignant melanoma (Clark et al., 1984; Rhodes, 1984; Rhodes and Melski, 1982). The syndrome of familial melanoma, B-K mole syndrome, and familial atypical multiple mole syndrome are associated with the presence of multiple dysplastic nevi (Greene and Fraumeni, 1979; Greene et al., 1985). Multiple melanomas develop in these individuals, often at an early age (Greene et al., 1985). Outside the familial setting, however, the risk associated with having dysplastic nevi is not fully known.

The incidence of malignant melanoma, like that of cutaneous carcinoma, increases with aging (Elwood and Lee, 1975; Silverberg, 1985). However, when subdivided into type of melanoma, superficial spreading melanoma (SSM), the most common pattern of this malignancy, occurs primarily in individuals between 40 and 60 years of age (Elwood and Lee, 1975). SSM is the pattern most often associated with a preexisting nevus (Greene and Fraumeni, 1979). Persons with the hereditary melanoma syndrome primarily develop SSM, usually on the trunk (Greene, 1985).

Older individuals tend to develop melanomas on the face and other chronically sun-damaged sites. These lesions have a distinct clinical and pathological appearance, referred to as lentigo maligna melanoma (LMM) (Clark and Mihm, 1969). Histological evidence of chronic photodamage, extensive solar elastosis, is the rule for these malignancies (Clark and Mihm, 1969). The prognosis for these lesions is no different, thickness for thickness, than it is for SSM (Koh et al., 1984). It is rare for an LMM to occur in association with a preexisting nevus. This may be a function of the decrease in nevus number and activity with aging (vide supra). The melanocytic hyperplasia and atypia seen in chronically photodamaged skin and at the margins of LMM may play a central role in the genesis of this tumor.

Although the biological behavior of LMM is similar to that of SSM, the etiology may be quite different. As first described by Clark et al. (1984), a stepwise progression from banal nevus to dysplastic nevus with progressive nevus cell hyperplasia and atypia can eventuate in malignant transformation, that is, SSM. The etiological factors responsible for the development of SSM are not entirely clear. Sunlight, endogenous promoters such as the intermediates in melanin synthesis (vide supra), and hormonal and genetic factors, all appear to play a role (Ershler et al., 1984; Greene, 1985; Holly and Roche, 1983). In contrast to SSM, the direct effect of UV radiation as an initiator and promoter, resulting in melanocytic hyperplasia and atypia on elderly sun-damaged skin (clonal expansion of an induced phenotype) and malignant conversion, is undoubtedly central to the development of LMM.

Role of Retinoids

Retinoids are a class of compounds that appears to have an influence on photoaging (Kligman, 1986) and photocarcinogenesis (Sporn et al., 1976). Isotretinoin (13-cis retinoic acid) orally and tretinoin (all-trans-retinoic acid) topically have been shown to inhibit the development of UV-induced tumors in some animals studies (Sporn and Roberts, 1983). In human subjects, topical tretinoin may have efficacy against premalignant actinic keratoses (Epstein, 1986) and isotretinoin appears to reduce the incidence of photocarcinogenesis in high-risk patients (Kraemer et al., 1988).

Retinoids appear to act by influencing cellular differentiation via their effect on the expression of oncogenes and peptide growth factors (Sporn and Roberts, 1983). In several tumor cell lines, retinoic acid induces terminal differentiation and suppression of c-*myc* or N-*myc* oncogene expression in vitro (Sporn et al., 1986). Thus, this class of vitamin A derivatives appears to have anticarcinogenic properties, although other studies indicate retinoic acid may also have a weak promoter effect (Epstein, 1986). Overall, these compounds hold great promise for undertanding and modulating the aging process and cutaneous carcinogenesis.

Summary

There is a wealth of new knowledge regarding mechanisms of carcinogenesis and their interaction with aging and environmental insults, particularly UV irradiation in the skin. Innovations and advances in tissue culture techniques now permit in vitro studies of keratinocytes, melanocytes, and other benign and malignant skin-derived cells. Thus, the aging process and cutaneous neoplasia can now be studied at the cellular level. New insights regarding the interrelationship of aging, the environment, and cutaneous neoplasia are close at hand.

References

Alper, J. C., and Holmes, L. B. 1983. The evidence and significance of birthmarks in a cohort of 4641 newborns. *Pediatric Dermatology* 1:58–68.

Androphy, E. J., and Lowy, D. R. 1984. Tumor viruses, oncogenes, and human cancer. *Journal of the American Academy of Dermatology* 10: 125–141.

Argyris, T. S. 1985. Promotion of epidermal carcinogenesis by repeated damage to mouse skin. *American Journal of Industrial Medicine* 8:329–337.

Auerbach, H. 1982. Geographic variation in incidence of skin cancer in the United States. *Public Health Report* 7(2):143–171.

Balmain, A. 1985. Transforming *ras* oncogenes and multistage carcinogenesis. *British Journal of Cancer* 51:1–7.

Balmain, A., Ramsden, M., Bowden, G. T., and Smith, J. 1984. Activation of the mouse cellular Harvey-*ras* gene in chemically induced benign skin papillomas. *Nature* 307:658–660.

Beadle, P. C., and Leach, J. F. 1982. Holidays, ozone and skin cancer. Skin cancer in Bristol—a comparison of theory with observation. *Archives of Dermatology Research* 274:47–56.

Beauregard, S., and Gilchrest, B. A. 1987. A survey of skin problems and skin care regimens in the elderly. *Archives of Dermatology* 123:1638–1643.

Boyle, J., MacKie, R. M., Briggs, J. D., Junor, B. J. R., and Aitchison, T. C. 1984. Cancer, warts and sunshine in renal transplant patients. *Lancet* 1:702–705.

Burnett, F. M. 1971. An immunologic approach to aging. *Lancet* 2:358–360.

Clark, W. M., Elder, D. E., Guerry D., Epstein, M. N., Greene, M. H., and
    Van Horn, M. 1984. A study of tumor progression: The precursor lesions
    of superficial spreading melanoma. *Human Pathology* 15:1147–1165.
Clark, W. M., Jr., and Mihm, M. C., Jr. 1969. Lentigo maligna and lentiga
    maligna melanoma. *American Journal of Pathology* 55:39–67.
de Gruijl, F. R., and Van der Leun, J. C. 1979. A dose-response model for skin
    cancer induction by chronic UV exposure of a human population. *Journal of
    Theoretical Biology* 83:487–504.
Diamond, L., O'Brien, T. G., and Baird, W. M. 1980. Tumor promoters and
    the mechanism of tumor promotion. *Advances in Cancer Research* 32:1–74.
Dion, K., Berscheid, E., and Walster, E. 1972. What is beautiful is good.
    Journal of Personality and Social Psychology 24:285–290.
Ebbesen, P. 1985. Papilloma development on young and senescent mouse skin
    treated with 12-0-tetradecanoylphorbol 13-acetate. *IARC Scientific Publica-
    tion* 58:167–170.
Elwood, J. M., and Lee, J. H. 1975. Recent data on the epidemiology of
    malignant melanoma. *Seminars in Oncology* 2:149–152.
Emmett, E. A. 1973. Ultraviolet radiation as a cause of skin tumors. *CRC
    Critical Reviews in Toxicology* 2:211–255.
Engel, A., Johnson, M. L., and Haynes, S. G. 1988. Health effects of sunlight
    exposure in the United States. *Archives of Dermatology* 124:72–79.
Epstein, J. H. 1970. Ultraviolet carcinogenesis. In Giese, A. (Ed.), *Photophys-
    iology* (Vol. 5). New York, Academic Press, pp. 235–273.
Epstein, J. H. 1983. Photocarcinogenesis, skin cancer and aging. *Journal of
    the American Academy of Dermatology* 9:487–502.
Epstein, J. H. 1986. All-trans-retinoic acid and cutaneous cancer. *Journal of
    the American Academy of Dermatology* 15:772–778.
Ershler, W. B., Stewart, J. A., Hacker, M. P., Moore, A. L., and Tindle, B. H.
    1984. B16 murine melanoma and aging: Slower growth and longer survival in
    old mice. *Journal of the National Cancer Institute* 72:161–164.
Farber, E. 1984. Pre-cancerous steps in carcinogenesis: Their physiological
    adaptive nature. *Biochimica et Biophysica Acta* 738:171–180.
Fears, T. R., and Scotto, J. 1983. Estimating increases in skin cancer morbidity
    due to increases in ultraviolet radiation exposure. *Cancer Investigation*
    1:119–126.
Fears, T., Scotto, J., and Schneiderman, M. A. 1977. Mathematical models
    of age and ultraviolet effects on the incidence of skin cancer among whites
    in the United States. *American Journal of Epidemiology* 105:420–427.
Fitzpatrick, T. B., and Sober, A. J. 1985. Letter: Sunlight and skin cancer.
    New England Journal of Medicine 313:818–820.
Gilchrest, B. A. 1987. Aging of the skin. In Fitzpatrick, T. B., Eisen, A. Z.,
    Wolff, K., Freedberg, I. M., and Austen, K. F. (Eds.), *Dermatology in
    General Medicine* (3rd ed.). New York, McGraw-Hill, pp. 147–153.
Gilchrest, B. A., Blog, F. B., and Szabo, G. 1979. Effects of aging and chronic
    sun exposure on melanocytes in human skin. *Journal of Investigative Der-
    matology* 73:141–143.

Gilchrest, B. A., Murphy, G. F., and Soter, N. A. 1982. Effects of chronologic aging and ultraviolet irradiation on Langerhans cells in human skin. *Journal of Investigative Dermatology* 79:85–88.

Gilchrest, B. A., Treloar, V. D., Grassi, A. M., Yar, M., Szabo, G., and Flynn, E. 1986. Characteristics of cultivated adult human neurocellular nevus cells. *Journal of Investigative Dermatology* 87:102–107.

Gilchrest, B. A., Vrabel, M. A., Flynn, E., and Szabo, G. 1984. Selective cultivation of human melanocytes from newborn and adult epidermis. *Journal of Investigative Dermatology* 83:370–376.

Gordon, D., and Silverstone, H. 1976. Worldwide epidemiology of premalignant and malignant cutaneous lesions. In Andrade, R. A. (Ed.), *Cancer of the Skin*. Philadelphia, W. B. Saunders, pp. 405–455.

Gordon, P. R., Treloar, V. D., Vrabel, M. A., and Gilchrest, B. A. 1986. Relative responsiveness of cultured human epidermal melanocytes and melanoma cells to selected mitogens. *Journal of Investigative Dermatology* 87:723–727.

Graham, J. H., and Helwig, E. B. 1966. Cutaneous premalignant lesions. In Montagna, W., and Dobson, R. L. (Eds.), *Advances in Biology of Skin: Carcinogenesis* (Vol. 7). Oxford, Pergamon Press, pp. 277–327.

Granstein, R. D., and Sober, A. J. 1982. Current concepts in ultraviolet carcinogenesis. *Proceedings of the Society for Experimental Biology and Medicine* 170:115–125.

Green Alex, E. S. 1978. Ultraviolet exposure and skin cancer response. *American Journal of Epidemiology* 107:277–280.

Green Alex, E. S., Findley, G. B., Klenk, K. F., Wilson, W. M., and Mo, T. 1976. The ultraviolet dose dependence of nonmelanoma skin cancer incidence. *Photochemistry and Photobiology* 24:353–362.

Green Alex, E. S., and Hedinger, R. A. 1978. Models relating ultraviolet light and nonmelanoma skin cancer incidence. *Photochemistry and Photobiology* 26:283–291.

Green Alex, E. S., and Mo, T. 1974. An epidemiological index for skin-cancer incidence. In *Third Conference on Climactic Impact of Atmospheric Pollutants*. Ann Arbor, University of Michigan Press, pp. 518–522.

Greenberg, L. J., and Yunis, E. J. 1975. Immunopathology of aging. *Human Pathology* 5:122–124.

Greene, M. H. 1985. Acquired precursors of cutaneous malignant melanoma, the familial dysplastic nevus syndrome. *New England Journal of Medicine* 312:91–95.

Greene, M. H., Clark, W. H., Jr., Tucker, M. A., Kraemer, K. H., Elder, D. E., and Fraser, M. C. 1985. High risk of malignant melanoma in melanoma-prone families with dysplastic nevi. *Annals of Internal Medicine* 102:458–465.

Greene, M. H., and Fraumeni, J. F. 1979. Hereditary variant of malignant melanoma. In Clark, W. H., Jr., Goldman, L. I., and Mastrangelo, M. J. (Eds.), *Human Malignant Melanoma*. New York, Grune and Stratton, p. 139.

Halaban, R., and Alfano, F. D. 1984. Selective elimination of fibroblasts from cultures of normal human melanocytes. *In Vitro* 20:447–450.

Hannan, M. A., Paul, M., Amer, M. H., and Al-Watban, F. H. 1984. Study of ultraviolet radiation and genotoxic effects of natural sunlight in relation to skin cancer in Saudi Arabia. *Cancer Research* 44:2192–2197.

Harper, J. R., Roop, D. R., and Yuspa, S. H. 1986. Transfection of EJ *ras*[H] gene into keratinocytes derived from carcinogen-induced mouse papillomas causes malignant progression. *Molecular and Cellular Biology* 6:3144–3149.

Harsanyi, Z. P., Post, P. W., Brinkman, J. P., Chedekel, M. R., and Deibel, R. M. 1980. Mutagenicity of melanin from human red hair. *Experientia* 36:291–292.

Hartley, J. A., Gibson, N. W., Zwelling, L. A., and Yuspa, S. H. 1985. The association of DNA strand breaks with accelerated terminal differentiation in mouse epidermal cells exposed to tumor promoters. *Cancer Research* 45:4864–4870.

Hennings, H., Shores, R., Mitchell, P., Spangler, E. F., and Yuspa, S. H. 1985. Induction of papillomas with a high probability of conversion to malignancy. *Carcinogenesis* 6:1607–1610.

Hennings, H., and Yuspa, S. H. 1985. Two-stage tumor promotion in mouse skin: An alternative interpretation. *Journal of the National Cancer Institute* 74:735–740.

Holly, A. H., and Roche, N. 1983. Cutaneous melanoma in relation to endogenous hormones and reproductive factors. *Journal of the National Cancer Institute* 70:827–830.

Hu, F. 1979. Aging and melanocytes. *Journal of Investigative Dermatology* 73:70–79.

Johnson, M. L., and Stern, R. S. 1979. Prevalence and ecology of skin cancer. In Fitzpatrick, T. B. (Ed.), *Dermatology in General Medicine* (2nd ed.). New York, McGraw-Hill, pp. 362–377.

Kligman, A. H., Grove, G. L., Hirose, R., and Leyden, J. J. 1986. Topical tretinoin for photoaged skin. *Journal of American Academy of Dermatology* 15:836–859.

Koh, H. K., Michalik, E., Sober, A. J., Lew, R. A., Day, C. L., Clark, W., Mihm, M. C., and Kopf, A. W. 1984. Lentigo maligna melanoma has no better prognosis than other types of melanoma. *Journal of Clinical Oncology* 2:1031–1039.

Kopf, A. W., Rigel, D. S., and Friedman, R. J. 1982. The rising incidence and mortality rate of malignant melanoma. *Journal of Dermatology and Surgical Oncology* 8:760–761.

Kraemer, K. H., DiGiovanna, J. J., Moshell, A. N., Tarone, R. E., and Peck, G. L. 1988. Prevention of skin cancer in xeroderma pigmentosum with the use of oral isotretinoin. *New England Journal of Medicine* 318:1633–1637.

Kripke, M. L., and Fisher, M. S. 1978. Immunologic aspects of tumor induction by ultraviolet radiation. *National Cancer Institute Monograph* 50:179–183.

Lin, A. N., and Carter, D. M. 1986. Skin cancer in the elderly. *Dermatology Clinics* 4:467–471.

Lutzner, M. A. 1985. Skin cancer in immunosuppressed renal transplant recipients. *Journal of the American Academy of Dermatology* 11:891–893.

MacKie, R. M., English, J., Aitchison, T. C., Fitzsimons, C. P., and Wilson, P. 1985. The number and distribution of benign pigmented moles (melanocytic naevi) in a healthy British population. *British Journal of Dermatology* 113:167–174.

Maize, J. C., and Foster, G. 1979. Age-related changes in melanocytic naevi. *Clinical and Experimental Dermatology* 4:49–58.

Marks, F., and Furstenberger, G. 1984. Stages of tumor promotion in skin. *IARC Scientific Publications* 56:13–22.

National Cancer Institute. 1981. Surveillance, Epidemiology, and End Results (SEER). Incidence and Mortality Data: 1973–1977. *National Cancer Institute Monograph* 57:98–101.

Norlund, J. J. 1986. The lives of pigment cells. *Dermatology Clinics* 4:407–418.

Ozato, K., and Wakamatsu, Y. 1983. Multi-step genetic regulation of oncogene expression in fish hereditary melanoma. *Differentiation* 24:181–190.

Parkinson, E. K. 1985. Defective responses of transformed keratinocytes to terminal differentiation stimuli: Their role in epidermal tumour promotion by phorbol esters and by skin wounding. *British Journal of Cancer* 52:479–493.

Pyle, J. A., and Derwent, R. G. 1980. Possible ozone reductions and UV changes at the earth's surface. *Nature* 286:373–375.

Quevedo, W. C., Jr., Szabo, G., and Virks, J. 1969. Influence of age and UV on the population of dopa-positive melanocytes in human skin. *Journal of Investigative Dermatology* 52:287–290.

Rhodes, A. R. 1984. The risk of malignant melanoma arising in congenital melanocytic nevi. An argument against the assignment of risk based on size alone. *American Journal of Dermatopathology* 6:184–188.

Rhodes, A. R., and Melski, J. W. 1982. Small congenital nevocellular nevi and the risk of cutaneous melanoma. *Journal of Pediatrics* 100:219–224.

Rundel, R. D. 1983. Promotional effects of ultraviolet radiation on human basal and squamous cell carcinoma. *Photochemistry and Photobiology* 38:569–575.

Rundel, R. D., and Nachtwey, D. S. 1983. Projections of increased nonmelanoma skin cancer incidence due to ozone depletion. *Photochemistry and Photobiology* 38:577–591.

Schottenfeld, D., and Fraumeni, J. 1982. *Cancer Epidemiology and Prevention*. Philadelphia, W. B. Saunders.

Scott, E. L., and Straf, M. L. 1977. Ultraviolet radiation as a cause of cancer. In *Origins of Human Cancer*. Cold Spring, NY, Cold Spring Harbor Laboratory, pp. 529–546.

Scott, R. E., and Maercklein, P. B. 1985. An initiator of carcinogenesis selectively and stably inhibits stem cell differentiation: A concept that initiation of carcinogenesis involves multiple phases. *Proceedings of the National Academy of Sciences* 82:2995–2999.

Scotto, J., Fears, T. R., and Fraumeni, J. F., Jr. 1983. *Incidence of Non-

melanoma Skin Cancer in the United States (Publication No. (NIH) 83-2433). Rockville, MD, U.S. Department of Health and Human Services.

Scotto, J., Fears, T. R., and Gori, G.. B. 1975. *Measurements of Ultraviolet Radiation in the United States and Comparisons with Skin Cancer Data* (Publication No. (NIH) 76-1029). Rockville, MD, U.S. Department of Health, Education and Welfare.

Scotto, J., Fears, T., Lisiecki, E., and Radosevich, S. 1980. *Incidence of Nonmelanoma Skin Cancer in the United States, 1977–78: Preliminary Report* (Publication No. (NIH) 80-2154). Bethesda, MD, National Cancer Institute.

Setlow, R. B. 1982. DNA repair, aging and cancer. *National Cancer Institute Monograph* 60:249–255.

Silverberg, E. 1985. Cancer Statistics. *CA—A Cancer Journal for Clinicians* 35:19.

Sloss, E. M., and Rose, T. P. 1985. *Possible Health Effects of Increased Exposure to Ultraviolet Radiation* (N-2330-EPA). Santa Monica, CA, RAND Corporation.

Sontheimer, R. D., Bergstresser, P. R., Gailiunas, P., Jr., Helderman, J. H., and Gilliam, J. N. 1984. Perturbation of human epidermal Langerhans cells in immunosuppressed human renal allograft recipients. *Transplantation* 37:168–174.

Sporn, M. B., Dunlop, N. M., Newton, D. L., and Smith, J. M. 1976. Prevention of chemical carcinogenesis by vitamin A and its synthetic analogies (retinoids). *Federation of American Societies for Experimental Biology* 35:1332–1338.

Sporn, M. B., and Roberts, A. B. 1983. Role of retinoids in differentiation and carcinogenesis. *Cancer Research* 43:3034–3040.

Sporn, M. B., Roberts, A. B., Roche, N. S., and Todaro, G. J. 1986. Mechanism of action of retinoids. *Journal of the American Academy of Dermatology* 15:756–764.

Stenback, F., and Arranto, A. 1985. Initiation and promotion in young and old animals. Implications for human tumor formation. *IARC Scientific Publications* 58:151–166.

Thiers, B. H., Maize, J. C., Spicer, S. S., and Cantor, A. B. 1984. The effect of aging and chronic sun exposure in human Langerhans cell populations. *Journal of Investigative Dermatology* 82:223–226.

Urbach, F., Forbes, P. D., and Davies, R. E. 1982. Modification of photocarcinogenesis by chemical agents. *Journal of the National Cancer Institute* 69:229–235.

Urbach, F., Rose, D. B., and Bonnem, M. 1972. Genetic and environmental interactions in skin carcinogenesis. In *Environment and Cancer*. Baltimore, MD, Williams & Wilkins, pp. 316–324.

Ward, J. M., Quander, R., Devor, D., Wenk, M. L., and Spangler, E. F. 1986. Pathology of aging female SENCAR mice used as controls in skin two-stage carcinogenesis studies. *Environmental Health Perspectives* 68:81–89.

Weary, P. E. 1979. Response to cosmetics; proposal for redefinition. *Journal of the American Academy of Dermatology* 1:151–162.

Yunis, E. J., and Lane, M. A. 1979. Cellular immunity and aging. *Journal of Investigative Dermatology* 73:24–28.

Yuspa, S. H. 1983. Cutaneous carcinogenesis: Natural and experimental. In Goldsmith, L. (Ed.), *Biochemistry and Physiology of the Skin*. New York, Oxford University Press, pp. 115–1138.

Yuspa, S. H. 1986. Cutaneous chemical carcinogenesis. *Journal of the American Academy of Dermatology* 15:1031–1044.

Yuspa, S. H. 1987. Cellular and molecular mechanisms of carcinogenesis in living epithelia. *Cancer Research* 39:3–15.

5

The Implications
of Age-Related Changes
in Immune Function and Toxicity

Richard M. Lewis, Ph.D.
Joy Cavagnaro, Ph.D.

The important factors in chemically induced toxic effects to the immune system, include not only the chemical structure and conditions of exposure but also host-related factors such as age, sex, genetic makeup, concurrent disease, and nutritional status (European Chemical Industry and Toxicology Center, 1987). A crucial issue in research on aging over the past several years has been the importance of distinguishing changes imposed by the environment from those intrinsic to the aging process (Kay, 1979).

The interaction of environmental chemicals with the immune system results in a variety of adverse conditions characterized by immunosuppression, uncontrolled proliferation, alterations in defense mechanisms against pathogens and neoplasia, allergy, or autoimmunity (Dean, Murray, and Ward, 1986). These primary changes in immunity are also related to many of the pathological processes that develop with age, that is, increased predisposition to malignancy, increased frequency and severity of infection, autoimmune diseases and damage caused by circulating immune complexes, and some forms of senile brain pathology. It has been postulated that the age-related changes in the immune system may actually represent an important intermediate link between functional aging and disease (Butenko, 1985).

Immune Cells and Their Function

Although it is commonly accepted that immunological changes associated with aging are intrinsic to the immune system, there are also interactions between other networks such as central nervous and endocrine systems. Of the characteristic alterations in structure and function to the many organs and systems that accompany aging, however, those to the immune system are the most pronounced. Changes occur in the immune system soon after puberty, when no decline in the functions of other systems has as yet become manifest, and increase progressively with age (Butenko, 1985).

Two major mechanisms are responsible for a functioning immune system: a nonspecific mechanism, which does not require prior exposure and lacks specificity, and a specific immune mechanism, which is directed against and is specific to the particular exposure. The specific immune reaction may impart immunological memory, allowing a more rapid and effective response on subsequent exposure.

Nonspecific resistance to environmental chemicals is achieved by mucous secretions, phagocytosis by mononuclear cells including blood monocytes and tissue macrophages and granulocytes, cytotoxic cells, or preexisting antibody. Lymphoid cells, namely, T lymphocytes and B lymphocytes as well as macrophages, are involved with specific host resistance. T lymphocytes migrate from the bone marrow, mature in the thymus, and migrate into the blood, lymph, and lymphoid tissue. They express antigen receptors and are further divided into helper, suppressor, and cytotoxic subpopulations. The various subpopulations are distinguished by the expression of specific cell surface glycoproteins (Boyd, 1987). B cells also originate in the bone marrow and migrate into blood, lymph, and lymphoid tissue. They express specific surface antibody and release antibody into the circulation. Interactions between these predominant cellular elements and other soluble components (e.g., the complement system, interleukins, interferons, etc.) form the basis of the immune response.

After exposure to an environmental compound (antigen) by an immunocompetent host, a series of complex events occur that are involved with specific host resistance. One of the two major types of immune responses is cell-mediated immunity, which is a response by specifically sensitized T lymphocytes and is generally associated with delayed-type hypersensitivity, graft rejection, and resistance to persistent infectious agents. The second type is humoral immunity, which involves the production of specific antibodies by B lymphocytes after sensitization by a specific antigen (Dean, Murray, and Ward, 1986).

Decreased Immunity Associated with Aging

The obvious physiological association with age and immune decline is the involution of the thymus gland (Boyd, 1932). The morphological and functional involution of the thymus gland is a particularly early and impressive precursor of immunological aging. In humans, the loss of cellular mass of the thymus begins soon after puberty and by the fifth decade retains only 5–10 percent of its maximal size (National Research Council, 1987). The involution of the thymus gland results in consistently observed decreases in T-dependent lymphocyte function (Anderson, Watson, and Yunis, 1985).

The effect of thymic decline on aging has been substantiated in several specific ways: by defective helper and effector functions, which may predispose an individual to infections or the emergence of neoplastic diseases, or by defective suppressor functions, which may predispose an individual to autoimmunity and antibody-mediated vascular diseases (MacKay, Whittingham, and Mathews, 1977). There is also statistical evidence that age-associated failure of the thymus-dependent immune functions predisposes individuals to earlier death (MacKay, Whittingham, and Mathews, 1977).

Although there is accumulating evidence to indicate the presence of functional abnormalities in T cells from aged, healthy humans, the cellular basis remains unclear. Because the thymus is responsible for T-cell maturation, it was presumed that age-related changes in T-cell numbers or subsets would be apparent. In fact, several studies found significant decreases in lymphocyte numbers that were attributable to decreases in the number of T cells (Ligthart, Schuit, and Hijmans, 1985; Makinodan, Lubinski, and Fong, 1987). Bender, Nagel, and Adler (1986), however, showed that lymphocyte numbers remained constant if the same individuals were measured at different times in their lives. The number and proportion of lymphocytes remained relatively constant throughout the human life span. By using functional assays, Ales-Martinez et al. (1988) showed that increases in natural killer (NK) cells masked an apparent T-lymphocyte reduction. The NK cells could not functionally substitute for the T lymphocytes that they replaced. NK cells belong to the group of large granular lymphocytes (LGL) that are capable of spontaneous lysis of nontumor and tumor target cells (Tilden et al., 1986). They are believed to play a vital role in the host immune defense system against infections and tumor growth. In mouse studies, it was shown that the number of lymphocytes in spleen, lymph node, and bone marrow did not change appreciably and that the small changes that did occur were not sufficient to account for the changes in immune function (Makinodan, Lubinski, and Fong, 1987; Stutman, 1974).

In a study involving a large number of human volunteers, cell-mediated immunity was measured by skin test reactivity (Maxwell and McCluskey, 1986). Decreases of cell-mediated immunity were evident in the aged population. The T-cell response to the nonspecific mitogens phytohemagglutinin (PHA) and concanavalin A (con A) has been shown to decrease with age but an age association has not been demonstrated for the B-lymphocyte mitogen pokeweed (Murasko et al., 1986).

The Decline of a Soluble Component with Age: Interleukin-2

Interleukin-2 (IL-2) is central to proper immune function, and its association with the age-related decline in cellular immunity must be emphasized. IL-2 is required for T-cell proliferation, cytotoxic T-cell differentiation, and initiation of B-cell responses. Decreased numbers of IL-2-producing cells in aged animals may account for deficiencies in these important immune functions (Thoman, 1985). Vissinga et al. (1987) reported a correlation between an age-related decline in delayed-type hypersensitivity and IL-2 production. Although both functions are mediated by T lymphocytes, the degree of loss in delayed-type hypersensitivity and IL-2 production suggested that it could not be entirely attributed to the decline in the proportion of these cells.

Thoman and Weigle (1985) reported that, when added to in vitro cultures, IL-2 enhanced cell-mediated immunity in splenocytes from aged mice. When administered along with antigen, IL-2 restored the cytotoxic T-lymphocyte response and T-dependent humoral immunity in aged mice. In other mouse experiments using fibrosarcoma (M-B6-1) cells as the target for cellular immunity, IL-2, when administered after immunization, resulted in a suppression of cytotoxic T-lymphocyte activity (Bruley-Rosset and Payelle, 1987). In vitro, IL-2 also enhanced cell-mediated immunity to fibrosarcoma cells in aged mice. The age-related decline in antitumor activity in the fibrosarcoma model was related to increases in suppressor T lymphocytes. T-lymphocyte transfer experiments also showed suppression of immunity in young mice. In experiments designed specifically to test the IL-2 effect on suppressor T lymphocytes, some aged animals showed a decrease in suppressor function that could be restored by addition of IL-2 (Gottesman, Walford, and Thorbecke, 1985). In animals that did not exhibit this decrease, IL-2 did not improve their responses. In related experiments, Vie and Miller (1986) demonstrated a decrease with age in the proportion of IL-2 receptor-bearing cells.

B Lymphocytes

Conflicting views concerning the T-cell involvement in the senescence of B-cell immunity have been presented by Habicht (1985) and Kim, Siskind, and Weksler (1985). The latter study showed that the ability to respond to T-independent antigens by formation of plaque-forming cells was not decreased in cultures of human lymphocytes from aged individuals; similarly, the ability of macrophages to produce stimulating factors was not diminished. They concluded that the reduced immunoglobulin (Ig) response in elderly subjects was a result of changes in the helper or suppressor functions of T cells. Cook et al. (1987), in a study of the response to hepatitis B vaccine in elderly patients, found that this population could be divided into responders and nonresponders. In vitro crossover experiments showed that T cells from responders were necessary for B-cell production of antihepatitis; B cells from responders alone and B cells from responders cultured with T cells from nonresponders were not sufficient for in vitro antibody production. Habicht (1985), in contrast, in experiments of tolerance induction in young and aged mice showed that low-dose treatment with cyclophosphamide to deplete suppressor cells did not block tolerance induction and that the defect of aging may be in the B-cell population.

Studies in the numbers of circulating B lymphocytes with age show that there is no change in absolute numbers, but the proportion may increase because of a fall in the proportion of T lymphocytes (Diaz-Jouanen, Stridkland, and Williams, 1975). In regard to B-lymphocyte-dependent functions, there appears to be an increase in IgG and IgA (Cassidy, Nordby, and Dodge, 1974). The capacity to produce specific antibody is well preserved in aged persons, although the thymus-dependent component (sustained IgG production) appears to decline. There is also an increase with age in abnormal serum components including monoclonal immunoglobulins and amyloid protein (MacKay, 1977).

Goodman and Weigle (1985) studied the T-dependent immunoglobulin response in young and aged mice. They showed that the B-cell mitogen lipopolysaccharide induced nonspecific Ig responses in cultures from young mice but not aged mice. The nucleoside 8-mercapto-guanosine (8-MeGuo) was shown to induce nonspecific Ig production in both young and aged mice, presumably as a result of its ability to cross the cell membrane. In the same report, it was shown that 8-MeGuo could substitute for a T-cell signal in specific antibody responses in aged mice. The authors suggested that senescence in the aged population was a result of changes in B-cell membrane receptors for T-cell signals and that 8-MeGuo bypassed that receptor (Goodman and Weigle, 1985).

In studies using bone marrow transplantation to young, lethally irradiated mice from either old or young donors, the Ig response was decreased when aged mice were used as donors (Ershler et al., 1986). Although the assays used measured the response of T-dependent antigens, their results could also be linked to changes in T-cell immunity. Studies of aged mice by Tsuda et al. (1988) demonstrated that if the bone marrow was partially shielded during irradiation the repopulated mouse responded to immunization by production of antibodies of the same affinity and number of plaque-forming cells as young, normal mice.

Mucosal Immunity

The immune function of the skin and the mucosal lining of the respiratory and gastrointestinal tracts also change with age. Alterations in mucosal immunity (mucosal defense) may render aged individuals susceptible to enteric infection and systemic infections in which the intestinal tract is the portal of entry; however, the changes seen do not parallel those observed in the systemic immune system (National Research Council, 1987).

Diseases Associated with the Age-Related Decline in Immune Function

The predominant health problem in aged individuals is the increased susceptibility to illness resulting from infection. The increased severity of infection in elderly people points to the progressive loss of immunological responsiveness with age (Phair, Hsu, and Hsu, 1988; Saltzman and Peterson, 1987).

Response to bacterial infection has been studied in a number of mouse models. Using *Mycobacterium tuberculosis* infection, Orme (1987) showed that whereas young mice were resistant to a standard immunizing dose of the bacteria, there was a notable increase in susceptibility with age. In passive cell transfer experiments, T cells from young immune individuals were shown to confer immunity to either young or old recipients. Although the macrophage is the effector cell in tuberculosis, the immunity apparently resides in the T cell. Orme (1988) suggested that the recurrence of tuberculosis in aged mice may result from the loss of an anamnestic response.

The ability to induce a suppressed response, low-dose paralysis, to pneumococcal polysaccharide was compared in young and old normal mice. McCoy et al. (1985) showed that suppression could be passively transferred from old to young mice by normal-sized suppressor T lymphocytes but not enlarged suppressor T lymphocytes or helper T lymphocytes. The suppressor T lymphocytes from primed young mice conferred low-dose paralysis to nonprimed young, but not old, recipients. A population of suppressor T lymphocytes presumably lost suppressor activity. In addition, B cells became unresponsive to suppression.

In contrast, in the *Listeria monocytogenes* model of mouse infection, Lovik and North (1985) reported the opposite effect: The LD_{50} was two to four times higher for old mice than young mice and the time to death was longer for old mice. In addition, if the inoculum was adjusted to equalize the groups, spleen cells capable of adoptive transfer were similar from old and young mice and the level of the anamnestic response was similar whether animals were tested at 4 or 17 weeks.

The reported age-related increase in susceptibility to viral infection prompted Rytel (1987) to compare interferon levels in young mice with those in adult animals. He demonstrated that aged animals had decreased circulating γ-interferon levels, relative to viral replication, in response to infection. The significance of lower levels of γ-interferon was described by Hayward and Herberger (1987) in studies on the reduced immunity to *Varicella zoster* virus as a consequence of aging. Whereas there was a small to moderate decline of T lymphocytes, particularly helper cells, in the blood with age, the number of NK T lymphocytes remained constant or rose (Hayward and Herberger, 1987). The proportionally greater loss of helper T lymphocytes compared with suppressor T lymphocytes in aging was consistent with the reduced responsiveness to *Varicella zoster* virus. These helper lymphocytes were responsible for releasing IL-2 and γ-interferon, which in turn activated NK cells to lyse intact cells or suppress virus replication within them.

Polymorphonuclear response to infection, in particular phagocytosis, is an important first response to microbial invasion. A decline in phagocytic ability of polymorphonuclear response has been shown to be correlated directly with age (Emanuelli et al., 1986). Unlike other immune parameters, there is no apparent threshold in the correlation, but a continuous decline in function.

It has been suggested that the ability of individuals to control body temperature is related to their ability to mount an immune response. Norman, Grahn, and Yoshibawa (1985) reviewed the correlation between age and the decreased ability to exhibit a proper fever response and discussed the clinical relevance in response to infection. They concluded that thermoregulation might have been related to the decreased production of the lymphokine IL-2.

Cancer

The age-specific incidence for many forms of neoplasia can be explained by the duration and degree of exposure to carcinogen, the

activity and inherent susceptibility of the exposed tissue, and immunological surveillance (MacKay, Whittingham, and Mathews, 1977).

Although the frequency of cancer in individuals with reduced normal immune function is higher than in those with normal immune functions, regardless of age or sex, this difference is most pronounced in
the aged (Makinodan, 1977).

NK cells are important in the immune surveillance of tumor immunity. Marked NK cell dysfunction has been demonstrated in patients
with various forms of neoplastic diseases and more recently in patients
with acquired immune deficiency syndrome (AIDS) (Forbes, Greco,
and Oldham, 1981; Rook et al., 1983).

Matsuoka, Takeichi, and Kobayashi (1987) showed that NK cell
activity was closely related to antitumor activity in the spontaneously
hypertensive rat (SHR) strain when injected with an adenocarcinoma.
At 1 month of age the NK activity was low; it increased until 3 months
of age, and it steadily declined until age 12 months. This activity was
inversely correlated to tumor growth. The injection of poly(I)-poly(C)
was shown to increase NK activity and significantly decrease tumor
growth. Sato et al. (1986), using the BALB/c mouse strain, showed
that there was a continuous correlation between age and the susceptibility to pristane-induced plasmacytomas. The increased susceptibility
also correlated not only with age but decreased NK activity as well as
decreased cellular immune function.

The age-associated loss of epidermal Langerhans cells is presumed
to impair recognition of foreign antigens, possibly including malignant
cells in the skin. The 10–20 percent loss of the residual cell population
of melanocytes per decade has been postulated to decrease the body's
protection against ultraviolet radiation. In combination with the age-
related decline in immunocompetence, this loss might predispose elderly individuals to photocarcinogenesis (National Research Council,
1987).

Autoimmunity

There is a good correlation between increased age of the population
and an increase in the prevalence of autoantibodies (MacKay, Whittingham, and Mathews, 1977). The regulatory mechanisms of the immune system normally prevent it from recognizing self-components as
antigens. However, when there is a breakdown in immune function,
the result is the production of antibodies that are self-reactive, that is,
autoantibodies.

In autoimmunity the regulatory mechanism allows the proliferation
of self-reactive immune cells. Autoimmunity in age partially affects

certain endocrine or exocrine tissues. Although not all autoantibodies are pathogenic, they are often associated with autoimmune disease. Autoimmune diseases are more commonly seen with advancing age, and also include hemolytic anemias, senile amyloidosis, maturity-onset diabetes, and various forms of periarteritis (Makinodan, Lubinski, and Fong, 1987). Since autoantibodies are associated with degenerative vascular disease, particularly in males, vascular degeneration appears to be mediated in part through autoimmune mechanisms. Circulatory immune complexes can contribute to vascular injury and thus to the increase in severity of atherosclerosis in elderly persons.

Altered Susceptibility to Immunotoxic Chemicals with Age

Alterations in the immune system by chemicals can result in immune suppression or enhancement, autoimmunity, and hypersensitivity. Not only may environmental agents with the potential to modulate immune functions be expected to affect the pattern of immunosenescence in later years, but also aged individuals with the associated immune deficiencies are potentially at greater risk to the effects of immunotoxic agents.

Immunologists and toxicologists began investigating the immunotoxic potential of prominent environmental chemicals such as the polychlorinated biphenyls and lead in the early 1970s (Koller, 1979; Vos, 1977). The results of these studies showed that chemicals present in the environment could compromise immunity in animals. The adverse immune effects exerted by chemicals were confirmed when exposure to these agents resulted in increased susceptibility to infectious agents, both in animals and humans (L. D. Koller, personal communication).

Exposure to environmental chemicals affects cell-mediated immunity more frequently than humoral immunity. Overall these changes in the immune response result in suppression rather than enhancement. Examples of chemicals affecting immunologic suppression or enhancement in rodents and/or humans include polyhalogenated aromatic hydrocarbons (2,3,7,8-tetrachlorodibenzo(p)dioxin, polybrominated biphenyl, polychlorinated biphenyl, hexachlorobenzene, and polychlorinated dibenzofurans), metals (lead and cadmium), aromatic hydrocarbons (benzene and toluene), polycyclic aromatic hydrocarbons (7,12-dimethylbenz(a)anthracene, benzo(a)pyrene, and malondialdehyde), pesticides (trimethylphosphothionate, carbofuran, and chlordane), organotins (tributyltin oxide), aromatic amines (benzidine and acetylfluorene), and others (asbestos, nitrosamide, and food additives (butylated hydroxyanisole)) (Luster, 1989).

Altered immune responses have been reported for factory workers with aplastic anemia and leukemia who were occupationally exposed to benzene. Suppressed cellular immune responses have also been reported in a number of cases of exposure to polyhalogenated aromatic hydrocarbons: Michigan residents and farmers exposed to polybrominated biphenyls from eating contaminated livestock and dairy products, Taiwanese and Japanese people exposed to a mixture of polychlorinated biphenyls and dibenzofurans in contaminated rice oil, and Missouri residents exposed to dioxin (Luster, 1989). The potential immunotoxic effects of trichloroethylene-polluted drinking wells in Massachusetts and aldicarb contamination of ground water in Wisconsin have also been investigated (Berman, 1987). Despite the reported changes in immune responsiveness, in most cases, there is as yet limited evidence (i.e., clinical significance) for the increased susceptibility to disease or incidence of tumors.

There is, however, overwhelming evidence linking asbestos exposure to subsequent development of several types of neoplasms. The most prominent are lung carcinoma and pleural and peritoneal malignant mesotheliomas (Lew et al., 1986). Although the pathogenesis of these forms of neoplasms is still unknown, the host immune system is considered to be an important factor. There is a high frequency of immune dysfunction (i.e., reduced helper/suppressor ratio and NK cell function) in asbestos workers and in patients with malignant mesothelioma. Lew et al. (1986) suggested that these changes among asbestos workers at high risk may be a direct consequence of asbestos exposure and might not be related to neoplastic processes. These findings led to the speculation that chronic immunosuppression associated with the presence of asbestos in the exposed workers may have caused the eventual breakdown of the host's surveillance system and the onset of neoplasia.

Environmental agents have also been implicated as causative agents in autoimmune disease. Chemicals may bind to tissue or serum proteins, thus generating an immune response against modified self-antigens resulting in cell injury or death. Examples of environmental chemicals and associated disease include the pesticide dieldrin in autoimmune leukocytic anemia and the metals gold and mercury in the induction of glomerular nephritis similar to that seen in Goodpasture's disease (Dean, Murray, and Ward, 1986).

Many environmental chemicals trigger hypersensitivity reactions by their repeated exposure. Sensitizers are usually small molecules that become antigenic when they attach to tissue or serum protein. Examples of environmental chemical structures that can act as sensitizers include epoxides, quinones, amines, metal salts, phenol ethers, and diazo compounds. Skin contact or inhalation of sensitizers can cause dermatitis or asthma, respectively (Luster, 1989).

Maintenance of Normal Immune Function

Intervention in immune deficiency has become an important aspect of aging and immunosenescence. In immune deficiencies such as cancer, AIDS, and malnutrition, a number of immunomodulatory approaches have been attempted with variable results (Hadden and Keskiner-Merriam, 1985). These therapies include the thymic hormones thymosin-alpha-1 and thymopentin, as well as interferons, IL-2, and others (Ershler et al., 1986; Frasca, Adorini, and Doria, 1987; Frasca et al., 1986; Kelley et al., 1986; Meroni et al., 1987). In addition, such chemical inducers as levamisole, isoprinosine, azimexon, and muramyl dipeptides have been applied (Hadden and Keskiner-Merriam, 1985). The concept of immunotherapy or immunomanipulation, therefore appears feasible (Busby and Caranasos, 1985).

Various approaches to therapeutic interventions in aging (i.e., maintenance of normal immune function) have included manipulation of the diet and body temperatures, drug treatments, and surgery. Dietary management has been employed in an attempt to selectively promote normal immune functions (e.g., antitumor cell immunity) and suppress abnormal immune functions (e.g., production of autoantibodies) (Jose and Good, 1971; Pierpaoli and Maestroni, 1988). Nutritional support may therefore be an important augmentation of immune responsiveness in aged people and of increasing importance after exposure of aged individuals to immunotoxic chemicals.

In a recent study in Nova Scotia the cell-mediated response in populations of elderly individuals who were living at home, living in a nursing home but were self-sufficient, living in a nursing home but were not self-sufficient, or hospitalized were compared (Marrie, Johnson, and Durant, 1988). The authors showed that cell-mediated immunity correlated with the individual's dependency. In a study of 96 elderly individuals, immune responsiveness was correlated not only with increased phagocytosis but with levels of serum prealbumin, a measure of malnutrition (Moulias et al., 1985).

Dietary fat content—the polyunsaturated fat/saturated (P/S) ratio—has been shown to affect suppressor cell activity as measured by contact photosensitivity (CPS) and plaque-forming cell assay in rats fed diets containing various P/S ratios. Animals were also treated with cyclophosphamide in order to determine the contribution of the suppressor cell to the decreased CPS. It was concluded that a low P/S diet increased suppressor activity, as shown by an age-related decline in CPS, and the animals fed on a high P/S diet showed no change in suppressor activity (Cinader et al., 1986). The opposite effects were observed for antibody production.

In a study of various diet conditions that ranged from unrestricted to a diet of reduced calories and proteins (vitamin and mineral enriched) it was demonstrated that mice from the groups on restricted diets lived 35–65% longer than those on unrestricted feed. In addition, the restricted mice showed lower incidence of tumor and increased T-cell proliferation (Thompson, Robbins, and Cooper, 1987). Fabris et al. (1986) suggested that the amino acids lysine and arginine when fed to humans may have important effects on mitogen responsiveness, T-cell marker expression, and production of thymic hormones. The authors proposed that the ingestion of lysine and arginine stimulated the neuro-endocrine system to reactivate the thymic release of immunologic hormones.

Dietary glutathione in mice has been shown to reverse decreases in splenic glutathione levels and augment T-cell immunity as determined by in vitro responses to con A and DTH assays (Furukawa, Meydani, and Blumber, 1987). The inosine analog, isoprinosine, was shown by Tsang et al. (1985) to improve the *in vitro* responses in aging humans in a number of T cell parameters tested. These functions included con A-induced lymphocyte proliferation, NK cell activity, polymorphonuclear chemotaxis, and IL-2 production. Further characterization by Delafuente and Panush (1988) showed that mitogen-induced mononuclear cell proliferation was significantly enhanced by isoprinosine but did not affect unstimulated cell growth.

Vitamin supplementation may also offer potential in improving the immune responsiveness of aged individuals. Vitamins E and C have been reported to induce positive effects. Meydani et al. (1986) described increased delayed-type hypersensitivity and response to con A and lipopolysaccharide after vitamin E administration. These responses also correlated with decreased prostaglandin synthesis. Studies of vitamin C did not show positive effects after a 3-week regimen or oral administration but seemed to improve responses when added to in vitro cultures (Delafuente, Prendergast, and Modigh, 1986).

Conclusion

The immune system is an intricate network of highly complex mechanisms involving multiple membrane interactions in numerous cell types and thereby offers many reactions in which lesions might occur (Nordin and Proust, 1988). The importance of the proper balance of the immune system is highlighted by the physiological changes associated with aging. Major factors in the age-related decline in the immune response are systemic influences that condition the characteristic changes of the immune and other systems. Environmental chemicals have also been implicated in effecting changes in immune responses, by immune dysregulation, similar to those associated with age.

Immunosenescence is usually characterized by the loss of thymus-dependent functions that are required by both cell-mediated immunity and the regulation of humoral immunity. Most of the evidence cited indicates that these two are interrelated and result in a defect in the T-lymphocyte response (including the helper/suppressor balance), effects of IL-2 produced by activated T lymphocytes, and reduction of thymic hormones. These results, however, could be predicted as a consequence of thymic involution. Nonspecific depression of immunity can cause serious complications with bacterial, fungal, and parasitic infections in certain malignancies. Clark et al. (1985) studied a number of mouse strains and varieties within strains and demonstrated that there were differences both in time of onset of age-related deficiencies and in the nature of these deficits. Similarly, Barcellini et al. (1988), in a study of healthy, elderly volunteers, concluded not only that immune deficiency is associated with aging but that there is a wide range of individuals with different deficiencies as well as different reactivities. The implications of the age-associated decline in immune responsiveness together with the variations in immune functions among the aged population will be important considerations in the evaluation of the potential susceptibility and risk of elderly people to the effect of potential immunotoxic chemicals.

Manipulation of the immune response by changing diet, body temperature, drugs, and/or surgery has been shown to be important in the maintenance of normal immune function. Immune intervention may ultimately result in alterations of immunosenescence or decreased susceptibility to the immunotoxic effects of environmental chemicals. Evidence also suggests a neuroendocrine control over the thymus and therefore offers many steps in the cascade where additional intervention might, in the future, be beneficial.

References

Ales-Martinez, J. E., Alvarez-Mon, M., Merino, F., Bonilla, F., Martinez, C., Durantez, A., and De la Hera, A. 1988. Decreased TcR-CD3+ T cell numbers in healthy aged humans. Evidence that T cell defects are masked by a reciprocal increase of TcR-CD3-CD2+ natural killer cells. *European Journal of Immunology* 18:1827–1830.

Anderson, W., Watson, A. L., and Yunis, E. J. 1985. Environmental and genetic factors that influence immunity and longevity in mice. *Basic Life Sciences* 35:231–240.

Barcellini, W., Borghi, M. O., Sguotti, C., Palmieri, R., Frasca, D., Meroni, P. L., Doria, G., and Zanusi, C. 1988. Heterogeneity of immune responsiveness in healthy elderly subjects. *Clinical Immunology and Immunopathology* 47:142–151.

Bender, B. S., Nagel, J. E., and Adler, W. H. 1986. Absolute peripheral blood lymphocyte count and subsequent mortality of elderly men. The Baltimore Longitudinal Study of Aging. *Journal of the American Geriatrics Society* 34:649–654.

Berman, C. L. 1987. United States moves toward immunotoxicity testing. *Spectrum Biotechnology Overview* 1:29–33.

Boyd, A. 1987. Human leukocyte antigens: An update on structure, function and nomenclature. *Pathology* 19:329–337.

Boyd, E. 1932. Progress in pediatrics: The weight of the thymus gland in health and in disease. *American Journal of Diseases in Children* 43:1162–1214.

Bruley-Rosset, M., and Payelle, B. 1987. Deficient tumor-specific immunity in old mice: In vivo mediation by suppressor cells, and correction of the defect by interleukin 2 supplementation in vitro but not in vivo. *European Journal of Immunology* 17:307–312.

Busby, J., and Caranasos, G. J. 1985. Immune function, autoimmunity, and selective immunoprophylaxis in the aged. *Medical Clinics of North America* 69:465–474.

Butenko, G. M. 1985. Aging of the immune system and diseases. In Likhachev, A., Anisimov, V., and Monesano, R. (Eds.), *Age-Related Factors in Carcinogenesis*. New York, Oxford University Press, pp. 71–83.

Cassidy, J. T., Nordby, G. L., and Dodge, H. J. 1974. Biologic variations of human serum immunoglobulin concentrations: Sex–age specific effects. *Journal of Chronic Diseases* 27:507–516.

Cinader, B., Clandinin, M. T., Koh, S. W., Brown, W. R., and Ramsay, C. A. 1986. Dietary fat alters progression of some age-related changes of the immune system. *Immunology Letters* 12:175–179.

Clark, D. A., Cinader, B., Rosenthal, K. L., Koh, S. Y., and Chaput, A. 1985. Strain-dependence and cellular aspects of the acceleration of age-dependent shift in class-specific helper and suppressor activity in the thymus of MRL/Mp mice by the LPR gene. *Cellular Immunology* 96:418–429.

Cook, J. M., Gualde, N., Hessel, L., Mounier, M., Michel, J. P., Denis, F., and Ratinaud, M. H. 1987. Alterations in the human immune response to the hepatitis B vaccine among the elderly. *Cellular Immunology* 109:89–96.

Dean, J. A., Murray, M. J., and Ward, E. C. 1986. Toxic responses of the immune system. In Haassen, C. D., Amdur, M. O., and Doull, J. (Eds.), *Casarett and Doull's Toxicology: The Basic Science of Poisons*. New York, Macmillan, pp. 245–285.

Delafuente, J., and Panush, R. S. 1988. Pharmacologic immunoenhancement in the elderly: In vitro effects of isoprinosine. *Clinical Immunology and Immunopathology* 47:363–367.

Delafuente, J. C., Prendergast, J. M., and Modigh, A. 1986. Immunologic modulation by vitamin C in the elderly. *International Journal of Immunopharmacology* 8:205–211.

Diaz-Jouanen, E., Stridkland, R. G., and Williams, R. D. 1975. Studies of human lymphocytes in the newborn and the aged. *American Journal of Medicine* 58:620–628.

Emanuelli, G., Lanzio, M., Anfossi, T., Romano, S., Anfossi, G., and Calcamuggi, G. 1986. Influence of age on polymorphonuclear leukocytes in vitro: Phagocytic activity in healthy human subjects. *Gerontology* 32:308–316.

Ershler, W. B., Rebert, J. C., Blow, A. J., Granter, S. R., and Lynch, J. 1985. Effect of thymosin alpha one on specific antibody response and susceptibility to infection in young and aged mice. *International Journal of Immunopharmacology* 7:465–471.

Ershler, W. B., Robbins, D. L., Moore, A. L., and Hebert, J. C. 1986. The age related decline in antibody response is transferred by old to young bone marrow transplantation. *Experimental Gerontology* 21:45–53.

European Chemical Industry and Toxicology Centre. 1987. *Identification of Immunotoxic Effects of Chemicals and Assessment of Their Relevance to Man* (Monograph 10). Brussels, European Chemical Industry and Toxicology Centre.

Fabris, N., Mocchegiani, E., Muzzioli, M., and Piloni, S. 1986. Recovery of age-related decline of thymic endocrine activity and PHA response by lys–arginine combination. *International Journal of Immunopharmacology* 8:677–685.

Forbes, J. T., Greco, F. A., and Oldham, R. K. 1981. Human natural cell mediated cytotoxicity. II. Levels of neoplastic diseases. *Cancer Immunology and Immunotherapy* 11:147–153.

Frasca, D., Adorini, L., and Doria, G. 1987. Enhanced frequency of mitogen-responsive T cell precursors in old mice injected with thymosin alpha 1. *European Journal of Immunology* 17:727–730.

Frasca, D., Adorini, L., Mancini, C., and Doria, G. 1986. Reconstitution of T cell functions in aging mice by thymosin alpha 1. *Immunopharmacology* 11:155–163.

Furukawa, T., Meydani, S. N., and Blumber, J. B. 1987. Reversal of age associated decline in immune responsiveness by dietary glutathione supplementation in mice. *Mechanisms of Ageing and Development* 38:107–117.

Goodman, M. G., and Weigle, W. O. 1985. Restoration of humoral immunity in vitro in immunodeficient aging mice by C8-derivatized guanine ribonucleosides. *Journal of Immunology* 134:3808–3811.

Gottesman, S. R., Walford, R. L., and Thorbecke, G. J. 1985. Proliferative and cytotoxic immune functions in aging mice. III. Exogenous interleukin-rich supernatant only partially restores alloreactivity in vitro. *Mechanisms of Ageing and Development* 31:103–113.

Habicht, G. S. 1985. Acquired immunological tolerance in aged mice. II. The cellular basis of the loss of tolerance sensitivity. *Mechanisms of Ageing and Development* 30:23–36.

Hadden, J. W., and Keskiner-Merriam, L. 1985. Immunopharmacologic basis of immunotherapy. *Clinical Physiology and Biochemistry* 3:111–119.

Hayward, A. R., and Herberger, M. 1987. Lymphocyte responses to *Varicella zoster* virus in the elderly. *Journal of Clinical Immunology* 7:174–178.

Jose, D. G., and Good, R. A. 1971. Absence of enhancing antibody in cell mediated immunity to tumor heterografts in protein deficient rats. *Nature* 231:645–649.

Kay, M. M. B. 1979. Effects of parainfluenza virus infection on immunologic aging. In Singhal, S. K., Sinclair, N. R., and Stiller, C. R. (Eds.), *Aging and Immunity*. Amsterdam, Elsevier-North Holland, pp. 117–134.

Kelley, K. W., Brief, S., Westly, H. J., Novakofski, J., Bechtel, P. J., Simon, J., and Waler, E. B. 1986. GH3 pituitary adenoma cells can reverse thymic aging in rats. *Proceedings of the National Academy of Sciences* 83:5663–5667.

Kim, Y. T., Siskind, G. W., and Weksler, M. E. 1985. Plaque-forming cell response of human blood lymphocytes. III. Cellular basis of the reduced immune response in the elderly. *Israel Journal of Medical Science* 21:317–322.

Koller, L. D. 1979. Effects of environmental chemicals on the immune system. *Advances in Veterinarian Science and Comparative Medicine* 23:367–395.

Lew, R., Tsang, P., Holland, J. F., Warner, N., Selidoff, I. J., and Bekesi, J. G. 1986. High frequency of immune dysfunctions in asbestos workers and in patients with malignant mesothelioma. *Journal of Clinical Immunology* 6:225–233.

Ligthart, G. J., Schuit, H. R. E., and Hijmans, W. 1985. Subpopulations of mononuclear cells in aging: Expansion of the null cell compartment and decrease in the number of T and B cells in human blood. *Immunology* 55:15–21.

Lovik, M., and North, R. J. 1985. Effect of aging on anti-microbial immunity: Old mice display a normal capacity for generating protective T cells and immunologic memory in response to infection with *Listeria* monocytogenes. *Journal of Immunology* 135:3479–3486.

Luster, M. 1989. Immunotoxicology and the immune system. *Health and Environment Digest* 3:1–3.

MacKay, I. R., Whittingham, S. F., and Mathews, J. D. 1977. The immunoepidemiology of aging. In Makinodan, T., and Yunis, E. (Eds.), *Immunology and Aging*. New York, Plenum Press, pp. 35–49.

Makinodan, T. 1977. Immunity and aging. In Finch, C. E., and Hayflick, L. (Eds.), *Handbook of the Biology of Aging*. New York, Van Nostrand Reinhold, pp. 379–408.

Makinodan, T., Lubinski, J., and Fong, T. C. 1987. Cellular, biochemical and molecular basis of T-cell senescence. *Archives of Pathology and Laboratory Medicine* 111:910–914.

Marrie, T. J., Johnson, S., and Durant, H. 1988. Cell-mediated immunity of healthy adult Nova Scotians in various age groups compared with nursing home and hospitalized senior citizens. *Journal of Allergy and Clinical Immunology* 81:836–843.

Matsuoko, T., Takeichi, N., and Kobayashi, H. 1987. Age-related changes of natural antitumor resistance in spontaneously hypertensive rats with T-cell depression. *Cancer Research* 47:310–313.

Maxwell, A. P., and McCluskey, D. R. 1986. Assessment of cell-mediated immunity in a British population using multiple skin test antigens. *Clinical Allergy* 16:365–369.

McCoy, K. L., Baer, P. J., Malik, T. R., and Chused, T. K. 1985. Enlargement of Lyt 2-positive cells is associated with functional impairment and autoimmune hemolytic anemia in New Zealand black mice. *Journal of Immunology* 135:232–237.

Meroni, P. L., Barcelline, W., Frasca, D., Squotti, C., Borghi, M. O., DeBartolo, G., Doria, G., and Zanussi, C. 1987. In vivo immunopotentiating activity of thymopentin in aging humans: Increase of IL-2 production. *Clinical Immunology and Immunopathology* 42:151–159.

Meydani, S. N., Meydani, M., Verdon, C. P., Shapiro, A. A., Blumberg, J. B., and Hayes, K. C. 1986. Vitamin E supplementation suppresses prostaglandin E1(2) synthesis and enhances the immune response of aged mice. *Mechanisms of Ageing and Development* 34:191–201.

Moulias, R., Devillechabrolle, A., Lesourd, B., Proust, J., Marescot, M. R., Doumerc, S., Favre-Berrone, M., Congy, F., and Wang, A. 1985. Respective role of immune and nutritional factors in the priming of the immune response in the elderly. *Mechanisms of Ageing and Development* 31:123–137.

Murasko, D. M., Nelson, B. J., Silver, R., Matour, D., and Kaye, D. 1986. Immunologic response in an elderly population with a mean age of 85. *American Journal of Medicine* 81:612–618.

National Research Council, Committee on Chemical Toxicity and Aging. Board on Environmental Studies and Toxicology, Commission on Life Sciences, 1987. *Aging in Today's Environment*. Washington, DC, National Academy Press.

Nordin, A. A., and Proust, J. J. 1988. Signal transduction mechanisms in the immune system. Potential implication in immunosenescence. *Endocrinology and Metabolism Clinics of North America* 16:919–945.

Norman, D. C., Grahn, D., and Yoshibawa, T. T. 1985. Fever and aging. *Journal of the American Geriatrics Society* 33:859–863.

Orme, I. M. 1987. Aging and immunity to tuberculosis: Increased susceptibility of old mice reflects a decreased capacity to generate mediator T lymphocytes. *Journal of Immunolgy* 138:414–418.

Orme, I. M. 1988. A mouse model of the recrudescence of latent tuberculosis in the elderly. *American Review of Respiratory Diseases* 137:716–718.

Phair, J. P., Hsu, C. S., and Hsu, Y. L. 1988. Aging and infection. *Ciba Foundation Symposium* 134:143–154.

Pierpaoli, W., and Maestroni, G. J. 1988. Melatonin: A principal neuroimmunoregulatory and anti-stress hormone: Its anti-aging effects. *Immunology Letters* 16:355–361.

Rook, A. H., Masur, H., Lane, C., Frederick, W., Kasahara, T., Macher, A. M., Djeu, J. Y., Manischewitz, J. F., Jackson, L., Fanci, A. S., and Quinnan, G. V., Jr. 1983. Interleukin-2 enhances the depressed natural killer and cytomegalovirus-specific cytotoxic activities of lymphocytes from patients with acquired immune deficiency syndrome. *Journal of Clinical Investigation* 72:398–403.

Rytel, M. W. 1987. Effect of age on viral infections: Possible role of interferon. *Journal of the American Geriatrics Society* 35:1092–1099.

Saltzman, R. L., and Peterson, P. K. 1987. Immunodeficiency of the elderly. *Reviews of Infectious Diseases* 9:1127–1139.

Sato, K., Bloom, E. T., Hirokawa, K., and Makinodan, T. 1986. Increased susceptibility of old mice to plasmacytoma induction. *Journal of Gerontology* 41:24–29.

Stutman, O. 1974. Cell mediated immunity and aging. *Federation Proceedings* 33:2028–2032.

Thoman, M. L. 1985. Role of interleukin-2 in the age-related impairment of immune function. *Journal of the American Geriatric Society* 33:781–787.

Thoman, M. L., and Weigle, W. O. 1985. Reconstitution of in vivo cell mediated lympholysis responses in aged mice with interleukin 2. *Journal of Immunology* 134:949–952.

Thompson, J. S., Robbins, J., and Cooper, J. K. 1987. Nutrition and immune function in the geriatric population. *Clinical Geriatric Medicine* 3:309–317.

Tilden, A. B., Grossi, C. E., Itoh, K., Cloud, G. A., Dougherty, P. A., and Balch, C. M. 1986. Subpopulations analysis of human granular lymphocytes: Associations with age, gender and cytotoxic activity. *Natural Immunity and Cell Growth Regulation* 5:90–99.

Tsang, K. Y., Pan, J. F., Swanger, D. L., and Fudenberg, H. H. 1985. In vitro restoration of immune responses in aging humans by isoprinosine. *International Journal of Immunopharmacology* 7:199–206.

Tsuda, T., Kim, Y. T., Siskind, G. W., and Weksler, M. E. 1988. Old mice recover the ability to produce IgG and high-avidity antibody following irradiation with partial bone marrow shielding. *Proceedings of the National Academy of Sciences (USA)* 85:1169–1173.

Vie, H., and Miller, R. A. 1986. Decline, with age, in the proportion of mouse T cells that express IL-2 receptors after mitogen stimulation. *Mechanisms of Ageing and Development* 33:313–322.

Vissinga, C. S., Dirven, C. J., Steinmeyer, F. A., Benner, R., and Boersma, W. J. 1987. Deterioration of cellular immunity during aging. The relationship between age-dependent impairment of delayed-type hypersensitivity, Thy-1+,Lyt-2− cells in C5BL/Ka and CBARij mice. *Cellular Immunology* 10:323–334.

Vos, J. G. 1977. Immune suppression as related to toxicology. *CRC Critical Reviews in Toxicology* 5:67–101.

6

The Impact of Aging
on Cardiovascular Function
and Reactivity

Christopher Lau, Ph.D.

It is generally thought that senescence in mammals is accompanied by an overall decline in the functional integrity of the organism and its ability to adapt to various environmental challenges. Indeed, a considerable body of evidence has shown that in both human and laboratory animals (mainly the rat), advancing age produces a number of significant alterations in the heart and circulatory hemodynamics. These include cardiac hypertrophy, slight decrease in heart rate and increase in the duration of contraction, loss of elasticity and distensibility in the arterial wall, elevated blood pressure, and altered responsivity to a host of physiologic and pharmacological stimuli. In recent years, a clearer picture has emerged not only to describe the physiological phenomena that take place in the aging heart and blood vessels but also to provide a better understanding of the cellular and biochemical mechanisms underlying these age-related changes. Several reviews on these topics have been published (Altura and Altura, 1977; Docherty, 1986; Fleg, 1986; Goldberg, Kreider, and Roberts, 1984; Goldberg and Roberts, 1976; Lakatta, 1985, 1987a, 1987b; Lakatta and Yin, 1982; Roberts and Goldberg, 1975; Rosenthal, 1987; Walsh, 1987; Weisfeldt, 1980.) and this chapter furnishes only a brief summary of the current understanding. Because of these findings, a fundamental issue of concern arises as to whether the cardiovascular system of an elderly individual is at an increased risk to toxic insults derived from drugs and hazardous environmental compounds. Surprisingly, this particular issue has thus far received scant attention, and only a few studies using diverse experimental approaches can be found in the literature. Despite the paucity of information available, this chapter nevertheless attempts to provide an overview of the current research findings.

Cardiovascular Structure and Aging

Data from several studies have indicated that the human heart undergoes a modest degree of hypertrophy with advancing age (Kannel, Gordon, and Offutt, 1969; Linzbach and Akuamoa-Boateng, 1973; Rosahn, 1941; Strandell, 1964). However, because the investigators in these studies did not exclude hearts from individuals with cardiovascular diseases, the possibility remains that these age-related changes of heart weight may in part reflect pathological processes. Myocardial hypertrophy was also detected in senescent rats maintained in the laboratory without any experimental manipulation, although these findings were similarly confounded with high incidence of pathological changes (Simms and Berg, 1957; Wilens and Sproul, 1938). The best evidence for enlargement of the aging heart in fact comes from an indirect measurement. Using the noninvasive echocardiographical technique, Sjogren (1972) reported a progressive increase in left ventricular posterior wall thickness in healthy human subjects ages 15–65. These findings were confirmed by Gerstenblith et al. (1977) and Gardin et al. (1979), who observed an increase (approximately 30 percent) in left ventricular wall thickness in healthy normotensive subjects ages 25–80. Similarly, thickening of the ventricular wall and enlargement of myocyte were also demonstrated in 18- to 24-month-old normotensive rats (Engelmann, Vitullo, and Gerrity, 1987). The precise stimulus for this apparent hypertrophy is unclear. Linzbach and Akuamoa-Boateng (1973) postulated that elevated mean blood pressure accompanying advancing age might induce cardiac hypertrophy, although Lakatta (1987c) recently suggested that the hypertrophic effects of hypertension on the myocardium might be distinguishable from those of aging.

Relatively few morphological changes in the senescent heart are associated exclusively with the aging processes. Lipofuscin accumulation and basophilic degeneration in cardiac muscle cells are commonly detected in elderly patients (Strehler et al., 1959) as well as in old animals (Topping and Travis, 1974; Travis and Travis, 1972). Mitochondrial structural abnormalities and significant reduction of mitochondrial coenzyme Q content have been found in the senescent rodent heart (Beyer and Starnes, 1985; Frenzel and Feimann, 1984), which may be associated with declines in myocardial oxidative metabolism (Abu-Erreish et al., 1977; Chen, Warshaw, and Sanadi, 1972; Frolkis and Bogatskaya, 1968; Hansford, 1978). Cardiac connective tissue components and collagen cross-linkage increase with aging (Engelmann, Vitullo, and Gerrity, 1987; Schabb, 1964; Weisfeldt, Loeven, and Shock, 1971), thus promoting ventricular stiffness and rendering the senescent heart less compliant than that of the young adult (Spurgeon et al., 1977; Werzar, 1969).

The effects of aging on vascular structure have been studied extensively, and comprehensive reviews of these findings were provided by Altura and Altura (1977) and Yin (1980). The structure of the vessel wall is essentially composed of three layers, the intima, media, and adventitia, each containing elastin, collagen, mesenchymal ground substance, smooth muscle, and other cells. Properties of the vasculature are determined by the composition of these components and the geometry of the vascular tree. The aging process affects essentially all properties of the blood vessels, including thickness of the arterial intima, which reduces the diameter of the arterial lumen; calcification and a decrease in inherent extensibility of elastin; and an increase of collagen content as a result of reduced turnover rate. Thus, the aging arteries and veins are generally characterized by a progressive loss of distensibility and an increase in rigidity; indeed, these structural modifications may be in part responsible for the rise of blood pressure as well as the altered responsiveness of vascular smooth muscle cells to vasoactive agents.

The Effects of Aging on Chronotropic and Inotropic Properties of the Myocardium

Small decreases in the heart rate of elderly humans and aged rats have been reported by several investigators (Bonaccorsi, Franco, and Garattini, 1977; Brandfonbrener, Landowne, and Shock, 1955; Fleg et al., 1982; Kostis et al., 1982; Posner et al., 1987; Rodeheffer et al., 1984). The intrinsic sinus rate (determined in the presence of both sympathetic and parasympathetic blockade) is also diminished significantly with advancing age (Jose, 1966). Indeed, one of the most noted characteristics of cardiac muscle obtained from senescent animals is a prolonged duration of isometric contraction relative to that of young adults. In general, the resting membrane potential of the isolated cardiac muscle preparation is unaltered with aging (Capasso et al., 1983; Wei, Spurgeon, and Lakatta, 1984). However, in cardiac tissue obtained from senescent animals, all phases of the transmembrane action potential, which include time to peak force, plateau phase, and relaxation time, are markedly prolonged during isometric contraction (Alpert, Gale, and Taylor, 1967; Froehlich et al., 1978; Lakatta, Gerstenblith, and Angell, 1975; Rumberger and Timmermann, 1976;

Templeton et al., 1978; Wei, Spurgeon, and Lakatta, 1984). The precise mechanism(s) responsible for the increased duration of contraction is unclear, although cardiac hypertrophy is unlikely to be associated with this age-related variation (Korecky, 1979; Spurgeon, Steinbach, and Lakatta, 1983; Wei, Spurgeon, and Lakatta, 1984; Yin et al., 1980). Rather, the changes in action potential are indicative of differences in ionic current flow subsequent to depolarization. The nature of these ionic alterations and their relationship with contractile parameters remain to be established. Nonetheless, Froehlich et al. (1978) and Lakatta (1985) suggested that a reduced rate of Ca^{++} sequestration by the sarcoplasmic reticulum from the myoplasm following an excitation may in part account for the delays in time peak force and electromechanical restitution time during the excitation–contraction cycle.

The inotropic state of cardiac muscle depends on several factors. A change in resting length may result in alteration of force production (Frank-Starling relation). In the rat, aging over the adult range has no appreciable effect on this relationship between length and developed force (Lakatta and Yin, 1982). In addition, the capacity of cardiac muscle to develop peak force in response to a wide range of extracellular calcium concentration does not appear to be impaired by the aging process (Gerstenblith et al., 1979; Lakatta et al., 1975; Spurgeon et al., 1977). These observations suggest that senescence is not likely associated with significant deficits in intrinsic contractile properties of the myofilaments.

Autonomic Modulation of Senescent Heart and Vasculature

A considerable body of evidence has suggested that autonomic nervous system control of cardiovascular function is compromised with aging. Deficits in adrenergic modulation of cardiovascular tissue performance in particular are among the most prominent alterations observed in senescent human and laboratory animals. Thus, physiological stresses such as exercise, hypoxia, and hypercarbia, which stimulate the sympathetic pathway and trigger release of catecholamines, produce less pronounced chronotropic responses in elderly individuals than in young people. These attenuated responses are likely associated with reduced reactivity of the baroreceptor reflex, decrease in cardiac catecholamine store, diminution of adrenergic receptor sensitivity to agonists, as well as deficiency in postsynaptic receptor coupling mechanisms. Comprehensive discussions of this subject have been provided in several recent reviews (Docherty, 1986; Goldberg, Kreider, and Roberts, 1984; Lakatta, 1987b; Roberts and Tumer,

1987); hence, this section covers only the salient features of these findings.

Myocardium

Although no difference in catecholamine storage vesicles could be detected (by histofluorescence technique) between cardiac tissues of 4- and 24-month-old rats (Santer, 1982), ample evidence has indicated significant decreases in norepinephrine content in both atria and ventricles of the senescent rodent (Frolkis et al., 1979; Gey, Burkard, and Pletscher, 1965; Martinez et al., 1981; Rappaport, Young, and Landsberg, 1981; Roberts and Goldberg, 1976; Thompson et al., 1974). The fall of catecholamine content in the aged rat heart appeared to be associated with reduced capacity of storage granules in the noradrenergic nerve terminals (Limas, 1975), as well as axonal degeneration (McLean, Goldberg, and Roberts, 1983). The influences of aging on catecholamine biosynthesis and metabolism are less consistent. Reduction in activities of the catecholamine-biosynthetic enzymes dopa decarboxylase and dopamine β-hydroxylase were reported in aged rat heart (Bender, 1970; Gey, Burkard, and Pletscher, 1965; Inagaki and Tanaka, 1974), although no significant change was detected in ^{14}C-tyrosine incorporation (Limas, 1975). Cardiac monoamine oxidase activity was found to increase with advancing age, but little or no alteration was seen in catechol-O-methyltransferase activity (Frolkis et al., 1979; Prange et al., 1967). Catecholamine release evoked by electrical stimulation of the cardioaccelerator nerve was diminished in senescent rats (Daly et al., 1984); however, the release of norepinephrine induced by tyramine, which acts indirectly by displacing the neurotransmitter from the presynaptic nerve terminals, was not affected by age (Kreider, Goldberg, and Roberts, 1986). Kreider, Goldberg, and Roberts deduced that since tyramine release of norepinephrine was not calcium dependent, the age-related deficiency in neurotransmitter release (*via* direct stimulation) might reflect defects in the calcium-dependent secretion coupling mechanisms in the noradrenergic nerve terminals of the heart.

Numerous studies have documented that cardiac β-adrenoceptor-mediated responses are compromised with aging. In humans, the dose of β-adrenergic agonists (isoproterenol, epinephrine, and norepinephrine) required to achieve an increment of chronotropic response was significantly larger in elderly individuals than in young people, indicating a decline of sensitivity to β-adrenergic stimulation (Bertel et al., 1980; Branconnier, Harto-Traux, and Cole, 1984; Hoffman et al., 1975; van Brummelen et al., 1981; Vestal, Woods, and Shand, 1979). In the rat, positive chronotropic and inotropic responses to isoproterenol and norepinephrine were diminished in the hearts from old rats (22–25 months) compared with those from younger animals (6–12 months) (Amerini et al., 1985; Guarnieri et al., 1980; Kreider, Goldberg, and Roberts, 1984; Lakatta et al., 1975). Although changes in β-adrenergic reactivity are well established in the senescent heart, the molecular basis for these alterations is not completely understood. Receptor binding studies using antagonist radioligands did not indicate any significant changes in β-adrenoceptor affinity or density (Abrass, Davis, and Scarpace, 1982; Fan and Banerjee, 1985; Guarnieri et al., 1980; Narayanan and Derby, 1982a; Scarpace, 1986). On the other hand, Narayanan and Derby (1982a) compared the ability of β-adrenergic agonists to compete for labeled antagonist ligand and showed an age-associated decline of affinity for agonist binding in the rat ventricle. Nonetheless, for the most part, diminution of cardiac responses to β-adrenergic stimulation does not appear to be associated with changes of β-adrenoceptor number or affinity. Alternatively, evidence from several studies has suggested that these age-related subsensitive responses may involve events linked distal to the adrenoceptor. Comparing 7- to 9- with 22- to 25-month-old rats, Guarnieri et al. (1980) showed that maximal contractile responses to isoproterenol and dibutryl cyclic adenosine monophosphate (cAMP) were 40–50 percent less in the cardiac septa of senescent rat, whereas no significant alteration was detectable in the isoproterenol-induced elevation of cAMP level and cAMP-dependent protein kinase activity between the two age groups of animals. In addition, both adult and senescent septa responded similarly to increased extracellular calcium concentration. These investigators surmised that the factors which limit cardiac responses to β-adrenergic stimulation lie distal to protein kinase activation but proximal to the calcium-troponin interaction. Results from several other studies also implicated age-related alterations in the efficiency of the catalytic subunit and the guanine nucleotide regulatory protein component of the adenylate cyclase complex coupled to the cardiac β-adrenoceptor (Fan and Banerjee, 1985; Kusiak and Pitha, 1983; Narayanan and Derby, 1982a; O'Conner, Scarpace, and Abrass, 1981). Thus, the diminished β-adrenergic sensitivity observed in the senescent heart appears to be correlated with deficient postreceptor coupling mechanisms, rather than changes in binding characteristics of the adrenoceptor itself.

Reductions in α_1-adrenoceptor density and α_2-mediated cardioinhibitory responsiveness have been reported in senescent rat heart (Dalrymple, Hamilton, and Reid, 1982; Docherty and Hyland, 1986; Partilla et al., 1982), although Amerini et al. (1985) observed an increase in positive inotropic response to the α-adrenergic agonist phenylephrine in old rats. An explanation to resolve these apparently conflicting results is not yet available and the significance of these age-related α-adrenergic changes in the modulation of cardiac function remains to be determined.

The effects of aging on parasympathetic control of myocardial function have also been investigated. In general, acetylcholine released from the vagus nerve acts on the cardiac muscarinic receptors to exert potent negative chronotropic and inotropic effects, and to attenuate the β-adrenergic influences on cardiac activity. Several studies with human subjects and laboratory animals have provided evidence that indicates that the cardiac responses to cholinergic stimulation are modified with advancing age. The positive chronotropic response resulting from vagotomy or blockade of muscarinic receptors with atropine has been reported to be minimal or absent in elderly humans (Dauchot and Gravenstein, 1971), and aged animals (Kelliher and Conahan, 1980). Indeed, direct stimulation of the vagal nerve and administration of cholinergic agonists also produced a smaller decrease in heart rate in aged rats compared with young adults (Kelliher and Conahan, 1980). In addition, an age-associated decrease in muscarinic-receptor-mediated inhibition of β-adrenergic activation of adenylate cyclase has also been demonstrated in the senescent rat heart (Narayanan and Tucker, 1986). Similar to observations with the β-adrenergic system, the diminished responsiveness of the aged heart to cholinergic stimulation does not appear to involve muscarinic receptor binding properties: The density and affinity of binding sites for muscarinic agonist and antagonist did not change with age (Elfellah, Johns, and Shepherd, 1986; Narayanan and Derby, 1982b). Rather, a significant decline in cholinergic control of the β-adrenergic–adenylate cyclase system at sites distal to the receptor has been proposed (Narayanan and Tucker, 1986).

Vasculature

Results derived from studies on aging and autonomic control of blood vessels have been quite variable (Fleisch, 1980; Fleisch and Hooker, 1976). Conflicting results were obtained from different species, strains, and substrains of laboratory animals, and differential changes were observed between arterial and venous tissues; indeed, even alterations found in one artery might not be identical to those found in another. Hence, cross-examination of multiple vessel types from several animal models is warranted to substantiate any simple generalization about the impact of aging on vascular smooth muscle function and reactivity.

An age-related decline in catecholamine content has been observed in blood vessels (mainly arteries) of the elderly human (Frewin et al., 1971; Gerke, Frewin, and Soltys, 1975; Neubauer and Christensen,

1978; Waterson, Frewin, and Soltys, 1974), rat (Embree et al., 1981; Santer, 1982), and rabbit (Saba et al., 1984). More recently, Duckles and co-workers (Duckles, 1987a; Handa and Duckles, 1987a) reported that with the exception of the superior mesenteric and caudal arteries, all other arteries examined in Fischer 344 rat (which included the renal, femoral, saphenous, superficial epigastric, and popliteal arteries) showed a significant decline in norepinephrine content with advancing age. Similarly, a significant reduction of norepinephrine was found in the tail artery of aging lvanos rats (Fouda and Atkinson, 1986). However, [^{3}H]norepinephrine accumulation, which was used as an index of noradrenergic nerve density, revealed little or no significant age-related differences (Duckles, Carter, and Williams, 1985). It is tempting to attribute these findings to a decline in metabolic activity (neurotransmitter biosynthesis, release, and degradation) of sympathetic neurons innervating the arterial smooth muscle in the senescent rat, rather than alteration of neuronal density per se. Additional studies are needed to clarify this point. On the other hand, the neurotransmitter content and accumulation in the renal, femoral, saphenous, and superior mesenteric veins remained constant at all ages. Hence, aging appears to have a differential impact on the sympathetic innervation of the arterial and venous smooth tissues.

A number of reports have produced conflicting findings on the effects of aging on α-adrenoceptor-mediated vasoconstriction, which suggest either reduced (Elliot et al., 1982; Fouda and Atkinson, 1986; Handa and Duckles, 1987b; Simpkins, Field, and Ress, 1983; Tuttle, 1966) or unaltered (Buhler et al., 1980; Duckles, 1987a, 1987b; Duckles, Carter, and Williams, 1985; Scott and Reid, 1982; Stevens, Lipe, and Moulds, 1982; Stevens and Moulds, 1981) responsiveness at senescence. Possible explanations for this inconsistency perhaps lie in differences among animal species, specific types of vessels examined, and experimental methodologies employed. In a recent study with Fischer 344 rats, Duckles, Carter, and Williams (1985) examined the influence of aging on vascular contractile responses of femoral and renal arteries and veins to norepinephrine and transmural nerve stimulation. In addition, norepinephrine sensitivity was compared between an innervated vessel (femoral artery) and a noninnervated vessel (carotid artery) at various ages. These investigators expressed their data as percentage of maximum contraction (to both potassium chloride and norepinephrine) that each tissue was capable of achieving, thereby rendering it possible to evaluate the adrenergic mechanisms independent of possible changes in blood vessel structure and composition. On the whole, no significant difference with age was found among the blood vessels studied in resting force, maximal contractile responses, or sensitivity to transmural nerve stimulation or exogenous norepinephrine.

Subsequent studies by Hynes and Duckles (1987) and Duckles (1987a, 1987b) confirmed these results. However, in the hindlimb of the same strain of rat (Fischer 344), vasoconstrictor responses to lumbar sympathetic nerve stimulation and intra-arterial administration of norepinephrine, phenylephrine and methoxamine (specific α_1-adrenergic agonist) were significantly diminished in the old animals (Handa and Duckles, 1987b). Similarly, divergent findings were reported when the effects of norepinephrine uptake blockade by cocaine were evaluated at various ages. Indeed, the cocaine-potentiated pressor responses to nerve stimulation or exogenous norepinephrine were attenuated (Docherty and Hyland, 1986), exaggerated (Handa and Duckles, 1987b), or unchanged (Duckles, 1987b) in the senescent rats. Possible factors contributing to these discrepencies remain to be elucidated. Using specific α-adrenergic agonists, Docherty and Hyland (1986) also reported little change in α_1-adrenoceptor-mediated pressor effects in the aged Sprague-Dawley rat, although the pressor and cardioinhibitory effects of the α_2-adrenergic agonist were significantly suppressed in the old animals. It would be interesting to determine if some of the conflicting findings described above might be attributable to differential impacts of aging on vascular α-adrenoceptor subtypes.

In humans, rats, and rabbits, there is a general agreement that sensitivity of β-adrenoceptor-mediated relaxation of arterial smooth muscle declines with advancing age, whereas that of the venous smooth muscle is well maintained through senescence (Duckles, and Hurlburt, 1985; Fleisch and Hooker, 1976; O'Donnell and Wanstall, 1983; Pan et al., 1986; Tsujimoto, Lee, and Hoffman, 1986). Furthermore, Strozzi et al. (1973) reported that vasodilation produced by metaproterenol, a β-adrenergic agonist, decreased with increasing age in human. Relaxation of the rat aorta induced by nitroglycerin did not change with advancing age, suggesting that the apparent effects of aging on the arterial vessels were not likely associated with alterations of aortic contractile tension (Fleisch and Hooker, 1976; Tsujimoto, Lee, and Hoffman, 1986). Tsujimoto, Lee, and Hoffman (1986) explored the mechanisms underlying these age-related alterations and reported that the loss in responsiveness of the mesenteric arteries to isoproterenol was not accompanied by any change in β-adrenoceptor number of binding affinity in these vessels. Instead, deficiencies at postreceptor loci such as cAMP accumulation and cAMP-dependent protein kinase activation might be involved in the reduced adrenergic responses. By comparing different arterial vessels (rat aorta and pulmonary artery), O'Donnell and Wanstall (1983) postulated that aging might affect β_2-

more than β_1-adrenoceptor-mediated responses, although Duckles and Hurlbert (1985) indicated that this hypothesis might not hold true with venous smooth muscle. Nonetheless, it remains to be determined whether this "receptor subtype" generalization might be applicable exclusively to arterial smooth muscle.

By and large, cholinergic control of vascular function does not appear to be modified at senescence. Kelliher and Conahan (1980) demonstrated that the response of muscarinic receptor in the peripheral vasculature was not altered by the aging process. Likewise, Tsujimoto, Lee, and Hoffman (1986) showed that the relaxation responses evoked by acetylcholine in rat mesenteric arteries were similar between 5- to 6-week-old and 10- to 12-month-old rats. These results were substantiated by Hynes and Duckles (1987), who extended the investigation to 20 months. In addition, although sensitivity of the endothelium to cholinergic stimulation appeared to increase with age in the aorta and caudal artery, these changes occurred primarily during growth and development rather than at old age.

Baroreceptor Reflex

A decline in baroreceptor sensitivity is generally observed with advanced age. Reflex bradycardic responses to phenylephrine-induced rise of blood pressure were smaller in elderly human subjects and rats than in their young adult counterparts (Gribbin et al., 1971; Rothbaum et al., 1974). Shimada et al. (1985, 1986) examined the cardiovascular responses to the Valsalva maneuver and concluded that the sympathetic vasoregulation and the baroreflex control of heart rate in the maneuver were impaired with advancing age. Indeed, Rowe and Troen (1980) postulated that reduction of baroreceptor sensitivity might be responsible for the age-related increases in plasma norepinephrine concentration and blood pressure.

Aging and Cardiovascular Pharmacology and Toxicology

It is well established that pharmacological action of drugs and xenobiotic compounds as well as their toxicity can be altered with age. Changes of pharmacokinetic factors (which include absorption, distribution, biotransformation, and elimination of a substance) in an elderly subject certainly may contribute to a different profile of bioavailability of an agent. A comprehensive discussion of this topic has been presented elsewhere in this volume. In addition, possible changes in sensitivity of the effector organ to drugs and chemicals per se may also play a role in these age-related alterations. For the cardiovascular system, although structural and functional changes have been noted in elderly humans and senescent laboratory animals, the influence of aging on reactivity of the myocardium and vasculature to drugs and xenobiotic chemicals has not come under vigorous investigation. A brief overview of information currently available is provided in this section.

It has long been recognized that tolerance to cardiac glycosides decreases with advanced age in both humans (Ewy et al., 1969; Irons and Orgain, 1966; Raisbeck, 1952; Schneider and Ruiz-Torres, 1978) and in experimental animals (Gerstenblith et al., 1979; Guarnieri et al., 1979; Hewett, Vulliemoz, and Rosen, 1982; Katano et al., 1984, 1985; Wollenberger, Jehl, and Karsh, 1953; also see review by Goldberg and Roberts, 1980). Clinically, ample evidence has shown that elderly patients are particularly prone to the toxic manifestations of digitalis therapy (Goldberg and Roberts, 1980). In addition, the toxic reactions observed in elderly people are subtly different from those seen in the average younger patient (Bender, 1964; Friend, 1961). Several factors may contribute to the enhanced toxicity of digitalis; these include compromised renal function, hypokalemia or other cation imbalance, altered thyroid status, and chronic cardiac and pulmonary diseases coexisting in the elderly patients (Doherty, 1968). Because digitalis is eliminated primarily by the kidney, reduced or impaired renal function due to aging would adversely increase circulating levels of the drug and prolong the duration of its action. On the other hand, although deficiencies of potassium and magnesium as well as high calcium levels are found to be linked to increased digitalis toxicity, there is no evidence to suggest that levels of these ions change with age; nor is there conclusive evidence to demonstrate that these alterations are involved directly in the increased drug toxicity.

Age-related changes of sensitivity to cardiac glycosides have also been reported in several animal studies. Dearing, Barnes, and Essex (1943) reported that digitalis was more likely to produce myocardial lesions in senescent cats than in younger ones. Chen and Robbins (1944a) showed that old rabbits (3–5 years of age) were more susceptible to ouabain-induced toxicity than were young adults (3–24 months of age). These findings were confirmed by Toda (1981). In the guinea pig, Wollenberger, Jehl, and Karsh (1953) found a decrease of tolerance to the toxic effects of ouabain as the animals reached adulthood. On the other hand, Guarnieri et al. (1979) reported that the toxicity of a rapid-acting cardiac glycoside, acetylstrophanthidin, remained unchanged in senescent beagle dogs, although the inotropic effect of the drug was significantly reduced. Similarly, using isolated ventricle trabeculae of Wistar rats, Gerstenblith et al. (1979) observed diminished inotropic responsiveness to ouabain in the aged animals (24 months), while Hewett, Vulliemoz, and Rosen (1982) also demonstrated greater responsiveness to the toxic effects of ouabain in Purkinje fibers from senescent canine hearts. The precise mechanisms responsible for these age-associated changes are not certain. The inotropic effect of the glycoside is dependent on transmembrane movements of potassium and sodium ions, which in turn are regulated by Na-K-activated ATPase (sodium pump) (Schwartz, Lindenmayer, and Allen, 1975). A number of studies (Akera, 1977; Hokin et al., 1973; Kyte, 1974; Lane et al., 1973) have shown that the sodium pump is associated with a receptor for glycoside. Thus, changes in the sodium pump and/or the glycoside receptor in the myocardium of aged animals may, in part, account for the altered sensitivity to digitalis. Indeed, Katano et al. (1984, 1985) reported lower Na-K-ATPase activity and fewer high-affinity ouabain binding sites in aged rat myocardium. These investigators postulated that these biochemical changes might be responsible for the senescent heart's reduced tolerance to the arrhythmogenic actions of digitalis. Alternatively, because sodium efflux is thought to be coupled to calcium influx, Goldberg and Roberts (1980) also proposed the possibility that age-related changes in the intracellular handling of calcium may be involved in alteration of cardiac glycoside action and toxicity. In addition, it should be noted that the cardiotoxic effects of digitalis may be mediated indirectly through actions of the drug on the autonomic nervous system (Gillis et al., 1972). Results from several studies suggest that cardiac glycosides might act on the sympathetic pathways, causing release of catecholamines to potentiate development of cardiac rhythm disturbances (Kelliher and Roberts, 1974; Roberts and Kelliher, 1972; Roberts, Kelliher, and Lathers, 1976; Roberts and Modell, 1961). Thus, changes in these neural functions with advanced age may also play a role in the altered reactivity of cardiac glycosides.

Clinical studies have shown that disorders of cardiac rhythm are common among elderly patients (Burch and DePasquale, 1969). Although there is little direct evidence to indicate that antiarrhythmic drugs may produce an altered profile of reactivity and toxicity in senescent subjects, cautions have been issued in the literature regarding the use of these agents (DeGroff, 1974). Because of the lipid solubility and plasma-protein-binding capacity of some of the antiarrhythmic drugs (e.g., lidocaine and phenytoin), potential changes in therapeutic sensitivity should be anticipated due to altered pharmacokinetic parameters in elderly patients. In the rat, Goldberg and Roberts (1975) and Goldberg, Cavato, and Roberts (1975) reported that the depressive effect of quinidine on atrial and ventricular pacemakers diminished with advancing age. Lidocaine had a similar effect on the ventricle with respect to aging; however, in the atria, the ability of lidocaine to decrease pacemaker activity appeared to be enhanced in the old animals. The cellular mechanisms to account for these paradoxical findings are yet to be clarified, although these investigators suggested alterations of drug–receptor interaction and/or transmembrane cation movements.

Because of changes in autonomic modulation of cardiovascular function in senescent human and laboratory animals, the impact of aging on reactivity of autonomic drugs has been studied extensively. Some of the findings involving sympathomimetics, parasympathomimetics, and their antagonists have been discussed in the previous section, and a brief review was also provided by Goldberg and Roberts (1980). Broadly speaking, sensitivity of the heart and vasculature to autonomic agents diminishes with senescence, although it should be noted that evidence currently available is by no means conclusive or uniformly agreeable. Several factors such as specific properties of the drugs tested, differential responses from various tissues examined, and animal species and strain differences may, in part, contribute to the conflicting results found in the literature. By comparison, the effects of aging on cardiotoxicity of autonomic drugs have received less attention, and studies in this area are fragmented. The LD_{50} of epinephrine decreased significantly with advancing age in mice (Frolkis, 1965), whereas that of ephedrine in rats decreased between 4 and 12 months of age, but increased somewhat by 24 months (Chen and Robbins, 1944b). The cardiotoxicity of the tricyclic antidepressant nortriptyline (which blocks reuptake of norepinephrine) appeared to be enhanced in the 24-month-old rats (compared with that of 7-week-old rats); however, these effects were primarily produced by a higher plasma concentration of the drug in the old animals (Bonaccorsi, Franco, and Garattini, 1977). Guideri et al. (1987) reported that the arrhythmogenic potential of isoproterenol increased markedly between 1–2 months and 10–12 months in rats, but remained relatively unchanged thereafter (up to 19–21 months). Thus, better focused investigation in this aspect of research is required in the future.

It is generally viewed that the aging process is accompanied by alterations of hormonal responses (Roth, 1979). Although the ability of thyroid hormones to evoke cardiac hypertrophy and adrenergic hyperreactivity has been well documented in developing and young adult animals, the impact of these hormones on the aging cardiovascular system has drawn considerably less attention. Florini, Saito, and Manowitz (1973) showed that thyroxine stimulated protein synthesis and induced cardiac hypertrophy to the same maximal levels in both young and old mice, although the time required to achieve these effects was prolonged in the aged animals. Similar findings of thyroxine-induced cardiac hypertrophy in mature (9–13 months) and senescent (22–24 months) rats were reported by Zitnik and Roth (1981). In addition, these authors also observed that thyroxine increased β-adrenoceptor binding (to [^{3}H]-dihydroalprenolol) to the same extent in both mature and senescent hearts. These data were confirmed subsequently by Tsujimoto, Hashimoto, and Hoffman (1987), who examined the effects of a different thyroid hormone (triiodothyronine, or T_3) and employed a different β-adrenoceptor ligand ([^{125}I]-cyanopindolol). On the other hand, the hemodynamic consequences of T_3 treatment were less prominent in the aged hyperthyroid rats compared with young hyperthyroid animals. The ability of isoproterenol to relax mesenteric arterial rings was markedly reduced in the old euthyroid rats; this deficit was partially restored by T_3 treatment. This effect of T_3 appeared to be unique to the older rats, because the hormone did not affect the isoproterenol-mediated relaxation in the arterial preparations from the young animals. These investigators concluded that the effects of thyroid hormones and age-related alterations of cardiovascular responsiveness to β-adrenergic stimulation might be interrelated in a complex fashion with a net attentuation of thyroid action in the older animals. In contrast to the findings with cardiac β-adrenoceptor, there was an age-related decrease in the number of myocardial $α_1$-adrenoceptor sites in the euthyroid rats. T_3 reduced the $α_1$-receptors in both young and old hearts, although the magnitude of reduction was diminished in the older animals (Tsujimoto and Hashimoto, 1987). However, it is noteworthy that in these two studies, 2-month-old rats were compared with 12-month-old animals. Thus, results observed may reflect maturational changes rather than alterations associated with senescence.

Although the impact of aging on cardiovascular reactivity to pharmacological agents has drawn considerable interest, only a few studies have focused on the interactions of aging and cardiotoxic effects of drugs of abuse (such as nicotine, alcohol and narcotics) and environmental toxic substances. Because long-term ethanol ingestion has been linked to development of cardiomyopathy and dysrhythmias (Bashour, Fahdul, and Cheng, 1975; Ferrans et al., 1965; Regan et al., 1977), several researchers have postulated that chronic alcohol intake at senescence might potentiate the age-related decline of cardiovascular functions. Morvai and Ungvary (1979) showed that chronic exposure to alcohol produced a greater fall of blood pressure and a more pronounced cardiac hypertrophy in aged rats than in their young cohorts. Posner et al. (1987) reported a decrease of heart rate and an increased incidence of arrhythmias in senescent rats, with chronic ethanol ingestion exacerbating these parameters. In addition, ethanol also reduced the basal tension of isolated atria of aged rats, as well as their inotropic responses to isoproterenol and calcium. It is of particular interest that the negative chronotropic and inotropic effects of ethanol were seen only in the senescent animals. These results prompted the authors to conclude that the aged heart was more vulnerable to the pathogenic effects of chronic alcohol consumption.

Several studies have also examined the effects of environmental agents on the aged heart. Kopp et al. (1983) evaluated the cardiovascular changes following chronic administration of low-level cadmium in the diet. Hypertension was evident in the cadmium-exposed rats 2 months after the commencement of treatment at postweaning age. The elevation of blood pressure persisted throughout the examination period (up to 18 months of age) but did not deviate appreciably with advancing age. Although heart rate in the cadmium-exposed rats did not differ from that of control, a reduction of cardiac contractile tension was observed in the treated animals at 18 months. Addition of lead to the cadmium-containing diet did not alter the changes produced by cadmium alone. These results suggest that chronic exposure to heavy metals approximating environmental levels may adversely affect cardiovascular function, although the issue of whether the senescent heart and vasculature are particularly vulnerable to these toxic effects remains to be addressed systemically. Watkinson (1985, 1986) also described the cardiotoxic effects of a formamidine pesticide, chlordimeform, in both geriatric and postweaning rats. Acute administration of the pesticide produced abrupt decreases of heart rate and blood pressure in both age groups, although the younger animals appeared to be more resistant to the toxic actions. However, it is unclear whether the differences seen between these two age groups reflect maturational changes or alterations due to senescence.

Concluding Remarks

From the preceding discussion, it is apparent that several aspects of the cardiovascular system are affected by the aging process. In general, minor structural changes are detectable in the heart and blood vessels of elderly humans and laboratory animals, although the overall resting function of the senescent cardiovascular system appears to be within the normal range for the young adult. However, autonomic control of cardiovascular function and cardiac responsivity to a variety of drugs and chemical compounds are profoundly compromised in aged individuals. Broadly speaking, cardiac β-adrenergic and muscarinic, vascular β- and α_2-adrenergic responses are attenuated with advancing age. Likewise, baroreflex sensitivity is also reduced. It should be noted that evidence supporting these findings is by no means definitive or even consistent in some cases. Considerable effort must be directed toward resolving the conflicting results currently found in the literature before general principles characterizing the aging cardiovascular system can be elaborated. Moreover, although central nervous system control of cardiovascular function has been under extensive investigation, possible interactions between this mode of control and aging have not been examined. In view of the well-documented age-related changes in the brain (e.g., senile dementia) and neurotoxic potentials of drugs and environmental substances, future research in this area may prove to be fruitful.

The effects of a few pharmacological agents and environmental toxic substances on the senescent myocardium are summarized in this review; however, our understanding of the interactions between aging and drug action/toxicity in the cardiovascular systems is strikingly lacking. Age-related changes in cellular mechanisms in the heart and blood vessels (such as drug–receptor interactions) as well as alterations of pharmacokinetic parameters may modify the therapeutic and/ or adverse effects of an agent significantly in the elderly patients. Thus, investigation of these potential deviations of drug actions in relation to aging becomes paramount in geriatric medicine. In addition, because of the ever-growing list of hazardous substances polluting our environment, the issue of whether the cardiotoxic potentials of these compounds might be enhanced in elderly individuals must be addressed in a more systematic fashion than what is presently available in the literature.

References

Abrass, I. B., Davis, J. L., and Scarpace, P. J. 1982. Isoproterenol responsiveness and myocardial beta adrenergic receptors in young and old rats. *Journal of Gerontology* 37:156–160.

Abu-Erreish, G. M., Neely, J. R., Whitmer, J. T., Whitman, V., and Sanadi, D. R. 1977. Fatty acid oxidation by isolated perfused working hearts of aged rats. *American Journal of Physiology* 232:E258–E262.

Akera, T. 1977. Membrane adenosine triphosphatase: A digitalis receptor? *Science* 198:569–574.

Alpert, N. R., Gale, H. H., and Taylor, N. 1967. The effect of age on contractile protein ATPase activity and the velocity of shortening. In Kavaler, K., Tanz, R. D., and Roberts, J. (Eds.), *Factors Influencing Myocardial Contractility*. New York, Academic Press, pp. 127–133.

Altura, B. M., and Altura, B. T. 1977. Some physiological factors in vascular reactivity. I. Aging in vascular smooth muscle and its influence on reactivity. In Carrier, O., and Shibata, S. (Eds.), *Factors Influencing Vascular Reactivity*. New York, Igaku-Shoin, pp. 169–188.

Amerini, S., Fusi, F., Piazzesi, G., Mantelli, L., Ledda, F., and Mugelli, A. 1985. Influences of age on the positive inotropic effect mediated by alpha-

and beta-adrenoceptors in rat ventricular strips. *Developmental Pharmacology and Therapeutics* 8:34–42.

Bashour, T. T., Fahdul, H., and Cheng, T. O. 1975. Electrocardiographic abnormalities in alcohol cardiomyopathy. A study of 65 patients. *Chest* 68:24–27.

Bender, A. D. 1964. Pharmacologic aspects of aging: A survey of the effect of increasing age on drug activity in adults. *Journal of the American Geriatrics Society* 12:114–134.

Bender, A. D. 1970. The influence of age on the activity of catecholamines and related therapeutic agents. *Journal of the American Geriatrics Society* 18:220–232.

Bertel, O., Buhler, F. R., Kiowski, W., and Lutold, B. E. 1980. Decreased beta-adrenoceptor responsiveness as related to age, blood pressure and plasma catecholamines in patients with essential hypertension. *Hypertension* 2:130–138.

Beyer, R. E., and Starnes, J. W. 1985. Coenzyme Q and myocardial function in aging and exercise. In Stone, H. L., and Weglicki, W. B. (Eds.), *Pathobiology of Cardiovascular Injury*. Boston, Martinus Nijhoff, pp. 489–511.

Bonaccorsi, A., Franco, R., and Garattini, S. 1977. Plasma nortriptyline and cardiac responses in young and old rats. *British Journal of Pharmacology* 60:21–27.

Branconnier, R. J., Harto-Traux, N. E., and Cole, J. O. 1984. The effect of aging on the positive chronotropic response to amitriptyline. *Psychopharmacology* 82:256–257.

Brandfonbrener, M., Landowne, M., and Shock, N. W. 1955. Changes of cardiac output with age. *Circulation* 12:557–566.

Buhler, F. R., Kiowski, W., van Brummelen, P., Amann, F. W., Bertel, O., Landmann, R., Lutold, B. E., and Bolli, P. 1980. Plasma catecholamines and cardiac, renal and peripheral vascular adrenoceptor mediated responses in different age groups in normal and hypertensive subjects. *Clinical and Experimental Hypertension* 2:409–426.

Burch, G. E., and DePasquale, N. P. 1969. Geriatric cardiology. *American Heart Journal* 78:700–708.

Capasso, J. M., Malhotra, A., Remily, R. M., Scheuer, J., and Sonnenblick, E. H. 1983. Effects of age on mechanical and electrical performance of rat myocardium. *American Journal of Physiology* 245:H72–H81.

Chen, K. K., and Robbins, E. B. 1944a. Influence of age of rabbits on the toxicity of ouabain. *Journal of the American Pharmacology Association* 33:61–62.

Chen, K. K., and Robbins, E. B. 1944b. Age of animals and drug action. *Journal of the American Pharmacology Association* 33:80–82.

Chen, J. C., Warshaw, J. B., and Sanadi, D. R. 1972. Regulation of mitochondrial respiration in senescence. *Journal of Cellular Physiology* 226:1293–1297.

Dalrymple, H. W., Hamilton, C. A., and Reid, J. L. 1982. The effect of age on peripheral α-adrenoreceptors in vivo and in vitro in the rabbit (abstract). *British Journal of Pharmacology* 77:322P.

Daly, R. N., Kreider, M. S., Goldberg, P. B., and Roberts, J. 1984. Changes in heart rate (HR) and norepinephrine (NE) outflow in response to electrical stimulation of the cardioaccelerator nerve in the rat as a function of age (abstract). *Pharmacologist* 26:175.

Dauchot, P., and Gravenstein, J. S. 1971. Effect of atropine on the electrocardiogram in different age groups. *Clinical Pharmacology and Therapeutics* 12:274–280.

Dearing, W. H., Barnes, A. R., and Essex, H. E. 1943. Experiments with calculated therapeutic and toxic doses of digitalis: Effects on the myocardial cellular structure. *American Heart Journal* 25:648–664.

DeGroff, A. C. 1974. Drug therapy of cardiovascular disease. *Geriatrics* 29:51–54.

Docherty, J. R. 1986. Aging and the cardiovascular system. *Journal of Autonomic Pharmacology* 6:77–84.

Docherty, J. R., and Hyland, L. 1986. α-adrenoceptor responsiveness in the aged rat. *European Journal of Pharmacology* 126:75–80.

Doherty, J. E. 1968. The clinical pharmacology of digitalis glycosides. A review. *American Journal of the Medical Sciences* 255:382–414.

Duckles, S. P. 1987a. Influence of age on vascular adrenergic responsiveness. *Blood Vessels* 24:113–116.

Duckles, S. P. 1987b. Effect of norepinephrine uptake blockade on contractile responses to adrenergic nerve stimulation of isolated rat blood vessels: Influence of age. *Journal of Pharmacology and Experimental Therapeutics* 243:521–526.

Duckles, S. P., Carter, B. J., and Williams, C. L. 1985. Vascular adrenergic neuroeffector function does not decline in aged rats. *Circulation Research* 56:109–116.

Duckles, S. P., and Hurlbert, J. S. 1985. Effect of age on beta adrenergic relaxation of the rat jugular vein. *Journal of Pharmacology and Experimental Therapeutics* 236:71–74.

Elfellah, M. S., Johns, A., and Shepherd, A. M. M. 1986. Effect of age on responsiveness of isolated rat atria to carbachol and on binding characteristics of atrial muscarinic receptors. *Journal of Cardiovascular Pharmacology* 8:873–877.

Elliott, H. L., Sumner, D. J., McLean, K., and Reid, J. L. 1982. Effect of age on the responsiveness of vascular alpha adrenoceptors in man. *Journal of Cardiovascular Pharmacology* 4:477–487.

Embree, L. J., Roubein, I. F., Jackson, D. W., and Ordway, F. 1981. Aging effect on the noradrenaline content of rat brain microvessels. *Experimental Aging Research* 7:215–224.

Engelmann, G. L., Vitullo, J. C., and Gerrity, R. G. 1987. Morphometric analysis of cardiac hypertrophy during development, maturation and senescence in spontaneously hypertensive rats. *Circulation Research* 60:487–494.

Ewy, G. A., Kapadia, G. G., Yao, L., Lullin, M., and Marcus, F. I. 1969. Digoxin metabolism in the elderly. *Circulation* 39:449–453.

Fan, T. H. M., and Banerjee, S. P. 1985. Age-related reduction of beta-adrenoceptor sensitivity in rat heart occurs by multiple mechanisms. *Gerontology* 31:373–380.

Ferrans, V. J., Hibbs, R. G., Weilbascher, D. G., Black, J., Walsh, J., and Burch, G. E. 1965. Alcoholic cardiomyopathy. A histochemical study. *American Heart Journal* 69:748–765.

Fleg, J. L. 1986. Alterations in cardiovascular structure and function with advancing age. *American Journal of Cardiology* 57:33C–44C.

Fleg, J. L., Rodeheffer, R. J., Gerstenblith, G., Becker, L. C., Weisfeldt, M. L., and Lakatta, E. G. 1982. Cardiac output does not decline with age in healthy, fit subjects (abstract). *Circulation* 66(Part II):185.

Fleisch, J. H. 1980. Age-related changes in the sensitivity of blood vessels to drugs. *Pharmacology and Therapeutics* 8:477–487.

Fleisch, J. H., and Hooker, C. S. 1976. The relationship between age and relaxation of vascular smooth muscle in the rabbit and rat. *Circulation Research* 38:243–249.

Florini, J. R., Saito, Y., and Manowitz, E. J. 1973. Effect of age on thyroxine induced cardiac hypertrophy in mice. *Journal of Gerontology* 28:151–162.

Fouda, A. K., and Atkinson, J. 1986. Sensitivity to noradrenaline and electrical stimulation decreases with age in the rat tail artery. *Naunyn-Schmiedebergs Archives of Pharmacology* 334:37–39.

Frenzel, H., and Feimann, J. 1984. Age-dependent changes in the myocardium of rats. A quantitative light- and electron-microscopic study on the right and left chamber wall. *Mechanisms of Ageing and Development* 27:29–41.

Frewin, D. B., Hume, W. R., Waterson, J. G., and Whelan, R. F. 1971. The histochemical localization of sympathetic nerve endings in human gingival blood vessels. *Australian Journal of Experimental Biology and Medical Sciences* 49:573–580.

Friend, D. 1961. Drug therapy and the geriatric patient. *Journal of Pharmacology and Experimental Therapeutics* 2:832–836.

Froehlich, J. P., Lakatta, E. G., Beard, E., Spurgeon, H. A., Weisfeldt, M. L., and Gerstenblith, G. 1978. Studies of sarcoplasmic reticulum function and contraction duration in young adult and aged rat myocardium. *Journal of Molecular and Cellular Cardiology* 10:427–438.

Frolkis, V. V. 1965. The sensitivity to and the endurance of pharmacological substances in aging of the organism. *Farmakologiya i Toksikologiya* 28:612–616.

Frolkis, V. V., and Bogatskaya, L. N. 1968. The energy metabolism of myocardium and its regulation in animals of various ages. *Experimental Gerontology* 3:199–210.

Frolkis, V. V., Shevtchuk, V. G., Verkhrastsky, N. S., Stupina, A. S., Karpova, S. M., and Lakiza, T. Y. 1979. Mechanisms of neurohumoral regulation of heart function in aging. *Experimental Aging Research* 5:441–477.

Gardin, J. M., Henry, W. L., Savage, D. D., Ware, J. H., Burn, C., and Borer J. S. 1979. Echocardiographic measurements in normal subjects evaluation of an adult population without clinically apparent heart disease. *Journal of Clinical Ultrasound* 7:439–447.

Gerke, D. C., Frewin, D. B., and Soltys, J. S. 1975. Adrenergic innervation of human mesenteric blood vessels. *Australian Journal of Experimental Biology and Medical Sciences* 53:241–243.

Gerstenblith, G., Frederiksen, J., Yin, F. C. P., Fortuin, N. J., Lakatta, E. G., and Weisfeldt, M. L. 1977. Echocardiographic assessment of a normal adult aging population. *Circulation* 56:273–278.

Gerstenblith, G., Spurgeon, H. A., Froehlich, J. P., Weisfeldt, M. L., and Lakatta, E. G. 1979. Diminished inotropic responsiveness to ouabain in aged rat myocardium. *Circulation Research* 44:517–523.

Gey, K. F., Burkard, W. P., and Pletscher, A. 1965. Variation of the norepinephrine metabolism of the rat heart with age. *Gerontologia* 11:1–11.

Gillis, R. A., Raines, A., Sohn, Y. J., Levitt, B., and Stranaert, G. 1972. Neuroexcitatory effects of digitalis and their role in the development of cardiac arrhythmias. *Journal of Pharmacology and Experimental Therapeutics* 183:154–168.

Goldberg, P. B., Cavato, F. V., and Roberts, J. 1975. Alterations in reactivity to antiarrhythmic agents produced by age (abstract). *Clinical Research* 23:185.

Goldberg, P. B., and Roberts, J. 1975. Age effects on atrial and ventricular sensitivity to quinidine and lidocaine (abstract). *Gerontologist* 15:1124.

Goldberg, P. B., and Roberts, J. 1976. Influence of age on the pharmacology and physiology of the cardiovascular system. In Elias, M. F., Eleftheriou, B. F., and Elias, P. K. (Eds.), *Special Review of Experimental Aging Research: Progress in Biology*. Bar Harbor, Maine, Experimental Aging Research, pp. 71–103.

Goldberg, P. B., and Roberts, J. 1980. Pharmacology. In Weisfeldt, M. L. (Ed.), *The Aging Heart*. New York, Raven Press, pp. 215–246.

Goldberg, P. B., Kreider, M. S., and Roberts, J. 1984. Effects of age on the adrenergic cardiac neuroeffector junction. *Life Sciences* 35:2585–2591.

Gribbin, B., Pickering, T. G., Sleight, P., and Peto, R. 1971. Effect of age and high blood pressure on baroreflex sensitivity in man. *Circulation Research* 29:424–431.

Guarnieri, T., Filburn, C. R., Zitnik, G., Roth, G. S., and Lakatta, E. G. 1980. Contractile and biochemical correlates of β-adrenergic stimulation of the aged heart. *American Journal of Physiology* 239:H501–H508.

Guarnieri, T., Spurgeon, H., Froehlich, J. P., Weisfeldt, M. L., and Lakatta, E. G. 1979. Diminished inotropic response but unaltered toxicity to acetylstrophanthidin in the senescent beagle. *Circulation* 60:1548–1554.

Guideri, G., Olivetti, G., Hiler, B., Ricci, R., and Anversa, P. 1987. Increased incidence of isoproterenol-induced ventricular fibrillation in aging rats. *Canadian Journal of Physiology and Pharmacology* 65:504–508.

Handa, R. K., and Duckles, S. P. 1987a. Influence of age on norepinephrine content in arteries and veins of Fischer 344 rats. *Neurobiology of Aging* 8:511–516.

Handa, R. K., and Duckles, S. P. 1987b. Age-related changes in adrenergic vasoconstrictor responses of the rat hindlimb. *American Journal of Physiology* 253:H1566–H1572.

Hansford, R. G. 1978. Lipid oxidation by heart mitochondria from young adult and senescent rats. *Biochemical Journal* 170:285–295.

Hewett, K., Vulliemoz, Y., and Rosen, M. R. 1982. Senescence-related changes in the responsiveness to ouabain of canine purkinje fibers. *Journal of Pharmacology and Experimental Therapeutics* 223:153–156.

Hoffman, V. H., Kiesewetter, R., Krohs, G., and Schmitz, E. 1975. Dependence on age of the effects of catecholamines in man. I. Effect of noradrenaline, adrenaline and isoprenaline on blood pressure and heart rate. *Zeitschrift fur die Gesamte Innere Medizin* 30:89.

Hokin, L. E., Dahl, J. L., Deupree, J. D., Dixon, J. F., Hackney, J. F., and Perdue, J. F. 1973. Studies on the characterization of the sodium–potassium transport adenosine triphosphatase. *Journal of Biological Chemistry* 248: 2593–2605.

Hynes, M. R., and Duckles, S. P. 1987. Effect of increasing age on the endothelium-mediated relaxation of rat blood vessels in vitro. *Journal of Pharmacology and Experimental Therapeutics* 241:387–392.

Inagaki, C., and Tanaka, C. 1974. Neonatal and senescent changes in *l*-aromatic amino acid decarboxylase and monoamine oxidase activities in kidney, liver, brain and heart of the rat. *Japanese Journal of Pharmacology* 24:439.

Irons, G. V., and Orgain, E. S. 1966. Digitalis-induced arrhythmias and their management. *Progress in Cardiovascular Diseases* 8:539–569.

Jose, A. D. 1966. Effect of combined sympathetic and parasympathetic blockade on heart rate and cardiac function in man. *American Journal of Cardiology* 18:476–478.

Kannel, W. B., Gordon, T., and Offutt, D. 1969. Left ventricular hypertrophy by electrocardiogram. Prevalence, incidence, and mortality in the Framingham study. *Annals of Internal Medicine* 71:89–105.

Katano, Y., Akera, T., Temma, K., and Kennedy, R. H. 1984. Enhanced ouabain sensitivity of the heart and myocardial sodium pump in aged rats. *European Journal of Pharmacology* 105:95–103.

Katano, Y., Kennedy, R. H., Stemmer, P. M., Temma, K., and Akera, T. 1985. Aging and digitalis sensitivity of cardiac muscle in rats. *European Journal of Pharmacology* 113:167–178.

Kelliher, G. J., and Conahan, S. T. 1980. Changes in vagal activity and response to muscarinic receptor agonist with age. *Journal of Gerontology* 35:842–849.

Kelliher, G. J., and Roberts, J. 1974. A study of the antiarrhythmic action of certain beta-blocking agents. *American Heart Journal* 87:458–467.

Kopp, S. J., Perry, H. M., Perry, E. F., and Erlanger, M. 1983. Cardiac physiologic and tissue metabolic changes following chronic low-level cadmium and cadmium plus lead ingestion in the rat. *Toxicology and Applied Pharmacology* 69:149–160.

Korecky, B. 1979. The effects of lead, internal environment, and age on cardiac mechanics. *Journal of Molecular and Cellular Cardiology* 11:33, suppl. 1.

Kostis, J. B., Moreyra, A. E., Amendo, M. T., Di Pietro, J., Cosgrove, N., and Kuo, P. T. 1982. The effect of age on heart rate in subjects free of heart disease. *Circulation* 65:141–145.

Kreider, M. S., Goldberg, P. B., and Roberts, J. 1984. Effects of age in adrenergic neuronal uptake in rat heart. *Journal of Pharmacology and Experimental Therapeutics* 231:367–372.

Kreider, M., Goldberg, P., and Roberts, J. 1986. The effect of age on the tyramine-sensitive intraneuronal pool of norepinephrine in rat heart. *Journal of Cardiovascular Pharmacology* 8:137–143.

Kusiak, J. W., and Pitha, J. 1983. Decreased response with age of the cardiac catecholamine sensitive adenylate cyclase system. *Life Sciences* 33: 1679–1686.

Kyte, J. 1974. The reaction of sodium and potassium ion-activated adenosine triphosphatase with specific antibodies. Implications for the mechanism of active transport. *Journal of Biological Chemistry* 249:3652–3660.

Lakatta, E. G. 1985. Heart and circulation. In Finch, C. E., and Schneider, E. L. (Eds.), *Handbook of the Biology of Aging*. New York, Van Nostrand Reinhold, pp. 377–413.

Lakatta, E. G. 1987a. Cardiac muscle changes in senescence. *Annual Review of Physiology* 49:519–531.

Lakatta, E. G. 1987b. Catecholamines and cardiovascular function in aging. *Endocrinology and Aging* 16:877–891.

Lakatta, E. G. 1987c. Do hypertension and aging have a similar effect on the myocardium? *Circulation* 75 (Suppl. I):169–177.

Lakatta, E. G., Gerstenblith, G., and Angell, C. S. 1975. Prolonged contraction duration in aged myocardium. *Journal of Clinical Investigation* 55: 61–68.

Lakatta, E. G., Gerstenblith, G., Angell, C. S., Shock, N. W., and Weisfeldt, M. L. 1975. Diminished inotropic response of aged myocardium to catecholamines. *Circulation Research* 36:262–269.

Lakatta, E. G., and Yin, F. C. P. 1982. Myocardial aging: Functional alterations and related cellular mechanisms. *American Journal of Physiology* 242:H927–H941.

Lane, L. K., Copenhaver, J. H., Lindenmayer, G. E., and Schwartz, A. 1973. Purification and characterization of a ^3H ouabain binding to transport adenosine triphosphatase from outer medulla of canine kidney. *Journal of Biological Chemistry* 248:7197–7200.

Limas, C. J. 1975. Comparison of the handling of norepinephrine in the myocardium of adult and old rats. *Cardiovascular Research* 9:664–668.

Linzbach, A. J., and Akuamoa-Boateng, E. 1973. Alternsversanderunger des menschlichen Herzens. I. Das Herzgewicht in Alter. *Klinische Wochenschrift* 51:156–163.

Martinez, J. L., Vasquez, B. J., Messing, R. B., Jensen, R. A., Liang, K. C., and McGaugh, J. L. 1981. Age-related changes in the catecholamine content of peripheral organs in male and female F344 rats. *Journal of Gerontology* 36:280–284.

McLean, M. R., Goldberg, P. B., and Roberts, J. 1983. An ultrastructural study of the effects of age on sympathetic innervation and atrial tissue in the rat. *Journal of Molecular and Cellular Cardiology* 15:75–92.

Morvai, V., and Ungvary, G. 1979. Effect of chronic exposure to alcohol on the circulation of rats of different ages. *Acta Physiologica Academiae Scientarium Hungaricae* 53:433–441.

Narayanan, N., and Derby, J. A. 1982a. Alterations in the properties of beta-adrenergic receptors of myocardial membranes in aging: Impairments in agonist–receptor interactions and guanine nucleotide regulation accompany diminished catecholamine-responsiveness of adenylate cyclase. *Mechanisms of Ageing and Development* 19:127–139.

Narayanan, N., and Derby, J. A. 1982b. Effects of age on muscarinic cholinergic receptors in rat myocardium. *Canadian Journal of Physiology and Pharmacology* 61:822–829.

Narayanan, N., and Tucker, L. 1986. Autonomic interactions in the aging heart: Age-associated decrease in muscarinic cholinergic receptor mediated inhibition of β-adrenergic activation of adenylate cyclase. *Mechanisms of Ageing and Development* 34:249–259.

Neubauer, B., and Christensen, N. J. 1978. The decrease in noradrenaline concentration in the posterior tibial artery with age. *Gerontology* 24: 299–303.

O'Connor, S. W., Scarpace, P. J., and Abrass, I. B. 1981. Age-associated decrease of adenylate cyclase activity in rat myocardium. *Mechanisms of Ageing and Development* 16:91–95.

O'Donnell, S. R., and Wanstall, J. C. 1984. Beta-1 and beta-2 adrenoceptor-mediated responses in preparations of pulmonary artery and aorta from young and aged rats. *Journal of Pharmacology and Experimental Therapeutics* 228:733–738.

Pan, H. Y. M., Hoffman, B. B., Pershe, R. A., and Blaschke, T. F. 1986. Decline in beta adrenergic receptor-mediated vascular relaxation with aging in man. *Journal of Pharmacology and Experimental Therapeutics* 239: 802–807.

Partilla, J. S., Hoopes, M. T., Ito, H., Dax, E. M., and Roth, G. S. 1982. Loss of ventricular alpha 1-adrenergic receptors during aging. *Life Sciences* 31:2507–2512.

Posner, P., Baker, S. P., Hunter, B., and Walker, D. W. 1987. Chronotropic and inotropic effects on atria of chronic ethanol ingestion in the aging rat. *Alcohol and Drug Research* 7:273–277.

Prange, A. J., White, J. E., Lipton, M. A., and Kinkead, A. M. 1967. Influence of age on monoamine oxidase and catechol-o-methyltranferase in the rat tissue. *Life Sciences* 6:581–586.

Raisbeck, M. J. 1952. The use of digitalis in the aged. *Geriatrics* 7:12–19.

Rappaport, E. B., Young, J. B., and Landsberg, L. 1981. Impact of age on basal and diet-induced changes in sympathetic nervous system activity of Fischer rats. *Journal of Gerontology* 36:152–157.

Regan, T. J., Ettinger, P. O., Haider, B., Ahmed, S. S., Oldewurtel, H. A., and Lyons, M. M. 1977. The role of ethanol in cardiac disease. *Annual Review of Medicine* 28:393–409.

Roberts, J., and Goldberg, P. B. 1975. Changes in cardiac membranes as a function of age with particular emphasis on reactivity to drugs. In Cristofalo, V. J., Roberts, J., and Adelman, R. C. (Eds.), *Advances in Experimental Medicine and Biology: Vol. 61. Explorations in Aging.* New York, Plenum Press, pp. 119–148.

Roberts, J., and Goldberg, P. B. 1976. Changes in basic cardiovascular activities during the lifetime of the rat. *Experimental Aging Research* 2:487–514.

Roberts, J., and Kelliher, G. J. 1972. The mechanisms of digitalis at the subcellular level. *Seminars in Drug Treatment* 2:203–220.

Roberts, J., Kelliher, G. J., and Lathers, C. M. 1976. Role of adrenergic influences in digitalis-induced ventricular arrhythmia. *Life Sciences* 18: 665–678.

Roberts, J., and Modell, W. 1961. Pharmacologic evidence for the importance of catecholamines in cardiac rhythmicity. *Circulation Research* 9:171–176.

Roberts, J., and Tumer, N. 1987. Age-related changes in autonomic function of catecholamines. In Rothstein, M. (Ed.), *Review of Biological Research in Aging.* New York, Alan R. Liss, pp. 257–289.

Rodeheffer, R. J., Gerstenblith, G., Becker, L. C., Fleg, J. L., Weisfeldt, M. L., and Lakatta, E. G. 1984. Exercise cardiac output is maintained with advancing age in healthy human subjects: Cardiac dilatation and increased stroke volume compensate for a diminishing heart rate. *Circulation* 69: 203–213.

Rosahn, P. D. 1941. Weight of the normal heart in adult males. *American Journal of Pathology* 17:595–596.

Rosenthal, J. 1987. Aging and the cardiovascular system. *Gerontology* 33 (Suppl. 1):3–8.

Roth, G. S. 1979. Hormone action during aging: Alterations and mechanisms. *Mechanisms of Ageing and Development* 9:497–514.

Rothbaum, D. A., Shaw, D. J., Angell, C. S., and Shock, N. W. 1974. Age differences in the baroreceptor response of rats. *Journal of Gerontology* 29:488–492.

Rowe, J. W., and Troen, B. R. 1980. Sympathetic nervous system and aging in man. *Endocrine Reviews* 1:167–179.

Rumberger, E., and Timmermann, J. 1976. Age-changes of the force-frequency-relationship and the duration of action potential of isolated papillary muscles of guinea pig. *European Journal of Applied Physiology* 35:277–284.

Saba, H., Cowan, T., Haven, A. J., and Burnstock, G. 1984. Reduction in noradrenergic perivascular nerve density in the left and right cerebral arteries of old rabbits. *Journal of Cerebral Blood Flow and Metabolism* 4:284–289.

Santer, R. M. 1982. Fluorescence histochemical observations on the adrenergic innervation of the cardiovascular system in the aged rat. *Brain Research Bulletin* 9:667–672.

Scarpace, P. J. 1986. Decreased beta-adrenergic responsiveness during senescence. *Federation Proceedings* 45:51–54.

Schabb, M. C. 1964. The aging of collagen in the heart muscle. *Gerontologia* 10:38–41.

Schneider, J., and Ruiz-Torres, A. 1978. Results concerning the sensitivity of old patients against digitalis. *Aktuelle Gerontologie* 8:159–165.

Schwartz, A., Lindenmayer, G. E., and Allen, J. C. 1975. The sodium potassium adenosine triphosphate: Pharmacological, physiological and biochemical aspects. *Pharmacological Reviews* 27:3–134.

Scott, P. J. W., and Reid, J. L. 1982. The effect of age on the responses of human isolated arteries to noradrenaline. *British Journal of Clinical Pharmacology* 13:237–239.

Shimada, K., Kitazumi, T., Ogura, H., Sadakane, N., and Ozawa, T. 1986. Effects of age and blood pressure on the cardiovascular responses to the Valsalva maneuver. *Journal of the American Geriatrics Society* 34:431–434.

Shimada, K., Kitazumi, T., Sadakane, N., Ogura, H., Ozawa, T. 1985. Age-related changes of baroreflex function, plasma norepinephrine, and blood pressure. *Hypertension* 7:113–117.

Simms, H. S., and Berg, B. N. 1957. Longevity and the onset of lesions in male rats. *Journal of Gerontology* 12:244–252.

Simpkins, J. W., Field, F. P., and Ress, R. J. 1983. Age-related decline in adrenergic responsiveness of the kidney, heart and aorta of male rats. *Neurobiology of Aging* 4:233–238.

Sjogren, A. L. 1972. Left ventricular wall thickness in patients with circulatory overload of the left ventricle. *Annals of Clinical Research* 4:310–318.

Spurgeon, H. A., Steinbach, M. F., and Lakatta, E. G. 1983. Chronic exercise prevents characteristic age-related changes in rat cardiac contraction. *American Journal of Physiology* 244:H513–H518.

Spurgeon, H. A., Thorne, P. R., Yin, F. C. P., Shock, N. W., and Weisfeldt, M. L. 1977. Increased dynamic stiffness of trabeculae carneae from senescent rats. *American Journal of Physiology* 232:H373–H380.

Stevens, M. J., Lipe, S., and Moulds, R. F. W. 1982. The effect of age on the responses of human isolated arteries and veins to noradrenaline. *British Journal of Clinical Pharmacology* 14:750–751.

Stevens, M. J., and Moulds, R. F. W. 1981. Heterogeneity of postjunctional alpha-adrenoceptors in human vascular smooth muscle. *Archives Internationales Pharmacodynie et de Therapie* 254:43–57.

Strandell, T. 1964. Heart volume and its relation to anthropometric data in old men compared with young men. *Acta Medica Scandinavica* 176:205–218.

Strehler, B. L., Mark, D. D., Mildvan, A. S., and Gee, M. V. 1959. Rate and magnitude of age pigment accumulation in the human myocardium. *Journal of Gerontology* 14:430–439.

Strozzi, C., Alboni, P., Pareschi, P. L., and Meduri, P. 1973. La risposta alla beta-stimolazione del circola periferico nell'anziano. *Acta Gerontologica* 23:245–257.

Templeton, G. H., Willerson, J. T., Platt, M. R., and Weisfeldt, M. 1978. Contraction duration and diastolic stiffness in aged canine left ventricle. In Kobayashi, T., Sano, T., and Dalla, N. S. (Eds.), *Recent Advances in Studies on Cardiac Structure and Metabolism: Vol. 2. Heart Function and Metabolism.* Baltimore, MD, University Park Press, pp. 169–173.

Thompson, J. H., Su, C., Shih, J., Aures, D., Choi, L., Butcher, S., Loskota,

W. S., Simon, M., and Silva, D. 1974. Effects of chronic nicotine administration and age on various neurotransmitters and associated enzymes in male Fischer 344 rats. *Toxicology and Applied Pharmacology* 24:41–59.

Toda, N. 1981. Cardiotoxic and inotropic effects of ouabain on atria isolated from rabbits of different ages. *British Journal of Pharmacology* 72:263–270.

Topping, T. M., and Travis, D. F. 1974. An electron cytochemical study of mechanisms of lysosomal activity in the rat left ventricular mural myocardium. *Journal of Ultrastructure Research* 46:1–22.

Travis, D. F., and Travis, A. 1972. Ultrastructural changes in the left ventricular rat myocardial cells with age. *Journal of Ultrastructure Research* 39:124–148.

Tsujimoto, G., and Hashimoto, K. 1987. Effects of triiodo-L-thyronine (T_3)-induced hyperthyroidism on the cardiovascular alpha-adrenoceptor system in young and older rats. *Japanese Journal of Pharmacology* 44:437–445.

Tsujimoto, G., Hashimoto, K., and Hoffman, B. B. 1987. Effects of thyroid hormone on β-adrenergic responsiveness of aging cardiovascular systems. *American Journal of Physiology* 252:H513–H520.

Tsujimoto, G., Lee, C. H., and Hoffman, B. B. 1986. Age-related decrease in beta adrenergic receptor-mediated vascular smooth muscle relaxation. *Journal of Pharmacology and Experimental Therapeutics* 239:411–415.

Tuttle, R. S. 1966. Age-related changes in the sensitivity of rat aortic strips of norepinephrine and associated chemical and structural alterations. *Journal of Gerontology* 21:510–516.

van Brummelen, P., Buhler, F. R., Kiowski, W., and Amann, F. W. 1981. Age-related decrease in cardiac and peripheral vascular responsiveness to isoprenaline: Studies in normal subjects. *Clinical Science* 60:571–577.

Vestal, R. E., Wood, A. J. J., and Shand, D. G. 1979. Reduced β-adrenoceptor sensitivity in the elderly. *Clinical Pharmacology and Therapeutics* 26:181–186.

Walsh, R. A. 1987. Cardiovascular effects of the aging process. *American Journal of Medicine* 82 (Suppl. 1B):34–40.

Waterson, J. G., Frewin, D. B., and Soltys, J. S. 1974. Age-related differences in catecholamine fluorescence of human vascular tissue. *Blood Vessels* 11:79–85.

Watkinson, W. P. 1985. Effects of chlordimeform on cardiovascular functional parameters: Part 1. Lethality and arrhythmogenicity in the geriatric rat. *Journal of Toxicology and Environmental Health* 15:729–744.

Watkinson, W. P. 1986. Effects of chlordimeform on cardiovascular functional parameters: Part 2. Acute and delayed effects following intravenous administration in the postweaning rat. *Toxicology and Environmental Health* 19:195–206.

Wei, J. Y., Spurgeon, H. A., and Lakatta, E. G. 1984. Excitation–contraction in rat myocardium. Alterations with adult aging. *American Journal of Physiology* 246:H784–H791.

Weisfeldt, M. L. 1980. *The Aging Heart.* New York, Raven Press.

Weisfeldt, M. L., Loeven, W. A., and Shock, N. W. 1971. Resting and active mechanical properties of trabeculae carneae from aged male rats. *American Journal of Physiology* 220:1921–1927.

Werzar, F. 1969. The stages and consequences of aging of collagen. *Gerontologia* 15:233–239.

Wilens, S. L., and Sproul, E. E. 1938. Spontaneous cardiovascular disease in the rat. I. Lesions of the heart. *American Journal of Pathology* 14:177–200.

Wollenberger, A., Jehl, J., and Karsh, M. L. 1953. The influence of age on the sensitivity of the guinea pig and its myocardium to ouabain. *Journal of Pharmacology and Experimental Therapeutics* 108:52–60.

Yin, F. C. 1980. The aging vasculature and its effects on the heart. In Weisfeldt, M. L. (Ed.), *The Aging Heart*. New York, Raven Press, pp. 137–213.

Yin, F. P. C., Spurgeon, H. A., Weisfeldt, M. L., and Lakatta, E. G. 1980. Mechanical properties of myocardium from hypertrophied rat hearts. A comparison between hypertrophy induced by aortic banding and senescence. *Circulation Research* 46:292–300.

Zitnik, G., and Roth, G. S. 1981. Effects of thyroid hormones on cardiac hypertrophy and β-adrenergic receptors during aging. *Mechanisms of Ageing and Development* 15:19–28.

7

Bone Metabolism, Structure, and Aging

Kenneth W. Lyles, M. D.

General toxicology textbooks describe bone as an inert tissue that is usually unaffected by toxic compounds and serves only as a storage depot or reservoir (Haley and Berndt, 1987). The effects of fluoride causing osteosclerosis and radiation causing osteosarcomas are well known. Less well appreciated are the effects of other toxicants on the skeleton, and considering the skeleton as only a repository for toxic compounds is incorrect.

Diseases of the skeleton increase with advancing age, the most common being osteoporosis and osteoarthritis. Because this chapter deals with the effects of environmental toxins on the skeleton, no further mention shall be made of arthritis, which is limited to specific joints or types of joints. Although *osteoporosis,* defined as a decrease in the amounts of both bone mineral and matrix per unit volume of skeletal tissue to a level at which fractures occur after minimal or no trauma (Lyles, 1989), is the most common metabolic bone disease caused by environmental toxins, other metabolic bone diseases have environmental factors in their pathogenesis. Such diseases are *osteomalacia,* a failure of mineralization of osteoid tissue; *osteosclerosis,* an increase in the volume of mineralized bone; *osteonecrosis,* death of areas of mineralized bone; and finally *bone neoplasms.* Before discussing how specific agents cause bone diseases, it is necessary to have a basic understanding of normal bone growth and the hormonal factors controlling it.

The skeleton serves two different and often competing functions (Raisz, 1981). It must be a strong, light, and mobile frame protecting organs and serving as sites for muscle insertions. This frame also must be capable of repair and remodeling in response to changing stresses. In contrast, the skeleton must also serve as the reservoir for most of the calcium and phosphorus in the body, as well as substantial amounts of magnesium, sodium, and carbonate. As part of its storage function the skeleton provides calcium and phosphorus when the supply of these minerals is deficient. The phosphate and carbonate of bone can also buffer excess acid in the diet. These metabolic functions may preempt the structural ones so that growth or remodeling are impaired and skeletal mass may decrease in states of calcium or phosphorus deficiency or chronic acidosis.

There are two types of bone: cortical and trabecular. Cortical bone, the compact layer that forms the outer shell of bone, makes up 80 percent of the adult skeleton. Trabecular bone, also known as spongy or cancellous bone, is a series of thin plates (trabeculae) forming the interior meshwork of bone and comprises 20 percent of the adult skeleton. Both cortical and trabecular bone contribute to skeletal strength. Trabecular bone is more sensitive to metabolic influences because of its greater surface-to-volume ratio (Snyder, 1975). Thus, conditions that produce rapid bone loss tend to affect trabecular bone more quickly than cortical bone.

Normally, growth of long bones ceases when epiphyses, or growth centers at the end of these bones, close; however, bone mass increases by radial growth until about age 30. After a period of stabilization, age-related bone loss begins in both sexes. Over their lifetime women lose approximately 35 percent of their cortical bone and 50 percent of their trabecular bone, whereas men lose about two-thirds of these proportions (Riggs and Melton, 1986). Two phases of bone loss have been identified for both cortical and trabecular bone—a prolonged slow phase that occurs in both sexes and a transient rapid phase that can occur in women after menopause and in men with androgen deficiency.

The skeleton is a dynamic tissue that undergoes continuous changes even after longitudinal bone growth has ceased. As long as bone growth is continuing in the cortical or trabecular envelopes, the process is known as *modeling*. Once the increase in bone volume ceases, further changes in the skeleton are known as *remodeling*. The process of remodeling involves bone formation and bone resorption, which are tightly coupled processes. At the beginning of each remodeling cycle, osteoclasts, cells derived from macrophages, appear on a previously inactive surface and, over a period of about 2 weeks, resorb a portion of cortical or trabecular bone. The osteoclasts are then replaced by osteoblasts, cells derived from bone marrow precursors, which fill in the resorption cavity with osteoid tissue. Over a period of 3–4 months the osteoid tissue is mineralized to create a new structural unit of bone. Failure of the osteoid matrix to mineralize results in osteomalacia. In children, this disease causes bowing of the legs. At the growing epiphyses the rachitic lesion occurs; hence the term *rickets*. In normal young adults, the resorption and formation phases are tightly coupled and bone mass is conserved. The mechanism for the coupling of bone resorption and formation is incompletely understood; however, numerous local regulators of bone growth are produced by osteoblasts, osteocytes, cartilage, and marrow cells. Their exact role as well as the role of systematically produced growth factors remain to be elucidated. Bone loss implies an uncoupling of the phases of bone remodeling, with a relative or absolute increase in resorption over formation. When such uncoupling occurs, bone turnover leads to net bone loss.

Thirty percent of the skeleton is composed of inorganic ions, the majority of which are calcium and phosphorus; the remaining 70 percent is composed of protein and collagen. The movement of these minerals in and out of the body and between bone and other compartments is largely controlled by three calcium regulators: parathyroid hormone (PTH), calcitonin, and vitamin D.

PTH maintains serum calcium concentration by stimulating bone resorption, by increasing reabsorption of filtered calcium in the kidney, and indirectly by increasing vitamin D activation, which in turn increases calcium absorption in the intestine. PTH has an additional important action in the kidney to decrease tubular reabsorption of phosphorus, thereby increasing phosphate excretion. This action decreases the serum phosphate concentration and helps to maintain the serum calcium concentration by limiting redeposition of calcium and phosphate back into bone.

Serum levels of immunoreactive PTH increase with aging, possibly in response to decreased gastrointestinal calcium absorption (Gallagher et al., 1980; Wiske et al., 1979). These data must be interpreted carefully because the reduction in glomerular filtration rate with aging may decrease the clearance of carboxy-terminal fragments of PTH. Thus, circulating levels of immunoactive PTH may be increased though these fragments may lack biological activity. However, urinary cyclic adenosine monophosphate (cAMP) and nephrogenous cAMP excretion, both measures of the biological actions of PTH, increase with age (Marcus, Madvig, and Young, 1984). Increased secretion of PTH with aging would increase bone turnover by increasing the number of bone remodeling units. Therefore, when bone resorption and formation are uncoupled, the increased amount of PTH would lead to increased bone loss.

Vitamin D functions as a hormone that can be synthesized and activated in the body in three steps. The ultraviolet rays in sunlight striking the skin convert 7-dehydrocholesterol to vitamin D_3 or cholecalciferol. In the liver, cholecalciferol is hydroxylated to 25-OH vitamin D, or calcifediol. A second hydroxylation occurs on the kidney to form 1,25-dihydroxy vitamin D, or calcitriol, which is the final active product of the vitamin D hormone system. The major effect of calcitriol is to increase the intestinal absorption of calcium and phosphorus, thus maintaining the supply of these ions for bone mineralization. Therefore, calcitriol is an essential hormone for bone growth.

Calcium absorption by the intestine decreases with aging, especially after age 70, and is even lower in patients with postmenopausal osteoporosis (Gallagher et al., 1979). Serum calcitriol concentrations decrease by about 50 percent with aging; this decrease is partly responsible for the decrease in calcium absorption, though age-related changes in the intestine may also play a role. A primary impairment of 25-hydroxy vitamin D-1-hydroxylase, the renal enzyme responsible for conversion of calcifediol to calcitriol, has been demonstrated indirectly by a blunting of the normal rise of serum calcitriol in response to infusion of PTH in elderly normal subjects and in elderly patients with hip or vertebral fractures (Slovik et al., 1981; Tsai et al., 1984). This impairment of calcitriol formation may be related to decreasing kidney function associated with aging.

Many other hormones affect bone metabolism and are important in the pathogenesis of metabolic bone diseases, though their mechanism(s) in affecting bone growth or loss may not be completely understood. Sex steroids are necessary during skeletal growth so that an individual may completely form his or her genetically determined amounts of cortical and trabecular bone.

Growth hormone is required for skeletal growth. Before puberty its major effect is on cartilage growth, and after puberty it stimulates bone and soft tissue growth. The effects of growth hormone on the skeleton are probably not direct but rather mediated through production of somatomedins or growth factors made in tissues such as the liver. These growth factors stimulate cartilage and bone cell growth. Also, bone cells and bone marrow cells produce growth factors that act in similar fashion locally to stimulate growth.

Many new hormones and humoral substances have been identified as having effects on the skeleton (Centrella and Canalis, 1985). Prostaglandins, osteoclast-activating factor, interleukin-1, lymphotoxin, tumor necrosis factor alpha, and other cytokines have been identified as agents that can cause bone resorption. Furthermore, γ-interferon has been shown to inhibit bone resorption. The mechanisms of action and precise role of these factors in causing or preventing osteoporosis await further study.

Osteoporosis

Osteoporosis is the most common form of metabolic bone disease and has become a major public health problem in Western civilizations, affecting Caucasian and oriental women. Generally the disease is silent and patients are unaware of the problem until they sustain a vertebral, wrist, or hip fracture with minimal trauma. Further evaluation will lead to the discovery of reduced amount of bone in trabecular or cortical bone envelopes. For a skeletal fracture to occur, a force must be delivered that the tissue cannot withstand without breaking. Certain forces such as those delivered in an automobile accident will result in a person of any age, whereas a fall from a standing height or out of bed may only cause a hip fracture in a person with a decreased bone mass. Thus unmarked or poorly lighted loose rugs, or scattered toys, can be an environmental hazard that result in a fractured wrist, hip, or vertebral body.

Most patients with osteoporosis are believed to have lost bone after their middle 30s, as a result of menopausal reduction of sex hormones or changes in the ability to absorb calcium from the diet and have osteoblasts incorporate it into bone. It probably takes 10–15 years of gradual bone loss to put a person at risk for osteoporotic fractures. Because there is such a latent period for the development of osteoporosis, it is not surprising that there are not a large number of environmental toxicants associated with the disease. A number of commonly used drugs do cause osteoporosis as a recognized side-effect. These drugs are glucocorticoid hormones, diphenylhydantoin, heparin, and certain alkylating agents used for cancer chemotherapy (Lyles, 1989).

Alcohol is a cause of osteoporosis, causing bone loss most probably by a direct toxic effect on osteoblasts (Bikle et al., 1985; Farley et al., 1985). It is unknown how much and how frequently alcohol must be consumed to cause osteoporosis. At present, we probably underestimate alcohol's direct toxic effect on the skeleton. In addition, impaired cognition and delayed reaction time from alcohol ingestion can lead to falls or motor vehicle accidents.

Cigarette smoking is associated with an increased risk for developing osteoporosis, but the mechanism for its effect is not completely clear (Daniell, 1976; Seeman et al., 1983). The most recent evidence suggests that female cigarette smokers have an increased rate of estrogen catabolism in the liver (Jensen, Christiansen, and Rodbro, 1985).

At present no data are available regarding the effect of passive inhalation of tobacco smoke on the selection.

In conclusion, there are no environmental toxicants associated with generalized osteoporosis. It is possible that some will be identified, but one difficulty in proving a causal relationship will be the long period of time required for development of symptoms from osteoporosis.

Localized areas of bone loss have been associated with environmental toxicants. Workers who are involved with polymerization of vinyl chloride develop acroosteolysis, a triad of Raynaud's phenomenon, sclerodermatous skin changes, and osteolysis (Destouet and Murphy, 1983). Although the triad may be the result of vascular occlusions, this mechanism or other ones may affect other skeletal sites. Hexachlorobenzene has been reported to cause loss of the distal tufts of the phalanges in affected subjects in Turkey (Cripps et al., 1984). Although the phalangeal bone loss may have been due to scarring of the skin from an acquired form of porphyria, a direct effect of hexachlorobenzene on the skeleton cannot be excluded. These agents are not thought to cause generalized osteoporosis, but the mechanisms for bone loss in the bones of the hands may be occurring in other skeletal areas with high trabecular bone content. Furthermore, no measurement of vertebral bone mineral content or search for vertebral fractures was made. Thus, when environmental toxicants are noted to cause bone loss in any portion of the skeleton, it is advisable to consider other skeletal areas that might have lost bone. With the ease of measuring bone mineral content in wrists, hips, and vertebrae (Avioli and Repa-Eschen, 1988), such studies are much easier to perform.

Osteomalacia

This form of metabolic bone disease occurs less frequently than osteoporosis, but usually has a more rapid onset. Therefore patients have a shorter latent period before seeking medical attention for their skeletal disease. Growing children with osteomalacia present with bowed legs and rickets, whereas adults present with bone pain and muscle weakness. The bone pain generally occurs because of stress on bones that are weakened by inadequate mineralization (Dent and Stamp, 1977). Pseudofractures or poorly healing fractures can also cause bone pain in osteomalacia. Muscle weakness is usually from a proximal myopathy and is usually caused by the frequently occurring hypophosphatemia.

The bisphosphonate etidronate is used to treat Paget's disease of bone. At its normal dose of 5 mg per kilogram of body weight, this drug is effective for treating Paget's disease. However, at doses of

20 mg per kilogram of body weight etidronate produces osteomalacia (Johnson, Khairi, and Meunier, 1980). Cessation of the drug reverses the osteomalacia.

A number of environmental toxicants cause an acquired defect in the proximal renal tubule, resulting in a syndrome known as "acquired Fanconi's syndrome." This syndrome is characterized by increased amounts of phosphate, glucose, and amino acids (DeFronzo and Thier, 1986). Less frequently bicarbonate, potassium, uric acid, and calcium can be lost. The toxins cause an injury to the proximal renal tubular epithelial cells so that they do not reabsorb the amino acids, glucose, bicarbonate, and phosphate from the glomerular filtrate. This failure to normally reabsorb substances is known as *renal tubular wasting* and the substances are found in increased quantities in the urine. Recent work has shown that with impairment of the proximal tubule and phosphate wasting there are low circulating serum 1,25-dihydroxy-vitamin D levels (Nogawa et al., 1987) This vitamin D metabolite is produced in the proximal renal tubule and the renal tubular defect in the acquired Fanconi syndrome most likely impairs production of 1,25-dihydroxy-vitamin D. Three environmental toxicants can cause this syndrome: cadmium, lead, and uranium (Bowley, 1984).

In the past, outdated and oxidized tetracycline was found to also cause an acquired Fanconi's syndrome (DeFronzo and Thier, 1986). The syndrome has also been associated with vitamin D intoxication when pharmacological doses of vitamin D have been administered.

Recently aluminum has been associated with a form of osteomalacia in patients with end-stage renal disease on long-term hemodialysis (Ott et al., 1982). The precise mechanism by which aluminum causes this osteomalacia is still under investigation.

Osteosclerosis

Osteosclerosis is characterized by increased amounts of bone per unit volume, and radiographs show increased density of both cortical and trabecular bones. The most common toxicant associated with osteosclerosis is fluoride. Abnormal exposure occurs from inhaling vapors or dust high in fluoride content or from drinking water containing greater than 8 ppm of fluoride. Affected subjects complain of back stiffness, vague aches, and joint pains. In addition to increased density of the bones, calcification of the insertion of tendons to bone is found (Grandjean and Thomsen, 1983; Singh et al., 1983). High concentration of fluoride in drinking water was found to cause staining of the enamel of teeth (Bowley, 1984). Subsequent work has shown that fluoride in small doses reduces caries by strengthening enamel, so fluoridization of water sources and toothpaste has become a public health measure. In large quantities fluoride has been shown to stimulate bone growth by a direct stimulation of osteoblasts (Farley, Werdedal, and Baylink, 1983). Sodium fluoride is now used to increase trabecular bone mass in certain patients with osteoporosis (Lyles, 1989).

Ingestion of more than 1 million units of vitamin A can cause an acute syndrome of increased intracranial pressure, bone pain, and alopecia. With chronic ingestion of large doses of vitamin A a more chronic syndrome develops with formation of new periosteal bone in the diaphysis of long bones in the extremities. Patients also develop hard tender masses in the extremities, anorexia, itching, dry skin, and hepatomegaly (Bowley, 1984). More recently a similar syndrome has been seen in patients with acne and severe refractory ichthyosis who receive retinoic acid (Pittsley and Yoder, 1983). These patients have bone pain, hypercalcemia, periosteal new bone formation, and hyperostosis. With increased use of vitamin A derivatives for severe acne and the possibility of using them for cancer prevention suggests that these drugs may be associated with other skeletal toxic manifestations. The signs and symptoms of vitamin A and retinoic acid derivative intoxication remit when the offending agent is stopped.

Radiation-Induced Bone Lesions

Two skeletal lesions, osteonecrosis and osteosarcomas, develop as a result of exposure to radiation, either externally by radiation used for therapeutic purposes or internally by implantation of a radioactive source or accidental ingestion of bone-seeking radioactive isotopes such as radium-226. Osteonecroses are areas of bone where osteocytes that have received the radiation are killed and the trabeculae become thin; bone can fracture if stress continues to be applied (Sharpe, 1983). Osteosarcomas can develop in areas of the skeleton that have received radiation and in cases of therapeutic radiation occur 5–10 years after exposure to 40–60 Gy (Hudson, 1987). The majority of radioisotope-induced osteosarcomas from environmental exposure have occurred in subjects around atomic bomb blasts, in radium dial-painters, and workers in the luminous paint industry. The time from exposure to the isotope until development of the neoplasm can vary widely, with 5–50 years reported from time of exposure to discovery of the neoplasm (Raabe, Book, and Parks, 1983).

Summary

The skeleton has previously been considered an inert tissue that generally serves only as a repository for environmental toxicants. Although in some cases this is an appropriate assessment of the interaction between host and toxicant, in other cases environmental toxicants do have a sufficient impact on the skeleton, which is a constantly changing, dynamic organ. With increased attention being paid to metabolic bone diseases, especially osteoporosis, and with new safe, accurate, and precise ways to assess bone mineral content, the number of environmental toxicants causing skeletal diseases is likely to grow.

References

Avioli, L. V., and Repa-Eschen, L. 1988. Increasing osteoporosis screening referrals. *Applied Radiology* (April) 25–35.

Bilke, D. D., Genant, H. K., Cann, C., Recker, R. R., Halloran, B. P., and Strewler, G. J., 1985. Bone disease in alcohol abuse. *Annals of Internal Medicine* 103:42–48.

Bowley, N. B. 1984. Various osteopathies. In Nordin, B. E. C. (Ed.), *Metabolic Bone and Stone Disease*. Edinburgh, Churchill Livingstone, pp. 234–270.

Centrella, M., and Canalis, E. 1985. Local regulators of skeletal growth: A perspective. *Endocrine Reviews* 6:544–551.

Cripps, D. J., Peters, W. A., Gocmen, A., and Dogramic, I. 1984. Porphyria turcica due to hexachlorobenzene: A 20 to 30 year follow-up on 204 patients. *British Journal of Dermatology* 111:413–422.

Daniell, H. W. 1976. Osteoporosis of the slender smoker: Vertebral compression fractures and loss of metacarpal cortex in relation to post-menopausal cigarette smoking and lack of obesity. *Archives of Internal Medicine* 136:298–304.

DeFronzo, R. A., and Thier, S. O. 1986. Inherited disorders of renal tubule function. In Brenner, B. M., and Rector, F. C. (Eds.), *The Kidney*. Philadelphia, W. B. Saunders, pp. 1297–1239.

Dent, C. E., and Stamp, T. C. B. 1977. Vitamin D, rickets and osteomalacia. In (Vol. 1), Avioli, L. V., and Krane, S. M. (Eds.), *Metabolic Bone Disease*. New York, Academic Press, pp. 237–306.

Destouet, J. M., and Murphy, W. A. 1983. Acquired acroosteolysis and acronecrosis. *Arthritis and Rheumatism* 26:1150–1154.

Farley, J. R., Fitzsimmons, R., Taylor, A. K., Jorch, U. M., and Lau, K-H. W. 1985. Direct effects of ethanol on bone resorption and formation in vitro. *Archives of Biochemistry and Biophysics* 238:305–314.

Farley, J. R., Werdedal, J. E., and Baylink, D. J. 1983. Fluoride directly stimulates proliferation and alkaline phosphatase activity of bone forming cells. *Science* 222:330–332.

Gallagher, J. C., Riggs, B. L., Eisman, J., Hamstra, A., Arnaud, S. B., and

DeLuca, H. F. 1979. Intestinal calcium absorption and serum vitamin D metabolites in normal subjects and osteoporosis patients: Effects of age and dietary calcium intake. *Journal of Clinical Investigation* 64:729–736.

Gallagher, J. C., Riggs, B. L., Jerpbak, C. M., and Arnaud, C. D. 1980. The effect of age on serum immunoreactive parathyroid hormone in normal and osteoporotic women. *Journal of Laboratory and Clinical Medicine* 95:373–385.

Grandjean, P., and Thomsen, G. 1983. Reversibility of skeletal fluorosis. *British Journal of Industrial Medicine* 40:456–461.

Haley, J. J., and Berndt, W. O. 1987. *Handbook of Toxicology.* New York, Harper and Row.

Hudson, T. M. 1987. *Radiologic–Pathologic Correlation of Musculoskeletal Lesions.* Baltimore, MD, Williams & Wilkins.

Jensen, J., Christiansen, C., and Rodbro, P. 1985. Cigarette smoking, serum estrogens and bone loss during hormone-replacement therapy early after menopause. *New England Journal of Medicine* 313:973–975.

Johnson, C. C., Jr., Khairi, M. R. A., and Meunier, P. J. 1980. Use of etidronate (EHDP) in Paget's disease of bone. *Arthritis and Rheumatism* 23:1172–1174.

Lyles, K. W. 1989. Osteoporosis. In Kelley, W. N. (Ed.), *Textbook of Internal Medicine.* Philadelphia, J. B. Lippincott, pp. 2601–2607.

Marcus, R., Madvig, P., and Young, G. 1984. Age-related changes in parathyroid hormone and parathyroid hormone action in normal humans. *Journal of Clinical Endocrinology and Metabolism* 58:223–230.

Nogawa, K., Tsuritani, I., Kido, T., Honda, R., Yamada, Y., and Ishizaki, M. 1987. Mechanism for bone disease found in inhabitants environmentally exposed to cadmium: Decreased serum 1 alpha 25 dihydroxyvitamin D level. *International Archives of Occupational and Environmental Health* 59:21–30.

Ott, S. M., Maloney, N. A., Coburn, J. W., Alfrey, A. C., and Sherrard, D. J. 1982. The prevalence of bone aluminum deposition in renal osteodystrophy and its relation to the response to calcitriol therapy. *New England Journal of Medicine* 307:709–713.

Pittsley, R. A. and Yoder, F. W. 1983. Skeletal toxicity associated with long-term administration of retinoic acid for refractory icthyosis. *New England Journal of Medicine* 308:1012–1014.

Raabe, O. G., Book, S. A., and Parks, N. J. 1983. Lifetime bone cancer dose response relationships in beagles and people from skeletal burden of [226]Ra and [90]Sr. *Health Physics* 44:33–48.

Raisz, L. G. 1981. Osteoporosis. *Journal of the American Geriatrics Society* 30:127–138.

Riggs, B. L., and Melton, L. J. 1986. Involutional osteoporosis. *New England Journal of Medicine* 314:1676–1684.

Seeman, E., Melton, L. J., III, O'Fallon, W. M., and Riggs, B. L. 1983. Risk factors for spinal osteoporosis in men. *American Journal of Medicine* 75:977–983.

Sharpe, W. D. 1983. Chronic radium intoxication: Radium osteonecrosis and cancer in relation to 226 Ra burdens. *Health Physics* 51:149–154.

Singh, A., Jelly, S. S., Bansal, B. C., and Mathur, C. C. 1963. Endemic fluorosis: Epidemiological, clinical and biochemical study of chronic fluoride intoxication in Punjab, India. *Medicine* 42:229–246.

Slovik, D. M., Adams, J. S., Neer, R. M., Holick, M. J., and Potts, J. T., Jr. 1981. Deficient production of 1,25 dihydroxyvitamin D in elderly osteoporotic patients. *New England Journal of Medicine* 305:372–364.

Snyder, W. 1975. *Report of the Task Group on Reference Manual*. Oxford, Pergamon.

Tsai, K-S., Heath, H., III, Kumar, R., and Riggs, B. L. 1984. Impaired vitamin D metabolism with aging in women: Possible role in pathogenesis of senile osteoporosis. *Journal of Clinical Investigation* 73:1668–1672.

Wiske, P. S., Epstein, S., Bell, N. H., Queener, S. F., Edmondson, J., and Johnston, C. C. 1979. Increases in immunoreactive parathyroid hormone with age. *New England Journal of Medicine* 300:1419–1421.

8

Xenobiotics
and Endocrine Function
in the Aging Organism

Jerome M. Goldman, Ph.D.
Ralph L. Cooper, Ph.D.

Hormones play an important, often critical, role in the regulation of a large number of physiological and behavioral processes, and their influence can be demonstrated throughout the life span. Some hormones have organizational effects in that their presence or absence during certain developmental periods will affect the way in which physiological and behavioral processes unfold or are expressed in adulthood. Through each portion of the life span, the maintenance of an appropriate endocrine milieu is essential to the numerous homeostatic processes required for survival. With advancing age, there are several, well-documented changes in the ability of organisms to synthesize and secrete a number of hormones. It is therefore likely that the typical age-related change in an organism's endocrine balance would result in, or at least contribute to, the impairment of homeostasis frequently observed in elderly individuals. Such impairments can be present in the rate with which elderly patients are able to recover from the insults of injury or disease. Consequently, it is quite plausible to reconsider the elderly as a population at risk, one that may exhibit marked alterations in its responsiveness to environmental challenges.

Whether they are derived from endogenous or exogenous sources, certain hormones may also play a significant role in the aging process. For example, age-related changes in several physiological functions appear to be closely linked to the level and pattern of hormonal stimulation present during adulthood. As such, different patterns of exposure to a hormonal environment may alter the rate of aging within a specific neuroendocrine system and, in turn, affect the organism's susceptibility to environmental insults at different segments of the life span.

Some environmental toxicants have also been shown to mimic the action of certain hormones. As a result, they then have the potential to alter normal physiological development and function in adulthood as well as the rate at which the organism ages. The incidence of such changes may be a consequence of long-term, low-level exposure. Alternatively, a brief exposure at certain critical developmental periods could have long-lasting effects on endocrine function and the maintenance of homeostasis.

The purpose of this chapter is to discuss evidence that demonstrates a role for hormonal status in the loss of physiological functions in the sensecent animal and the effect that age-related endocrine changes have on the animal's response to environmental toxicants. A second purpose is to review evidence suggesting that some toxicants may be able to influence the normal progression of aging, or the appearance of age-related events, by an interference with normal endocrine homeostasis.

It is not our intention to provide a detailed and comprehensive overview of all of the known activational roles of hormones in young adult and aged animals. Rather, this chapter focuses on some of the better known alterations in the hormonal milieu that occur during maturity and aging that can influence the overall physiology of the animal. Sex differences are not explicitly considered. Although it is commonly understood that there are disparities in endocrine status between males and females (especially in the young adult) that presumably could affect an organism's response to toxic insult, we are concerned more with discussions of aging and the xenobiotic–hormone relationship in both sexes.

Age-Related Changes in Endocrine Function: Implications for Assessment of Toxicity

There are a number of different ways in which endocrine systems and the hormonal signaling operations that they use may undergo alterations with age and exposure to a toxicant. These can be categorized as changes in (1) the availability of hormones for binding to the target tissues, (2) the reception of the pertinent transmitter or hormonal signal by the target cells, and (3) the nature of the hormonal message.

Changes in Hormonal Availability with Age

At any point in time, the concentration of a hormone in the blood is a consequence of both its metabolism and secretion. Age-related or toxicant-induced shifts in synthesis, rate of clearance, and rate of secretion will all function to alter hormonal concentrations. Such changes in the size of the available signal pool may have corresponding effects on the magnitude of the response by the target tissue. In rats and humans, declines with age in a variety of hormones have been reported, including luteinizing hormone (LH) (e.g., Karpas et al., 1983; Meites, Steger, and Huang, 1980; Winters and Troen, 1982), follicle-stimulating hormone (FSH) (Meites, Steger, and Huang, 1980), and growth hormone (Sonntag, Hylka, and Meites, 1983).

These changes may reflect declines with age in the homeostatic controls, which rely heavily on endocrine feedback relationships within organ systems. Falls in LH in the female rat, for example, have been attributed to alterations in signals between the central nervous system (CNS) and the pituitary (Steger et al., 1980) and have been linked to reductions in gonadal activity. Gray, Smith, and Davidson (1980), on the other hand, believe that a decline in serum LH seen in middle-aged male rats is due to an increase in the sensitivity of the pituitary gonadotrope to the inhibitory feedback effects of testosterone. Regardless of the triggering site, the net effect is a diminution of homeostatic control.

A variety of toxicants have also been observed to cause changes in circulating hormonal levels (Cooper, Goldman, and Rehnberg, 1986). Significant reductions in serum testosterone, for example, have been seen following short-term exposure to the plasticizer dinitrobenzene (Rehnberg et al., 1988b) and the pesticide chlordimeform (Goldman et al., 1990), the latter also causing reductions in serum LH, thyroid-stimulating hormone (TSH), thyroxine, and triiodothyronine. The effects, moreover, may be remarkably specific. Following 3 days of exposure in male rats, the pesticide linuron, for instance, was reported to decrease serum thyroxine in a dose–response manner, while leaving triiodothyronine and the pituitary and gonadal hormones unaffected (Rehnberg et al., 1988a).

There is also a growing body of evidence that demonstrates a hormonal influence on toxicant metabolism. A sizeable number of xenobiotics, including both pharmaceutical compounds and environmental toxicants, are metabolized by the hepatic cytochrome P-450 monooxygenase system (Nebert and Gonzalez, 1987). Components of this system have been found to be under glucocorticoid (Schuetz et al., 1984; Simmons, McQuiddy, and Kasper, 1987) and sex steroid (Kamataki et al., 1985; Kato et al., 1986) regulation and markedly affected by growth hormone (MacGeoch, Morgan,and Gustafsson, 1985; Yamazoe et al., 1987). Consequently, persistent shifts in the circulating levels of such hormones, as have been reported for the aging animal, could affect the manner in which xenobiotics are metabolized following exposure.

Serum hormonal levels, as a rule, are not maintained at constant levels. They tend to fluctuate, sometimes markedly, throughout a 24-hr period. In the young adult man, peaking morning testosterone values can fall by one-third to an early evening nadir, before rising again through the late evening and early morning hours (Bremmer, Vitiello, and Prinz, 1983; Resko and Eik-Nes, 1966). A similar circadian rhythm in circulating levels of testosterone is prevalent in the rat (e.g., Ellis and Desjardins, 1982; Kinson and Liu, 1973). Human cortisol (Bilchert-Toft, 1978) and rat corticosterone (Kato, Saito, and Suda, 1980; Moberg, Bellinger, and Mendel, 1975) concentrations also exhbit well-known rhythmic fluctuations, as do thyrotropin (Leppaluoto, Ranta, and Tuomisto, 1974; Vanhaelst et al., 1972) and growth hormone (Millard et al., 1985).

Reported attenuations with age in the rhythms of human and rat serum testosterone (Bremner, Vitiello, and Prinz, 1983; Steiner et al., 1984; Tenover et al., 1988), LH (Vermeulen, Deslypere, and Kaufman, 1989), and growth hormone (Sonntag et al., 1980), among other hormones, can present differences in comparisons of young versus old subjects, depending on when such sampling is performed. Furthermore, such typical rhythmic changes also indicate that normal homeostasis need not function to maintain an invariance with a system. Thus, in these situations declines may well involve dysfunctions in rhythmicity that are expressed as minimally variant conditions. Comparable effects on hormonal rhythms have been reported to occur in response to toxicant exposure. For example, single injections of 2,3,7,8-tetrachlorodibenzo-p-dioxin (TCDD) showed some evidence in rats of alterations in prolactin and corticosterone rhythms (Jones et al., 1987). It may be then that an aging system, which is still exhibiting rhythmic hormonal changes typical of the normal young adult, may be increasingly sensitive to their disruption by low toxicant levels.

Although observable changes in hormonal rhythms or significant differences in circulating hormone concentrations may reflect disturbances in the overall functional integrity of the associated organ system, the absence of such changes should not be necessarily assumed to indicate a corresponding absence of a functional alteration. The notion of a "system at risk" presupposes an increase in the susceptibility to disruption of the homeostatic controls. In other words, an aging system that may be undergoing a subtle erosion in its endocrine balance could be more likely to exhibit alterations in its response to toxic insult. This may have particular importance considering that various toxicants have already been mentioned to induce significant endocrine changes. For example, age-related differences have already been observed in ovarian failure following chemotherapeutic treatment for Hodgkin's disease (Schilsky et al., 1981). Also, in comparisons be-

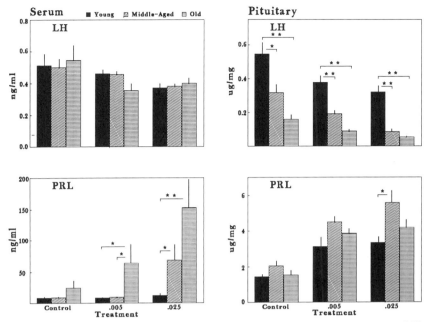

Figure 8.1. Age-related changes in rat serum and pituitary luteinizing hormone (LH) and prolactin (PRL) following 2 weeks of exposure to diethylstilbestrol (DES). DES treatment groupings (in micromoles) are listed along the horizontal axis. Group sizes for the young adult (Y, 3–5 months), middle aged (MA, 12 months), and old (0, 24 months) males were as follows: for control, Y = 9, MA = 7, O = 6; for 0.005 μmoles, Y = 9, MA = 6, O = 6; for 0.025 μmoles, Y = 8, MA = 7, O = 6. Significant main effects of age (serum LH, $p < .05$; serum PRL, $p < .01$; pituitary LH, $p < .01$; pituitary PRL, $p < .01$) and DES treatment (serum PRL, $p < .01$; pituitary LH, $p < .01$; pituitary PRL, $p < .01$) were found, and there was a significant age-dose interaction ($p = .01$) for measures of serum PRL.
* $p < .05$; ** $p < .01$ for age comparisons within treatment conditions.

tween current cigarette smokers and people who have never smoked, there is a reported advancement in the age of menopause for the former group (Jick, Porter, and Morrison, 1977).

Figure 8.1 summarizes hormonal data from young adult (3–5 months), middle-aged (12 months), and old (24 months) Long-Evans hooded male rats that had been given continuous subcutaneous doses (0, .005, or .025 μmoles/kg, by implanted minipump) of the nonsteroidal estrogen diethylstilbestrol (DES) for 2 weeks. On Day 14, animals were killed and serum and pituitary tissue collected for measurement of LH and prolactin. In the young adult group, neither of these two low doses affected the circulating levels of these hormones. Immunoreactive LH in the pituitary showed declines with age. But, although a dose-related fall in pituitary LH was also present, there was no interaction of age with dose; all ages were comparably susceptible to DES exposure. In contrast, a marked interaction effect was noted for measures of immunoreactive prolactin in serum. At higher doses of DES, an elevation in prolactin is a well-documented effect. These low doses, although ineffective in raising serum prolactin levels of animals in the younger age group, were considerably more potent in the older rats. The aging animals, then, were at increased risk, at least in terms of their prolactin response to an estrogen challenge.

Changes with Age in the Reception of the Signal by the Target Cells

One of the influences contributing to age-related alterations in endocrine activity appears to be a modulation in the activity of specific transmitter systems that function to regulate hormonal release (e.g., Barraclough and Wise, 1982; Goldman, Walker, and Cooper, 1985). The releasing hormones that trigger the secretion of the gonadotropins, TSH, growth hormone, and adrenocorticotropic hormone (ACTH) from the pituitary all reside in the hypothalamus, and their release is controlled by adrenergic transmitter activity (e.g., Al-Damluji, 1988; Kalra and Kalra, 1983; Krulich et al., 1977; Martin, 1976). Also, the secretion of prolactin is under the tonic inhibitory control of dopamine (e.g., Ben-Jonathan, 1985), and there appears to be both serotonergic and cholinergic involvement in pituitary hormone release (e.g., Chihara, Arimura, and Schally, 1979; Smythe, Brandstater, and Lazarus, 1975; Walker, 1983).

There are numerous studies showing impairments of adrenergic, dopaminergic, and serotonergic activity in the senescent animal (Roth and Joseph, 1988; Telford et al., 1988; Trabucchi et al., 1982; Zhou et al., 1984). One of the underlying causes of these alterations seems to be an overall loss of receptors (e.g., Greenberg and Weiss, 1983; Roth and Joseph, 1988; Weiss, Clark, and Greenberg, 1984). Consequently, a general decline in the transmitter regulation of hormonal function may also place an aging animal at increased risk for toxicant exposure (Govoni et al., 1988), given that various environmental toxicants (e.g., the solvents vinyltoluene, ethylbenzene, and styrene; the halogenated hydrocarbon TCDD, and certain heavy metal cations) have been reported to interact with catecholaminergic systems (Arfini et al., 1987; Govoni et al., 1978, 1979; Jason and Kellogg, 1981; Lucci et al., 1981; Mutti et al., 1988; Russell et al., 1988). Work with manganese acetate has already provided some evidence that induced depletions of dopamine within the brain striatal region are much greater in 2- to $2\frac{1}{2}$-year-old rats than in 2- to 3-month-old animals (Silbergeld, 1982).

A consideration of alterations with age or toxicant exposure in the reception of a hormonal (or transmitter) message by the target cells concerns not only effects on receptor number per se, but changes in the membrane itself. It is well known that cell membranes are not rigid in structure, but exist as dynamic assemblies whose internal environments are normally maintained at a relatively constant state of fluidity. As a consequence, many of the lipids and proteins comprising the membrane are able to move in both lateral (within the membrane plane) and transverse (one side of the membrane to the other) directions. This is true for receptors as well as for other membrane components and is acknowledged to play an important role in receptor-associated functions of the cell. For example, shifts in membrane fluidity appear to mask or unmask binding sites (Danforth, Wells, and Stouffer, 1985; Dave and Witorsch, 1984; Wesemann, Weiner, and Hoffman-Bleihauer, 1986).

In aging tissue, there is evidence for a progressive decrease in membrane fluidity (Hershkowitz, 1983; Nagy et al., 1983; Samuel et al., 1982). This is at least partially attributable to alterations in the lipid composition, which is close to 50% of membrane material. Since protein activity in the membrane is influenced by the fluidity of the lipid microenvironment, any alterations with age in membrane viscosity can affect not only receptor functions, but enzymatic activity as well (Sanderman, 1978). Such changes, in turn, could alter the normal process of membrane building that involves the addition of previously assembled units of proteins and lipids that are consistent with existing membranes in composition and distribution. This process ensures an overall functional compatibility between new and old segments and is controlled by the activity and synchrony of a variety of intracellular enzymes. Consequently, alterations in this process in the aging animal can influence membrane composition and fluidity. For example, with age there are reported elevations in cholesterol, sphingolipids and saturated fatty acid chains, all leading to increases in rigidification (Rouser, Kritchevsky, and Yamamoto, 1972).

In addition to normal age-related shifts in membrane composition and fluidity, any insult to the membrane that is capable of altering its composition or configuration has the potential to alter its fluidity and functional capability. Endotoxin administration, for instance, has been found to decrease the fluidity of dog liver plasma membranes, apparently by triggering phospholipase-induced changes in membrane phospholipid composition (Liu, Ghosh, and Yang, 1983). Various environmental toxicants have been reported to cause peroxidative damage to the membrane (e.g., Litov et al., 1978; Tappel, 1973), resulting in cross-linkages among lipid and/or protein components that may impair overall membrane activity. Moreover, there are reports of increases in general peroxidative phenomena with age that diminish the fluidity of the membrane (Hegner, 1980; Schroeder, 1984). It may be then that the normal age-related processes of membrane rigidification (i.e., shifts in membrane lipid composition and peroxidative cross-linking) increase the levels of vulnerability of the aging membrane to toxicant-induced disruptions in function. Such a possibility, discussed in greater detail in Chapter 2, is particularly relevant to such perturbations in the mechanisms of hormonal signal transduction at the target cell membrane.

Changes in the Nature of the
Hormonal Message with Age

The relationship between hormonal immunoactivity and bioactivity has been of concern to endocrine scientists ever since immunoassay methods entered the endocrine armamentarium and markedly increased the ease with which quantitative hormone measures are obtained. The antigenic site(s) on a hormone recognized by antibodies can be quite distinct from those regions that bind to the receptors that trigger a physiological response in the target tissue. The distinction takes on added importance for studies in aging, because alterations with age in peptide hormone structure have been reported (Conn et al., 1980) that indicate effects on posttranslational processes. These effects, moreover, may be influenced by shifts in the steroid hormonal milieu in the older animal (Ulloa-Aguirre et al., 1988). A number of hormones are glycosylated to varying degrees and such differences in their carbohydrate residues may alter biological activity (Ulloa-Aguirre and Chappel, 1982; Warner, Dufau, and Santen, 1985) and/or plasma half-life (Morrell et al., 1971). Consequently, hormonal measures based solely on immunoreactivity per se may potentially offer a somewhat inaccurate picture of endocrine alterations with age.

The Effects of Hormones on the Aging Process

The preceding section addressed the role that age-related changes in neuroendocrine function may play in modifying the responsiveness of the aged organism to environmental toxicants. An alternate consideration in environmental toxicology concerns the effects that toxicants, acting through neuroendocrine mechanisms, can have on the rate of aging, or the rate at which those changes associated with aging typically appear. These changes fall into two general categories: (a) organizational effects that occur in the developing organism and (b) alterations induced by toxicants in the adult.

Organizational Effects of Hormones

Manipulations of the early hormonal environment have been shown to have a marked influence on the development and subsequent function of a wide range of physiological and behavioral processes in adulthood. Often these organizational effects depend on the presence or absence of hormonal stimulation during restricted developmental stages or critical periods (Goy and Goldfoot, 1973). Furthermore, these effects tend to be irreversible and may be permanent, although their expression is often temporally delayed. More specifically, alterations of the typical levels of thyroid, adrenal, or gonadal hormones during certain early developmental stages have been shown to have lasting effects on physiological and behavioral functions in adulthood and late life (Eayrs, 1960; Levine and Mullins, 1966; Phoenix et al., 1959).

Experimentally induced hypothyroidism during the perinatal period leads to lethargy in adulthood (Levine and Mullins, 1966), alterations in CNS development including decreases in axonal growth and synaptic formation (Verity et al., 1976; Weichsel and Dawson, 1976), and lasting changes in the animal's metabolic rate (Balazs et al., 1971) that persist into adulthood. Experimental manipulation of adrenal cortical hormone concentration in the developing organism has also been shown to influence the function of the pituitary–adrenal axis, CNS development (Howard, 1968), and behavior (Joffe, Milkovic, and Levine, 1972; Nyakas and Endroczi, 1972), in the adult. It is also important to note that changes in the typical organizational effects of the adrenal hormones may have broad consequences for other homeostatic processes. Recent evidence shows a clear interrelationship between the function of the immune system and the pituitary–adrenal hormones (Bateman et al., 1989).

Perhaps the most dramatic, or at least the most studied, endocrine manipulations are those that affect adult reproduction physiology and behavior. In several species, the presence of androgens during particular "critical periods" of development will "masculinize" the central nervous system. This neonatal or perinatal exposure results in identifiable morphological differences between the male and female brain, as well as distinct differences in the ways in which the two sexes respond behaviorally to gonadal hormones in adulthood (Gorski, 1986).

Because many xenobiobtics alter endocrine function, brief exposure of the organism to certain environmental toxins could dramatically modify subsequent developmental and aging processes. For example, it has been shown that exposure to DES and other estrogenic pesticides will alter the normal development and aging of the female rat's reproductive system (Gorski, 1971). These effects are discussed in more detail in Chapter 9. In addition, it is likely that exposure to agents that alter thyroid (e.g., urea-based compounds) or adrenal function (e.g., dexamethasone) could alter normal development of the organism and how that organism subsequently ages.

Alterations of the Aging Process Induced by Toxicants in the Adult Animal

Several compounds have been shown to disrupt normal endocrine function in the adult animal. Treatment with many of these compounds results in an endocrine alteration that is similar to that observed in the aged animal. For example, compounds that affect the release of LH from the pituitary of the young adult female rat can induce a pattern of persistent estrus that is the endocrine state typically present in the aged female (Cooper, McNamara, and Linnoila, 1986). This change in the endocrine profile can have broad-reaching sequelae at both the physiological and behavioral levels (e.g., altered immune and metabolic function [Grossman, 1984; Gustafsson et al., 1983; Luebke et al., 1984]).

Treatment with synthetic adrenal corticoids has been shown to alter the rate of age-related changes within the hippocampus (Finch and Landfield, 1985). Similarly, compounds such as dexamethasone that bind to the adrenal steroid receptors cause changes within the CNS that are similar to those seen in the older organism (Finch and Landfield, 1985; Sapolsky, Krey, and McEwen, 1986). The hippocampal region is known to bind corticosterone (Gerlach and McEwen, 1972) and appears to be involved in the inhibitory regulation of ACTH by the hypothalamus (Keller-Wood and Dallman, 1984). Any damaging effects of cumulative corticoid feedback on the hippocampus could then alter the regulation of pituitary ACTH secretion in the older animal (Sapolsky, Krey, and McEwen, 1985). Such observations have led to a more generalized hypothesis that many of the alterations present in the older organism are attributable to accrued damage from the lifelong exposure to endogenous hormones. Accordingly, it has been demonstrated that sustained exposure to the gonadal steroid estradiol results in alterations of the hypothalamic feedback mechanisms involved in the pituitary's control of ovulation. Cumulative damage to CNS tissue has been noted in intact female rats and in rats that are ovariectomized in adulthood and implanted with extradiol-containing capsules (Brawer, Schipper, and Robaire, 1983). This would suggest that during the reproductive life span of the female each preovulatory elevation of plasma estradiol destroys a fraction of the axonal connections within the hypothalamic regions associated with the control of neuroendocrine function until the accumulated damage eventually disrupts the feedback regulation of ovarian function (Brawer, Schipper, and Robaire, 1983). Conversely, preventing the typical pattern of exposure to estradiol to the organism (by ovariectomy) delays or blocks the occurrence of many of the conditions (see below) present in late life (Brawer and Finch, 1983).

The effect of estradiol exposure on tumor development provides another example of how imbalances in the endocrine milieu may contribute to age-associated pathologies. Mammany gland tumors are typical in the old female rat, and the probability that an animal will develop such a tumor increases with age (Cooper, 1983; Meites, Goya, and Takahashi, 1987). These tumors begin to appear in females between 15 and 20 months, and their incidence can be dramatically reduced by ovariectomy in adulthood. For example, it was found that when females were ovariectomized at 4 months and observed until 32 months of age, no mammary tumors were present (Cooper, 1983).

The significance of estrogen to the development of such tumors is underscored by the fact that mammary gland tumors were present in 100 percent of animals ovariectomized at 4 months and observed at 12 months of age, if the animals were implanted with capsules containing estradiol at the time of ovariectomy. Because several compounds have inherent estrogenic activity (e.g., dichloro-diphenyl-trichloroethane, methoxychlor, and zearalenone [Bulger and Kupfer, 1985]), chronic exposure to low levels of these compounds or brief exposure at doses sufficient to alter permanently reproductive cycling in the rat could have significant impact on the pathophysiological condition of the aging animal.

The pituitary gland and the gonadal and adrenal steroids also are known to affect immune function. The extent to which the functions of the endocrine and immune system are interdependent is only now becoming evident (Bateman et al., 1989; Buzzetti et al., 1988; Grossman, 1984). Estrogens depress most, if not all, of the major functions attributed to the cell-mediated immune system, although the precise mechanism(s) remains unclear (Myers, Butler, and Peterson, 1986). Serum estrogen levels are correlated with the production of natural killer cells and the ability to ward off infection (Luebke et al., 1984). Thus, it may be anticipated that immune function could be compromised with advancing age if the adrenal and gonadal hormone titers are altered. Similarly, any perturbation of steroid secretion resulting from exposure to a toxic compound might be expected to influence immune function in late life.

The pituitary and gonadal hormones also have been implicated in the maintenance of a number of other functions. Because there is steroid hormonal feedback to the CNS, alterations in serum levels could have a direct effect on a number of neurotransmitter and behavioral functions (Lofstrom et al., 1977). Also, pituitary hormones alter monoamine oxidase activity and could thus affect both central and peripheral metabolic function (Illsley, Kita, and Lamartiniere, 1980). Such alterations would obviously influence the response to numerous xenobiotics known to modify neurotransmitter function and would likely contribute to any age differences in response. Similarly, estrogens have recently been implicated in the regulation of extrapyramidal functions in rats and humans, and it has been hypothesized that age-related changes in the concentrations of these hormones may be involved in the development of certain age-related extrapyramidal disorders (Van Hartesveldt and Joyce, 1986). Gonadal steroids also are known to affect liver enzyme function. Sex differences exist in steroid and xenobiotic metabolism within the liver of a number of species. In the rat, these metabolic differences appear to be regulated through the hypothalamic–pituitary axis (Gustafsson et al., 1983; Kamataki et al., 1985). The extent to which age differences in hypothalamic–pituitary–gonadal or adrenal function contribute to age-dependent changes in liver function remains to be explored.

Finally, embedded within the category of endocrine-induced effects on the rate of aging is a consideration of aging per se versus the changes associated with the endocrine status as it exists at the time. For example, the pattern of estrogen secretion present in the aged female rat may alter a variety of physiological responses compared with the young adult female. These altered responses are most often attributed solely to the difference in age between the two groups. But, when the pattern of estrogen secretion in the young is matched to that present in the old female, some of the reported "age differences" are no longer present (Cooper et al., 1984). In terms of risk assessment, however, it may not be necessary to tease apart these factors, since age-related alterations in the endocrine milieu can be considered an integral part of the "package" of changes that comprise the aging process.

Summary

Much of the evidence in support of an increase in the susceptibility of the aging organism to toxic insult is still presumptive. We are dealing with separate relationships to endocrine homeostasis as a common factor. Declines in endocrine homeostasis occur with age, and a large number of toxicants are able to affect the endocrine milieu either directly or indirectly. The logical presumption, then, is that there is an alteration in the susceptibility of the endocrine system to toxicant exposure late in life, during a time when the system is already giving evidence of homeostatic deterioration. Although this is a very real possibility, it should be understood that even the existence of such a relationship within one endocrine-associated organ system does not necessarily mean that other systems are at comparable risk from insult. Considerable variability may exist. Nevertheless, given the widespread influence of endocrine factors, the potential for impact is clear.

This diversity and extent of the endocrine influence throughout the body also mean that the scope of this chapter had to be balanced against considerations of economy. Consequently, discussions of such important age-related issues as late-onset diabetes (and the numerous effects on the individual's physiological well-being), among others, were not included. It is evident, however, that our understanding of the relationships between a changing endocrine environment and the sensitivity of the aging organism to toxicant exposure is just beginning to emerge.

References

Al-Damluji, S. 1988. Adrenergic mechanisms in the control of corticotrophin secretion. *Journal of Endocrinology* 119:5–14.

Arfini, G., Mutti, A., Vescovi, P., Ferroni, C., Ferrari, M., Giaroli, C., Passeri, M., and Franchini, I. 1987. Impaired dopaminergic modulation of pituitary secretion in workers occupationally exposed to styrene: Further evidence from PRL response to TRH stimulation. *Journal of Occupational Medicine* 29:826–830.

Balazs, R., Cocks, W. A., Eayrs, J. R., and Kovacs, S. 1971. Biochemical effects of thyroid hormones on the developing brain. In Hamburgh, M., and Barrington, E. J. W. (Eds.), *Hormones in Development*. New York, Appleton-Century-Crofts, pp. 357–379.

Barraclough, C. A., and Wise, P. M. 1982. The role of catecholamines in the regulation of pituitary LH and FSH secretion. *Endocrine Reviews* 3:91–119.

Bateman, A., Singh, A., Kral, T., and Solomon, S. 1989. The immune–hypothalamic–pituitary–adrenal axis. *Endocrine Reviews* 10:92–112.

Ben-Jonathan, N. 1985. Dopamine: A prolactin-inhibiting hormone. *Endocrine Reviews* 6:564–589.

Bilchert-Toft, M. 1978. The adrenal glands in old age. In Greenblatt, R. B. (Ed.), *Geriatric Endocrinology: Vol. 5. Aging*. New York, Raven Press, pp. 81–102.

Brawer, J. R., and Finch, C. E. 1983. Normal and experimentally altered aging processes in the rodent hypothalamus and pituitary. In Walker R. F., and Cooper, R. L. (Eds.), *Experimental and Clinical Interventions in Aging*. New York, Marcel Dekker, pp. 45–65.

Brawer, J., Schipper, H., and Robaire, B. 1983. Effects of long term androgen and estradiol exposure on the hypothalamus. *Endocrinology* 112:194–199.

Bremner, W. J., Vitiello, M. V., and Prinz, P. N. 1983. Loss of circadian rhythmicity in blood testosterone with aging in normal men. *Journal of Clinical Endocrinology and Metabolism* 56:1278–1281.

Bulger, W. H., and Kupfer, D. 1985. Estrogenic activity of pesticides and other xenobiotics on the uterus and male reproductive tract. In Thomas, J. A., Korach, K. S., and McLachlan, J. A. (Eds.), *Endocrine Toxicology*. New York, Raven Press, pp. 1–33.

Buzzetti, R., McLoughlin, L., Scavo, D., and Rees, L. H. 1988. A critical assessment of the interactions between the immune system and the hypothalamo–pituitary–adrenal axis. *Journal of Endocrinology* 120:183–187.

Chihara, K., Arimura, A., and Schally, A. V. 1979. Effect of intraventricular injection of dopamine, norepinephrine, acetylcholine, and 5-hydroxytryptamine on immunoreactive somatostatin release into rat hypophyseal portal blood. *Endocrinology* 104:1656–1662.

Conn, P. M., Cooper, R. L., McNamara, M. C., Rogers, D. C., and Shoenhardt, L. 1980. Qualitative change in gonadotropin during normal aging in the male rat. *Endocrinology* 106:1549–1553.

Cooper, R. L. 1983. Pharmacological and dietary manipulations of reproductive aging in the rat. Significance to central nervous system aging. In Walker, R. F., and Cooper, R. L. (Eds.), *Experimental and Clinical Interventions in Aging*. New York, Marcel Dekker, pp. 27–44.

Cooper, R. L., Goldman, J. M., and Rehnberg, G. L. 1986. Pituitary function following treatment with reproductive toxins. *Environmental Health Perspectives* 70:177–184.

Cooper, R. L., McNamara, M. C., and Linnoila, M. 1986. Catecholaminergic serotonergic balance in the CNS and reproductive cycling in aging rats. *Neurobiology of Aging* 7:9–16.

Cooper, R. L., Roberts, B., Rogers, D. C., Seay, S. G., and Conn, P. M. 1984. Endocrine status versus chronological age as predictors of altered luteinizing hormone secretion in the aging rat. *Endocrinology* 114:391–396.

Danforth, D. R., Wells, M. A., and Stouffer, R. L. 1985. Modulation of membrane fluidity in the primate (*Macaca mulatta*) corpus luteum: Correlation with changes in gonadotropin binding. *Endocrinology* 117:755–761.

Dave, J. R., and Witorsch, R. J. 1984. Modulation of prolactin binding sites in vitro by membrane fluidizers. II. Age-dependent effects on rat ventral prostatic membranes. *Biochimica et Biophysica Acta* 772:321–327.

Eayrs, J. T. 1960. Influence of the thyroid on the central nervous system. *British Medical Bulletin* 16:122–126.

Ellis, G. B., and Desjardins, C. 1982. Male rats secrete luteinizing hormone and testosterone episodically. *Endocrinology* 110:1618–1627.

Finch, C. E., and Landfield, P. W. 1985. Neuroendocrine and autonomic functions in aging mammals. In Finch, C. E., and Schneider, E. L. (Eds.), *Handbook of the Biology of Aging* (2nd ed.), New York, Van Nostrand Reinhold, pp. 645–691.

Gerlach, J. L., and McEwen, B. S. 1972. Rat brain binds adrenal steroid hormone: Radioautography of hippocampus with corticosterone. *Science* 175:1133–1136.

Goldman, J. M., Cooper, R. L., Laws, S. C., Rehnberg, G. L., Edwards, T. L., McElroy, W. K., and Hein, J. F. 1990. Chlordimeform-induced alterations in endocrine regulation within the male rat reproductive system. *Toxicology and Applied Pharmacology* 104:25–35.

Goldman, J. M., Walker, R. F., and Cooper, R. L. 1985. Aging in the rat hypothalamic–pituitary–ovarian axis: The involvement of biogenic amines in the loss of reproductive cyclicity. In Parvez, H., Parvez, S., and Gupta, D. (Eds.), *Neuroendocrinology of Hormone–Transmitter Interactions.* Utrecht, VNU Science Press, pp. 127–152.

Gorski, R. A. 1971. Gonadal hormones and the perinatal development of neuroendocrine function. In Martini, L., and Ganong, W. F. (Eds.), *Frontiers in Neuroendocrinology.* New York, Oxford University Press, pp. 237–290.

Gorski, R. A. 1986. Sexual differentiation of the brain: A model for drug-induced alterations of the reproductive system. *Environmental Health Perspectives* 70:163–175.

Govoni, S., Memo, M., Spano, P. F., and Trabucchi, M. 1979. Chronic lead treatment differentially affects dopamine synthesis in various rat brain areas. *Toxicology* 12:343–349.

Govoni, S., Montefusco, O., Spano, P. F., and Trabucchi, M. 1978. Effect of chronic lead treatment on brain dopamine synthesis and serum prolactin release in the rat. *Toxicology Letters* 2:333–337.

Govoni, S., Rius, R. A., Battaini, F., Magnoni, M. S., Lucchi, L., and Trabucchi, M. 1988. The central dopaminergic system: Susceptibility to risk factors for accelerated aging. *Gerontology* 34:29–34.

Goy, R. W., and Goldfoot, D. A. 1973. Hormonal influences on sexually dimorphic behavior. In *Handbook of Physiology. Endocrinology II, Part 1.* Washington, DC, American Physiological Society, 169–186.

Gray, G. D., Smith, E. R., and Davidson, J. M. 1980. Gonadotropin regulation in middle-aged male rats. *Endocrinology* 107:2021–2026.

Greenberg, L. H., and Weiss, B. 1983. Neuroendocrine control of catecholaminergic receptors in aging brain. In Agnoli, A., Crepaldi, G., Spano, P. F., and Trabucchi, M. (Eds.), *Aging Brain and Ergot Alkaloids.* New York, Raven Press, pp. 37–52.

Grossman, C. J. 1984. Regulation of the immune system by sex steroids. *Endocrine Reviews* 5:435–455.

Gustafsson, J-A., Mode, A., Norstedt, G., and Skett, P. 1983. Sex steroid induced changes in hepatic enzymes. *Annual Review of Physiology* 45:51–60.

Hegner, D. 1980. Age-dependence of molecular and functional changes in biological membrane properties. *Mechanisms of Ageing and Development* 14:101–118.

Hershkowitz, M. 1983. Mechanisms of brain aging—the role of membrane fluidity. In Gispen, W. H., and Traber, J. (Eds.), *Aging of the Brain.* New York, Elsevier, pp. 85–98.

Howard, E. 1968. Reductions in size and total DNA of cerebrum and cerebellum in adult mice after corticosterone treatment in infancy. *Experimental Neurology* 22:191–208.

Illsley, N. P., Kita, E., and Lamartiniere, C. A. 1980. Role of pituitary in modulating hepatic monoamine oxidase activity. *Endocrinology* 106:798–804.

Jason, K. M., and Kellogg, C. K. 1981. Neonatal lead exposure: Effects on development of behavior and striatal dopamine neurons. *Pharmacology, Biochemistry and Behavior* 15:641–649.

Jick, H. Porter, J., and Morrison, A. S. 1977. Relation between smoking and age of natural menopause. *Lancet* 1:1354–1355.

Joffee, J. M., Milkovic, K., and Levine, S. 1972. Effects of changes in maternal pituitary–adrenal function on behavior of rat offspring. *Physiology and Behavior* 8:277–288.

Jones, M. K., Weisenburger, W. P., Sipes, I. G., and Russell, D. H. 1987. Circadian alterations in prolactin, corticosterone, and thyroid hormone levels and down-regulation of prolactin receptor activity by 2,3,7,8-tetrachlorodibenzo-p-dioxin. *Toxicology and Applied Pharmacology* 87:337–350.

Kalra, S. P., and Kalra, P. S. 1983. Neural regulation of luteinizing hormone secretion in the rat. *Endocrine Reviews* 4:311–351.

Kamataki, T., Shimada, M., Maeda, K., and Kato, R. 1985. Pituitary regulation of sex-specific forms of cytochrome P-450 in liver microsomes of rats. *Biochemical and Biophysical Research Communications* 130:1247–1253.

Karpas, A. E., Bremner, W. J., Flifton, D. K., Steiner, R.A., and Dorsa, D. M. 1983. Diminished luteinizing hormone pulse frequency and amplitude with aging in the male rat. *Endocrinology* 112:788–792.

Kato, H., Saito, M., and Suda, M. 1980. Effect of starvation on the circadian adrenocortical rhythm in rats. *Endocrinology* 106:918–921.

Kato, R., Yamazoe, Y., Shimada, M., Murayama, N., and Kamataki, T. 1986. Effect of growth hormone and ectopic transplantation of pituitary gland on sex-specific forms of cytochrome P-450 and testosterone and drug oxidations in rat liver. *Journal of Biochemistry* 100:895–902.

Keller-Wood, M. W., and Dallman, M. F. 1984. Corticosteroid inhibition of ACTH secretion. *Endocrine Reviews* 5:1–106.

Kinson, G. A., and Liu, C. 1973. Diurnal variation in plasma testosterone of the male laboratory rat. *Hormone and Metabolic Research* 5:233–234.

Krulich, L. A., Giachetti, A., Marchlewska-Koj, A., Hefco, E., and Jameson, H. E. 1977. On the role of the central noradrenergic and dopaminergic systems in the regulation of TSH secretion in the rat. *Endocrinology* 100:496–505.

Leppaluoto, J., Ranta, T., and Tuomisto, J., 1974. Diurnal variations of serum immunoassayable thyrotropin (TSH) concentration in the rat. *Acta Physiologica Scandinavica* 90:699–702.

Levine, S., and Mullins, R. F. 1966. Hormonal influences on brain organization in infant rats. *Science* 156:1585–1592.

Litov, R. E., Irving, D. H., Downey, J. E., and Tappel, A. L. 1978. Lipid peroxidation: A mechanism involved in acute ethanol toxicity as demonstrated by in vivo pentane production in the rat. *Lipids* 13:305–307.

Liu, M.-S., Ghosh, S., and Yang, Y. 1983. Changes in membrane fluidity induced by phospholipase A activation: A mechanism of endotoxic shock. *Life Sciences* 33:1995–2002.

Lofstrom, A., Enroth, P., Gustafsson, J.-A., and Skett, P. 1977. Effects of extradiol benzoate on the catecholamine levels and turnover in discrete areas of the median eminence and the limbic forebrain, and on serum luteinizing hormone, follicle-stimulating and prolactin concentrations in the ovariectomized female rat. *Endocrinology* 101:1559–1569.

Lucci, L., Memo, M., Airaghi, M. L., Spano, P. F., Trabucchi, M. 1981. Chronic lead treatment induces in rat a specific and differential effect on dopamine receptors in different brain areas. *Brain Research* 213:397–404.

Luebke, R. W., Luster, M. I., Dean, J. H., and Hayes, H. T. 1984. Altered host resistance to *Trichinella spiralis* infection following subchronic exposure to diethylstilbestrol. *International Journal of Immunopharmacology* 6:609–617.

MacGeoch, C., Morgan, E. T., and Gustafsson, J. A. 1985. Hypothalmo–pituitary regulation of cytochrome P-450$_{15\beta}$ apoprotein levels in rat liver. *Endocrinology* 117:2085–2092.

Martin, J. B. 1976. Brain regulation of growth hormone secretion. In Martini, L., and Ganong, W. F. (Eds.), *Frontiers in Neuroendocrinology* (Vol. 4). New York, Raven Press, pp. 129–168.

Meites, J., Goya, R., and Takahashi, S. 1987. Why the neuroendocrine system is important in aging processes. *Experimental Gerontology* 22:1–15.

Meites, J., Steger, R. W., and Huang, H. H. 1980. Relation of neuroendocrine system to the reproductive decline in aging rats and human subjects. *Federation Proceedings* 39:3168–3172.

Millard, W. J., O'Sullivan, D. M., Fox, T. O., and Martin, J. B. 1985. Sexually dimorphic patterns of growth hormone secretion in rats. In Crowley, W. F., Jr., and Hofler, J. G. (Eds.), *The Episodic Secretion of Hormones*. New York, John Wiley, pp. 287–304.

Moberg, G. P., Bellinger, L. L., and Mendel, V. E. 1975. Effect of meal feeding on daily rhythms of plasma corticosterone and growth hormone in rat. *Neuroendocrinology* 19:160–169.

Morrell, A. G., Gregoriadis, G., Scheinberg, I. H., Hickman, J., and Ashwell, G. 1971. The role of sialic acid in determining the survival of glycoproteins in the circulation. *Journal of Biological Chemistry* 246:1461–1467.

Mutti, A., Falzoi, M., Romanelli, A., Bocchi, M. C., Ferroni, C., and Franchini, I. 1988. Brain dopamine as a target for solvent toxicity: Effects of some monocyclic aromatic hydrocarbons. *Toxicology* 49:77–82.

Myers, M. J., Butler, L. D., and Peterson, B. H. 1986. Estradiol-induced alteration in the immune system. II. Suppression of cellular immunity in the rat is not the result of direct estrogenic action. *Immunopharmacology* 11:47–55.

Nagy, K., Zs.-Nagy, V., Bertoni-Freddari, C., and Zs.-Nagy, I. 1983. Alterations of the synaptosomal membrane "microviscosity" in the brain cortex of rats during aging and centrophenoxine treatment. *Archives of Gerontology and Geriatrics* 2:23–29.

Nebert, D. W., and Gonzalez, F. J. 1987. P450 Genes—structure, evolution and regulation. *Annual Review of Biochemistry* 56:945–993.

Nyakas, C., and Endorczi, E. 1972. Effect of neonatal corticosterone administration on behavioral and pituitary–adrenocortical responses in the rat. *Acta Physiologica Academiae Scientiarum Hungaricae* 42:231–241.

Phoenix, C. H., Goy, R. W., Gerall, A. A., and Young, W. C. 1959. Organizing action of prenatally administered testosterone propionate on the tissues mediating mating behavior in the female guinea pig. *Endocrinology* 65:369–382.

Rehnberg, G. L., Goldman, J. M., Cooper, R. L., Hein, J. F., McElroy, W. K., Booth, K. C., and Gray, L. E. 1988a. Effect of linuron on the brain–pituitary–testicular reproductive axis in the rat (abstract). *The toxicologist* 8:121.

Rehnberg, G. L., Linder, R., Goldman, J. M., Hein, J. F., McElroy, W. K., and Cooper, R. L. 1988b. Changes in testicular and serum hormone concentrations in the male rat following treatment with m-dinitrobenzene. *Toxicology and Applied Pharmacology* 95:255–264.

Resko, J. A., and Eik-Nes, K. B. 1966. Diurnal testosterone levels in peripheral plasma of human male subjects. *Journal of Clinical Endocrinology and Metabolism* 26:573–576.

Roth, G. S., and Joseph, J. A. 1988. Peculiarities of the effect of hormones and transmitters during aging: Modulation of changes in dopaminergic action. *Gerontology* 34:22–28.

Rouser, G., Kritchevsky, G., and Yamamoto, A. 1972. Lipids in the nervous system of different species as a function of age: Brain, spinal cord, peripheral nerve, purified whole cell preparations and subcellular particulates: Regulatory mechanisms and membrane structure. *Advances in Lipid Research* 10:261–360.

Russell, D. H., Buckley, A. R., Shah, G. N., Sipes, I. G., Blask, D. E., and Benson, B. 1988. Hypothalamic site of action of 2,3,7,8-tetrachlorodibenzo-p-dioxin (TCDD). *Toxicology and Applied Pharmacology* 94:496–502.

Samuel, D., Heron, D. S., Hershkowitz, M., and Shinitzky, M. 1982. Aging, receptor binding, and membrane microviscosity. In Giacobini, E., Filogamo, G., Giacobini, G., and Vernadakis, A. (Eds.), *The Aging Brain: Cellular and Molecular Mechanisms of Aging in the Nervous System* (Vol. 20). New York, Raven Press, pp. 93–97.

Sandermann, H., Jr. 1978. Regulation of membrane enzymes by lipids. *Biochima et Biophysica Acta* 515:209–237.

Sapolsky, R. M., Krey, L. C., and McEwen, B. S. 1985. Prolonged glucocorticoid exposure reduces hippocampal neuron number: Implications for aging. *Journal of Neuroscience* 5:1221–1226.

Sapolsky, R. M., Krey, L. C., and McEwen, B. S. 1986. The neuroendocrinology of stress and aging: The glucocorticoid cascade hypothesis. *Endocrine Reviews* 7:284–301.

Schilsky, R. L., Sherins, R. J., Hubbard, S. M., Wesley, M. N., Young, R. C., and DeVita, V. T. 1981. Long-term follow-up of ovarian function in women treated with MOPP chemotherapy for Hodgkin's disease. *American Journal of Medicine* 71:552–556.

Schroeder, F. 1984. Role of membrane lipid asymmetry in aging. *Neurobiology of Aging* 5:323–333.

Schuetz, E. G., Wrighton, S. A., Barwick, J. L., and Guzelian, P. S. 1984. Induction of cytochrome P-450 by glucocorticoids in rat liver. I. Evidence that glucocorticoids and pregnenolone 16α-carbonitrile regulate de novo synthesis of a common form of cytochrome P-450 in cultures of adult rat hepatocytes and in the liver in vivo. *Journal of Biological Chemistry* 259:1999–2006.

Silbergeld, E. K. 1982. Current state of neurotoxicology, basic and applied. *Trends in Neuroscience* 5:291–294.

Simmons, D. L., McQuiddy, P., and Kasper, C. B. 1987. Induction of the hepatic mixed-function oxidase system by synthetic glucocorticoids—transcriptional and post-transcriptional regulation. *Journal of Biological Chemistry* 262:326–332.

Smythe, G. A., Brandstater, J. F., and Lazarus, L. 1975. Serotonergic control of rat growth hormone secretion. *Neuroendocrinology* 17:245–257.

Sontag, W. E., Hylka, W., and Meites, J. 1983. Impaired ability of old male rats to secrete GH in vivo but not in vitro in response to hpGRF 1-44. *Endocrinology* 113:2305–2307.

Sonntag, W. E., Steger, R. W., Forman, L. J., and Meites, J. 1980. Decreased pulsatile release of growth hormone in old male rats. *Endocrinology* 107:1875–1879.

Steger, R. W., Huang, H.-H., Hafez, E. S. E., and Meites, J. 1980. Changes in control of gonadotropin secretion in the transcription period between regular cycles and constant estrus in aging female rats. *Biology of Reproduction* 22:595–603.

Steiner, R. A., Bremmer, W. J., Clifton, D. K., and Dorsa, D. M. 1984. Reduced pulsatile luteinizing hormone and testosterone secretion with aging in the male rat. *Biology of Reproduction* 31:251–258.

Tappel, A. L. 1973. Lipid peroxidation damage to cell components. *Federation Proceedings* 32:1870–1874.

Telford, N., Mobbs, C. V., Osterburg, H. H., and Finch, C. E. 1988. Alterations in hypothalamic serotonergic–catecholaminergic relationships in aging C57BL/6J female mice. *Experimental Gerontology* 23:481–489.

Tenover, J. S., Matsumoto, A. M., Clifton, D. K., and Bremner, W. J. 1988. Age-related alterations in the circadian rhythms of pulsatile luteinizing hormone and testosterone secretion in healthy men. *Journal of Gerontology* 43:M163–169.

Trabucchi, M., Spano, P. F., Govoni, S., Riccardi, F., and Bosio, A. 1982. Dopaminergic function during aging in rat brain. In Giacobini, E., Filogamo, G., Giacobini, G., and Vernadakis, A. (Eds.), *The Aging Brain: Cellular and Molecular Mechanisms of Aging in the Central Nervous System* (Vol. 20). New York, Raven Press, pp. 195–201.

Ulloa-Aguirre, A., and Chappel, S. C. 1982. Multiple species of follicle-stimulating hormone exist within the anterior pituitary of male golden hamsters. *Journal of Endocrinology* 95:257–266.

Ulloa-Aguirre, A., Espinoza, R., Damian-Matsumura, P., and Chappel, S. C.

1988. Immunological and biological potencies of the different molecular species of gonadotrophins. *Human Reproduction* 3:491–501.

Vanhaelst, L., Van Cauter, E., Degaute, J. P., and Golstein, J. 1972. Circadian variations of serum thyrotropin levels in man. *Journal of Clinical Endocrinology and Metabolism* 35:479–482.

Van Hartesveldt, C., and Joyce, J. N. 1986. Effects of estrogen on the basal ganglia. *Neuroscience and Biobehavioral Reviews* 10:1–14.

Verity, M. A., Brown, W. J., Cheung, M., Huntsman, H., and Smith, R. 1976. Effects of neonatal hypothyroidism on cerebral and cerebellar synaptosome development. *Journal of Neuroscience Research* 2:323–335.

Vermeulen, A., Deslypere, J. P., and Kaufman, J. M. 1989. Influence of antiopioids on luteinizing hormone pulsality in aging men. *Journal of Clinical Endocrinology and Metabolism* 68:68–72.

Walker, R. F. 1983. Quantitative and temporal aspects of serotonin's facilitatory action on phasic secretion of luteinizing hormone in female rats. *Neuroendocrinology* 36:468–474.

Warner, B. A., Dufau, M. L., and Santen, R. J. 1985. Effects of aging and illness on the pituitary testicular axis in men: Qualitative as well as quantitative changes in luteinizing hormone. *Journal of Clinical Endocrinology and Metabolism* 60:263–268.

Weichsel, M. E., Jr., and Dawson, L. 1976. Effect of hypothyroidism and undernutrition on DNA content and thymidine kinase activity during cerebellar development in the rat. *Journal of Neurochemistry* 26:675–681.

Weiss, B., Clark, M. B., and Greenberg, L. H. 1984. Modulation of catecholaminergic receptors during development and aging. In Lajtha, A. (Ed.), *Handbook of Neurochemistry:* Vol. 6. *Receptors in the Nervous System.* New York, Plenum Press, pp. 595–627.

Wesemann, W., Weiner, N., and Hoffmann-Bleihauer, P. 1986. Modulation of serotonin binding in rat brain by membrane fluidity. *Neurochemistry International* 9:447–454.

Winters, S. J., and Troen, P. 1982. Episodic luteinizing hormone (LH) secretion and the response of LH and follicle-stimulating hormone to LH-releasing hormone in aged men—evidence for co-existent primary testicular insufficiency and an impairment in gonadotropin secretion. *Journal of Clinical Endocrinology* 55:560–565.

Yamazoe, Y., Shimada, M., Murayama, N., and Kato, R. 1987. Suppression of levels of phenobarbital-inducible rat-liver cytochrome B-450 by pituitary hormone. *Journal of Biological Chemistry* 262:7423–7428.

Zhou, L-W., Weiss, B., Freilich, J. S., and Greenberg, L. H. 1984. Impaired recovery of alpha$_1$- and alpha$_2$-adrenergic receptors in brain tissue of aged rats. *Journal of Gerontology* 39:538–546.

9

Delayed Effects on Reproduction following Exposure to Toxic Chemicals during Critical Periods of Development

Leon Earl Gray, Jr., Ph.D

Although it has been widely recognized since the thalidomide "incident" of the 1950s that exposure to toxic chemicals during gestation can adversely affect fetal outcome, it is becoming increasingly apparent that the consequences of exposure in utero may include functional deficits in the absence of gross morphological malformations (Hutchings, 1978). Organ systems that differentiate during the fetal or early neonatal periods but do not function until after birth cannot be adequately evaluated using standard test procedures that examine the morphology of the near-term fetal rodent or rabbit. For this reason, the detection of functional alterations of the central nervous system (CNS), reproductive, immune, and kidney function, for example, requires an evaluation of the postnatal development of the pups.

In addition to functional alterations of these organ systems, chemical carcinogens ingested by a pregnant female have been shown to induce tumors in the offspring later in life (Rice, 1981). These observations are of concern because similar developmental abnormalities have been observed in humans following exposure in utero to xenobiotic chemicals and drugs. For example, reproductive tract lesions and reduced reproductive capacity have been noted in men and women exposed in utero to diethylstilbestrol (DES) (Schmidt et al., 1980), behavioral problems have been reported in children of heroin and cocaine addicts and alcoholics (Hutchings, 1978), and accidental contamination of the food of pregnant women in Japan with methyl mercury altered CNS and behavioral development of the children. In addition to causing reproductive problems, prenatal DES is a transplacental carcinogen in humans.

   This chapter discusses the phenomena and mechanisms of perinatal reproductive development and relates alterations of this process to infertility and reproductive senescence.

Perinatal Reproductive Development

During the past 50 years, it has been held that steroids can modify development during a short period of early life. During this critical period, it was proposed, steroids either sensitize or organize the structure and function of steroid-sensitive tissues, including the brain, reproductive tract, liver, and kidney. The critical period for these permanent steroid effects was thought to be restricted to prenatal life in long-gestation mammals and to continue into postnatal life in the short-gestation species, including most rodents. Female rats, mice, and hamsters are sterilized and behaviorally masculinized by exposure to testosterone or estradiol during the first few days after birth (vom Saal and Finch, 1988). In contrast to the effects of neonatal steroid exposure seen in rodents, exposure to androgens during prenatal sex differentiation does not result in sterility in primates, although there are marked effects on morphology and behavior (Goy and McEwen, 1980).

   Sexual development of the male or female phenotype from an indifferent state, entails a complex series of events. Genetic sex is determined at fertilization and the sex chromosomes direct the differentiation of gonadal sex. At this stage of embryonic development the male and female are morphologically identical and the reproductive tract and external genitalia have bisexual potential. Primordial germ cells (PGCs) migrate to the future genital ridges, increasing in numbers as they migrate. Gonadal sex differentiation occurs after the arrival of the PGCs and, subsequently, gonadal secretions induce the further differentiation of the sexual phenotype. At this stage of development the morphological and physiological development of the two sexes diverges, resulting in the formation of the male and female phenotypes. The development of phenotypic sex includes persistence of either the Wolffian (male) or Mullerian (female) duct system and differentiation of the external genitalia and the CNS. The male phenotype arises as a result of the action of testicular secretions, testosterone, and Mullerian regression factor. In the absence of these secretions, the female phenotype is expressed (whether or not an ovary is present). In the human embryo the onset of testosterone synthesis by the testis occurs 65 days after fertilization, just prior to the development of the male phenotype. Testosterone induces the differentiation of the Wolffian duct system into the epididymis, vas deferens, and seminal vesicles while its metabolite, dihydrotestosterone (DHT), induces the development of the prostate and male external genitalia. In the CNS testosterone is metabolized to both estradiol and DHT, and it has been suggested that all three hormones may play a role in masculinization of the CNS. In the rat, mouse, and hamster the aromatization of testosterone to estradiol is partly responsible for CNS sex differentiation, whereas in certain other mammals (e.g., rhesus monkey) the androgenic (DHT) pathway appears to be essential (McEwen, 1980). In primates the role, if any, of estrogens in the CNS sex differentiation process has yet to be defined.

Reproductive Senescence

Although reproductive senescence lies at the other end of the developmental spectrum from sex differentiation, it is clear from data from rodent studies that the timing of this event late in life can, in some cases, be influenced by events that took place in utero.

The onset of infertility with age differs markedly between females and males with regard to mechanisms and consequences. In most species females lose the capacity to ovulate during middle age, whereas some males remain fertile at ages approaching their maximum life span. In men there are a number of morphological, physiological, and behavioral changes during aging that can lead to infertility; in women the exhaustion of ovarian oocytes is the main cause of reproductive senescence. Healthy men do not have a similar loss of testicular germ cells.

Women

In women the loss of menstrual cycles at menopause is associated with a nearly complete loss of oocytes. The exhaustion of the follicles is considered the pacesetter of reproductive senescence in women. Women generally have a 25-year reproductive life span with a drop in fecundity before age 35, at which time the menstrual cycles are the least variable (vom Saal and Finch, 1988). The menstrual cycles become less variable up to about 7 years before menopause, at which time the cycles become irregular. Some cycles are shortened because of a short follicular phase, whereas others are lengthened because of a failure of ovulation. The decline in fertility after age 35 is associated with an increased incidence in spontaneous abortions and abnormal fetuses. In women, such aging is considered "eugeric," that is, it is not necessarily related to any disease or pathological condition. The age at reproductive senescence is relatively consistent in women as compared with men, with the average age of the last birth being about 40 and the oldest documented birth at 57.

The progression of reproductive senescence in women can be altered by environmental events. Social cues have been shown to improve cyclicity and restore ovulatory cycles in premenopausal women, and precocious infertility is associated with malnutrition, genitourinary tract infections, delayed effects of childhood mumps, autoimmune disorders (vom Saal and Finch, 1988), and treatment with ionizing radiation or alkylating agents (Mattision, 1985).

Female Rodent

In the female rodent there are changes in all aspects of the reproductive system during reproductive senescence. There are characteristic age-related changes in the brain–pituitary axis that accompany the depletion of ovarian follicles, and at this time there is an increase in the frequency of genetic and morphological abnormalities of oocytes, an increase in fetal resorption, and an increase in stillbirths and in incidence of nonlethal malformations in the offspring. There is also an increased variability in estrous cyclicity in rodents with age, just as the menstrual cycles increase in variability in women as they approach menopause. Along with the altered cyclicity, the fertility rate declines, and there is a decrease in litter size with age.

The initial state of acyclicity in the rat and mouse is associated with periods of persistent estrus, tonic serum levels of estrogen and low levels of progesterone, and persistent vaginal cornification (PVC). The state of PVC is often followed by repetitive pseudopregnancy (RPP) and finally by persistent anestrus. During aging the pituitaries of female rats and mice often develop prolactin-secreting tumors as a function of time after they entered PVC, which in turn induce the state of RPP. Although PVC and RPP do not typically occur in primates, persistent anestrus resembles the human changes after menopause in that levels of ovarian estradiol and progesterone are low. Since the ovulatory cycle of rodents does not include menstruation, menopause (the last menstrual cycle) does not occur in these species. Although it is evident that oocyte depletion is related to reproductive senescence in rodents, it is clear that there are other important extragonadal factors regulating this process as well. The fact that rats contain substantial oocyte reserves at the time that cycles end suggests that hypothalamic–pituitary aging is an important mediator of reproductive senescence in the rat (Cooper, Goldman, and Rehnberg, 1986), while in some strains of mice it appears that the progressive loss of oocytes is a major factor in reproductive senescence. In contrast to the rat, mice have very few oocytes remaining at the age when regular cycles cease (vom Saal and Finch, 1988).

Men

In men the decline in reproductive function during middle age is both pathogeric (related to diseases of aging) and eugeric (a general feature of aging not related to any disease state). Typically, less than 35 percent of men older than 80 years are sexually active. The decline in fertility in men is complex and often related to age-related diseases. Impotence occurs in about 50 percent of diabetic adults and is a common side effect of alcoholism and drugs used to treat hypertension. Impotence is also common after prostate surgery. Studies have found that there are no major changes in luteinizing hormone, follicle-stimulating hormone, prolactin, or testosterone in healthy men, although the human chorionic gonadotropin response of the testes is slightly reduced with age. Function of the Leydig cell has been reported to be reduced with aging in some studies, although others have associated this with disease (vom Saal and Finch, 1988). It is known that paternal age contributes to the incidence of some congenital malformations in the offspring.

Male Rodent

In rodents there is considerable variability within and between species, but, in general, there are subgroups of healthy, fertile males, while others suffer from pathological lesions and are infertile. In male rats and mice, but not in hamsters, there is general decline in fertility and libido with aging. Fewer sperm are present in the testes and epididymides of 2.5-year-old male mice compared with 6-month-old mice. The older males also had lower ejaculated sperm counts, but there was no decrease in litter size in the old mice. Male rats show similar age-related changes in sperm counts, but, unlike mice, they sire smaller litters (vom Saal and Finch, 1988).

Compound-Induced Alterations of Reproductive Development

In general, the normative data on reproductive senescence suggest that perinatal treatments that alter neuroendocrine function or deplete fetal oocyte numbers have the potential to accelerate reproductive senescence in females. The following data from studies using rodents clearly demonstrate that perinatal alterations of the neuroendocrine function and germ cell numbers accelerate the onset of reproductive senescence; however, there are no comparable data for the human female. In the rodent and human male it would appear that chemicals, like DES, that increase the incidence of diseases or pathological lesions of the reproductive system are likely to accelerate reproductive aging, but few studies have actually tested this hypothesis.

Effects in Women

Diethylstilbestrol   The pathological effects that develop as a consequence of exposure in utero to DES are well established. DES causes clear cell adenocarcinoma of the vagina and gross structural abnormalities of the cervix, uterus, and fallopian tubes, and increases chances for an adverse pregnancy outcome, including spontaneous abortions, ectopic pregnancies, and premature delivery (Steinberger and Lloyd, 1985). It appears, however, that psychological and biological milestones of pubertal development in young women are not altered by prenatal DES exposure (Meyer-Bahlburg et al., 1984), and to date there have been no reports suggesting that DES accelerates reproductive senescence in women as it does in rodents.

In addition to DES, the use of other synthetic estrogens, like dienestrol and hexestrol, is counterindicated during pregnancy because they have the potential to induce delayed precancerous and cancerous changes in the reproductive tract.

Androgens and Progestins   Other hormonally active chemicals have been shown to induce alterations of sexual differentiation of the external genitalia. Women given androgens during pregnancy risk masculinization of the female offspring (Schardein, 1985). Female masculinization has been associated with the androgens danazol, methandriol, methyltestosterone, and normethandrone. The degree of masculinization appears related to the dosage of the drug administered, but, in general, the anomaly is less severe than the pseudohermaphrodites with congenital virilizing adrenal hyperplasia. The type of anomaly is also correlated with the time of treatment in gestation. Treatment between the 8th and 13th weeks of gestation causes labioscrotal fusion, whereas phallic enlargement can result from either gestational or neonatal treatment. There is almost total regression of most of the cases of phallic enlargement, and simple surgical procedures correct the labioscrotal fusion and the offspring eventually mature as fertile women.

As is the case with androgens, female offspring are masculinized by exposure to certain synthetic progestins during pregnancy. The progestins ethisterone and norethindrone are the most active.

Potential Effects in Women: The Central Nervous System

In contrast to the well-studied effects of hormonally active chemicals on human morphological sex differentiation, the effects of such exposure on the CNS have received little consideration to date. Although CNS effects were initially thought to be rodent specific, a number of recent studies have found behavioral alterations in women prenatally exposed to DES, androgenized women, and androgenized nonhuman female primates. In the rhesus monkey prenatal administration of testosterone or DHT defeminizes (Pomerantz et al., 1985) and masculinizes (Goy, 1978) some of the reproductive behaviors and the rough-and-tumble play of the androgenized female. The evidence accumulated so far suggests that in children physical energy expenditure during play is influenced by prenatal androgens, albeit to a limited degree (Ehrhardt and Meyer-Bahlburg, 1981). Meyer-Bahlburg et al. (1985) reported that women exposed to DES were found to have less well-established sexual relationships and to be lower in sexual desire and enjoyment, sexual excitability, and coital functioning. In addition, it was recently established that a morphological difference exists between men and women in the size of the preoptic area, reminiscent of the sex dimorphism present in the rat. Swaab and Fliers (1985) found that the preoptic area of the human hypothalamus is 2.5 times as large in men as in women and contains 2.2 times as many cells. Although the functional importance of this area in humans is still somewhat unclear, in other mammals (e.g., the rat) it contains a neuronal network that is essential for gonadotropin release and sexual behavior (Leranth et al., 1985).

In summary, it is clear that prenatal exposure to DES, estrogens, androgens, and progestins causes abnormalities of morphological development in human female offspring. Little is known about the effects of such treatments on the effects of prenatal hormones on the development sex dimorphisms in CNS structure and function. However, scientists have recently found sexual dimorphisms in the human brain, suggesting that differentiation of this organ might be altered by androgenic treatments.

Effects on Sexual Differentiation in Female Rodents

In the earlier discussion of reproductive aging in rodents it was stated that changes in the neuroendocrine axis and depletion of oocytes are both important mediators of reproductive senescence in female rats and mice. This dichotomy becomes even more apparent during an examination of the effects of prenatal exposure to toxic chemicals on reproductive function and aging in the female rodent. The first group of treatments, which includes hormonally active chemicals, alters neuroendocrine and hypothalamic–pituitary function during the critical stages of CNS sex differentiation and accelerates the onset of PVC and anestrus. The second group appears to induce infertility and accelerate the onset of reproductive senescence by depleting the pool of oocytes during the perinatal period. In most cases, the morphological and physiological consequences of treatments that deplete the germ cells are quite different from those that alter sex differentiation. Depletion of germ cell reserves does not alter the behavioral and morphological sexual phenotype of the offspring, whereas treatments that alter sex differentiation can induce infertility and accelerate reproductive senescence without affecting germ cell numbers.

Androgens/Progestins/Estrogens/Diethylstilbestrol Neonatal testosterone administration at high dosage levels in female rodents induces the development of PVC, polycystic ovaries, and infertility at puberty. Lower doses of testosterone shorten the reproductive life span of the treated females (Gerall, Dunlap, and Sonntag, 1980). These females also develop PVC and stop ovulating. This condition has been called the "delayed anovulatory syndrome" (DAS). It was proposed that neonatal steroid treatment accelerated neural and endocrine age-related changes in the hypothalamus (Swanson and van der Werff ten Bosch, 1964). Concurrent with the onset of DAS are changes in catecholaminergic system regulating gonadotropin-releasing hormone secretion that occur in response to estradiol (Barraclough and Wise, 1982). The DAS females do not show the dramatic changes in norepinephrine in the hypothalamus after ovariectomy and estrogen treatment that are seen in untreated females. The loss of cyclicity during normal aging has also been related to changes in dopaminergic and noradrenergic systems. These androgenized females also have elevated serum levels of prolactin and estradiol and lower levels of progesterone than do untreated females (Mennin and Gorski, 1975).

Additional studies have shown that testosterone's effects on these processes, at least in the rat and hamster, appear to be mediated by the aromatization of testosterone to estradiol. A single injection at 5 days of age of 5 μg of estradiol benzoate was the minimum dose required to induce DAS in the rat (Gorski, 1963). The aromatizable androgens testosterone and androstenedione induced PVC at doses of 200 μg and above (injected on Days 2, 3, and 4), while the nonaromatizable androgen DHT was ineffective. In contrast, all three androgens effectively masculinized the external genitalia of treated females (Luttge and Whalen, 1970). It is now known that the volume of the sexually dimorphic nucleus in the preoptic area of the rat brain is severalfold larger in adult male rats than adult female rats. This sex difference is due to the influence of androgenic and estrogenic steroids during the perinatal period.

Whereas the role of androgens and estrogens in sexual differentiation has been extensively studied, less is known about the role of progestins on this process. However, fetal tissues contain progesterone receptors and exposure to progestins during the perinatal period can cause changes in adult sex behavior and genital morphology and can lead to acyclicity in the female rat (Hull, 1981). For example, Kincl and Dorfman (1962) gave pregnant rats oral doses of methyl acetoxyprogesterone on Days 15–20 of gestation and found that this progestin masculinized females such that they displayed clitoral hypertrophy, increased anogenital distance, urethrovaginal fistulas, and blind vaginas. Holzhausen, Murphy, and Birke (1984) reported that medroxyprogesterone acetate (5 μg/g) given subcutaneously to lactating dams on postnatal Day 1 altered the proestrus LH surge in the female pups.

It is important to note that the effect of perinatal administration of chemicals to rodents also causes a number of lesions of the reproductive tract in addition to its effects on the CNS. For example, the administration of DES to pregnant mice on Days 9–16 of gestation reduced fertility in a dose-related manner and produced structural abnormalities of the oviduct, uterus, cervix, and vagina (McLachlan et al., 1982; Newbold et al., 1983). Huseby and Thurlow (1982) found that dietary administration of 0.2 μg of DES per gram of diet during pregnancy reduced fertility and doubled the incidence of mammary carcinomas in the treated female offspring. Neonatal injection of 20 μg of estradiol for 5 days also produced mammary gland abnormalities in female mice (Bern, Mills, and Jones, 1983). Ennis and Davies (1982) found two types of reproductive tract abnormalities in rats treated neonatally with DES (3 μg subcutaneously for 5 days): Squamous metaplasia was found in the uteri of DES-treated rats, and part of the cervix was nonexistent in DES-treated rats. Prenatal exposure (administered on Days 16–20 of gestation) to the synthetic estrogen, RU 2858 (moxestrol at 0.4, 2, 10, or 50 μg/rat) altered the genital tract of rat offspring more markedly than did estradiol (50, 250, or 1,250 μg/rat) (Vannier and Raynaud, 1980). At adulthood most treated females had a cleft clitorine urethra, and with higher doses a well-developed vagina was lacking, the ovaries were small, and two females had persistent Wolffian ducts. In this study fertility was reduced for both estrogens below the doses that resulted in morphological changes.

Antiestrogens   The administration of antiestrogens during the perinatal period also results in abnormal reproductive development in rodents. A number of these antiestrogens act as estrogen agonists rather than antagonists in the neonatal female, and for this reason they induce estrogen-like alterations of reproductive development. The neonatal administration of the antiestrogens tamoxifen, clomiphene, and nafoxidine to female mice resulted in estrogen-like growth on the columnar epithelium in cervicovaginal preparations. MER-25, another antiestrogen, was without affect (Forsberg, 1985). The antiestrogens tamoxifen, nafoxidine, and clomiphene also cause gross abnormalities of reproductive development as a consequence of neonatal exposure (Chamness et al., 1979; Clark and McCormack, 1977). Vaginal opening was early, cycles were absent at 4 months of age, all ovaries and uteri were atrophic, and oviducts showed squamous metaplasia. Female offspring, exposed in utero to the antiestrogen LY117018, had cleft phallus and oviduct malformations, as did rats treated with DES and estradiol (Henry and Miller, 1986). Interestingly, perinatal treatment of female rats with the antiestrogen tamoxifen resulted in permanent anovulatory sterility, but tamoxifen did not influence differentiation of the sexually dimorphic nucleus in the preoptic area (Dohler et al., 1986).

Environmental Estrogens   Aware of the potential reproductive alterations that develop after perinatal administration of potent estrogens, a number of investigators evaluated the perinatal toxicity of the estrogenic pesticides Kepone (chlordecone), dichloro-diphenyl-trichloroethane (DDT), and methoxychlor. Perinatal administration of these pesticides accelerates vaginal opening, and induces PVC and DAS in female rats. DDT (1 mg) was administered subcutaneously on the second, third, and fourth days of life to female rat pups. DDT treatment advanced vaginal opening by 3 days, PVC was present in all the treated rats by 120 days, and the ovaries contained follicular cysts and lacked corpora lutea (Heinrichs et al., 1971). Gellert (1978) found that subcutaneous administration of Kepone (0.2 or 1.0 mg/pup) advanced vaginal opening by more than 10 days and accelerated the onset of PVC in a dose-related manner. PVC was detected in some of the high-dose rats at 4 months and was present in the low-dose group at 6 months. Ovarian weight was reduced in the group that received 1 mg/day as a result of lack of corpora lutea. Feeding Kepone during gestation (Days 14–20, 15 mg/kg/day) by gavage also induced PVC, anovulation, reduced ovarian weight, and tonic serum levels of estradiol at 6 months of age (Gellert and Wilson, 1979). Female hamsters neonatally injected with Kepone or estradiol at 2 days of age displayed masculine sex behavior as adults whereas the untreated females did not. These females were not defeminized by the treatments because they all displayed normal estrous cycles and feminine sex behavior. It is known that hamsters are easily masculinized by steroid exposure during the critical neonatal period of CNS sex differentiation, but, unlike rats, female hamsters are difficult to defeminize. For this reason, DAS is seen only at doses two orders of magnitude above those that masculinize female hamsters.

The administration of another weakly estrogenic pesticide, methoxychlor, in utero and during lactation to the rats at 50 mg/kg/day, accelerated vaginal opening by 6 days and induced PVC in the female offspring (Gray et al., 1989). Females were bred from weaning until 11 months of age at which time they were necropsied. The treated pups were all in PVC at 10 months and produced less than half as many pups as did the control females.

In addition to estrogenic pesticides, there are many other classes of "environmental estrogens" that have the potential to alter sex differentiation. This includes a number of plant estrogens and fungal toxins. The effects of neonatal exposure to the fungal toxin zearalenone on the female rat and hamster reproductive system has been investigated. A single subcutaneous injection of 1.0 mg of zearalenone to 3- or 5-day-old female rats caused PVC in adulthood (Kumagai and Shimizu, 1982). Ovaries in these animals were smaller and contained many large follicles but not newly formed corpora lutea. PVC was observed in 6 of 9 rats injected at 5 days of age and in all rats dosed at 3 days of age. Irregular estrous cycles with prolonged estrus preceded the onset of PVC. Neonatal female hamsters, injected at 2 days of age with 1 mg/pup of zearalenone, displayed accelerated vaginal opening as neonates and abnormal malelike sex behavior as adults. The treated females, however, were not defeminized and ovarian weights were normal (Gray, Ferrell, and Ostby, 1985b).

Neuroactive Drugs Additional studies have found that nonsteroidal treatments can also alter the process of CNS sex differentiation. Arai and Gorski (1968) found that neonatal treatment with the tranquilizing agents reserpine and chlorpromazine partially blocked the sterilizing effect of testosterone on the female rat, while the barbiturates pentobarbital and phenobarbital provided marked protection against testostereone. They also found that coadministration of the antibarbiturate pentylentetrazol blocked the protective action of pentabarbital. Prenatal morphine treatment disrupted the development of reproductive function of the female rat, but had only minor effects on male reproductive function (Vathy, Etgen, and Barfield, 1985). Dams were exposed to morphine sulfate during gestational Days 11–18 (5–10 mg/kg twice a day). The female offspring displayed precocious vaginal opening and there was a substantial inhibition of feminine sexual behavior. This effect was linked to the emergence of opiate receptors in the fetal brain.

The preceding discussions of compound-induced alterations of sex differentiation in females demonstrate that homologous alterations of morphological sex differentiation occur in women and female rodents. Androgenic treatments masculinize the external genitalia in all mammalian species and DES is a transplacental carcinogen in mice, rats, and women. The organizational role of hormones in the process of sex differentiation of the CNS in humans has only recently been reported, whereas, in contrast, numerous studies using rodents have demonstrated that morphological sex differences in the brain and spinal cord of rodents develop during sex differentiation.

Effects on Germ Cells in Female Rodents

Radiation   Awareness of the potential for adverse treatment effects on germ cells began with studies of ionizing radiation in the late 1900s (see Erickson, 1985), and the effects of ionizing radiation on the ovary have been extensively investigated. The primary germ cells (PGCs), which arise outside of the embryo, are highly sensitive to damage by ionizing radiation. Oogonia are also highly sensitive to irradiation, but unlike the PGCs, they are not capable of restoring the population with an increase in the rate of mitosis. Oocytes at the early stage of meiotic prophase become increasingly resistant to the effects of irradiation. It has been shown that a dose of 100 R reduced the number of pups produced by mice prenatally exposed to X rays by half compared with untreated mice after they were exposed on Day 13.5 of gestation, when most of the germ cells were oogonia. By Day 16.5, when most of the germ cells are in the pachytene stage of meiosis, there was only a slight effect (Baker, 1985). It has been determined that oocytes of calf, monkey, and human fetuses are far more resistant to radiation than those of mice and rats (Baker and Neal, 1977). In fetal monkeys a dose of 1,000 R was required to severly reduce the population of germ cells, while in human fetal ovaries, maintained in organ culture, an X-ray dose of 4,000 R was required to induce a 65 percent reduction in the population of germ cells. It is important to note that a dramatic reduction in the numbers of germ cells in the fetus is required to produce an effect on postnatal fertility and reproductive senescence because of the compensatory ability of the stem cells. Erickson (1985) estimated that it is necessary to kill more than half the gonocytes with irradiation to affect gamete production. In addition, Mattison (1985) has mathematically predicted that premature menopause in women (less than 35 years) would occur only in individuals born with only 20 percent of the normal complement of oocytes. As the following studies demonstrate, even though robust effects on prenatal germ cell numbers are required to accelerate reproductive senescence, this effect has been achieved in rodents using a variety of chemicals.

Drugs   When mouse fetuses were exposed to the common antineoplastic agent procarbazine (160 mg/kg subcutaneously) on Days 10, 12, or 17 of gestation, the subsequent fertility of the females was decreased (McLachlan and Dixon, 1973). The strongest effect was obtained in the group dosed on Day 12, during the peak of oocyte DNA synthesis. McLachlan and Dixon reported that these effects were obvious later in life but were not apparent during the first few matings. Similar effects have been obtained with busulfan, another agent that alters DNA synthesis (Merchant, 1975). Polycyclic aromatic hydrocarbons are also known to deplete PGCs in fetal rodent ovaries, and exposure in utero to dimethylbenzanthracene or benzo(a)pyrene depletes germ cells and causes infertility after maturation (McLachlan, 1981).

Azo Dyes   We have induced similar reproductive alterations with the diazo dye congo red. Gestational administration of congo red to mice on Days 8–12 at a dose of 1 g/kg/day accelerated reproductive senescence in the female offspring. Even though nearly 80 percent of females treated with congo red bred when paired with an untreated male, they produced about 40 percent fewer pups and litters over an 11-month period than did the untreated females. Histologic examination of the ovaries of the females treated with congo red indicated an increased incidence of ovarian atrophy, the ovaries having fewer maturing follicles (Gray et al., 1983).

Thymectomy   An example of an indirect treatment effect that dramatically accelerates the loss of oocytes is provided by the finding that removal of the thymus gland between 2 and 4 days after birth results in autoimmune ovarian dysgenesis in most mice (Michael, 1983). This is reminiscent of the premature ovarian failure in women with thymic hypoplasia (vom Saal and Finch, 1988).

The preceding discussion of compound-induced alterations of reproductive development in the female rodent clearly demonstrates that reproductive senescence can be accelerated by a number of treatments in rodents. Two basic mechanisms appear to be involved. A number of chemicals deplete oocyte reserves in utero, resulting in infertility or shortened reproductive life span, whereas chemicals with hormonal activity induce DAS via an alteration of neuroendocrine and hypothalamic sex differentiation. In women, precocious infertility is associated with malnutrition, genitourinary tract infections, autoimmune disorders, and treatment with ionizing radiation or alkylating agents. Prenatal exposure to hormonally active compounds alters the morphology of the reproductive tract, but effects on the CNS and DAS-like conditions, seen in rodents, have not been reported

Effects in Men

Diethylstilbestrol   The potent estrogenic substance DES is now widely known to be a reproductive teratogen and transplacental carcinogen in humans. Some of the pathologic effects that develop in fetal males following DES exposure appear to result from an inhibition of androgens (hypospadias and underdevelopment or absence of the vas deferens, epididymis, and seminal vesicles) and antimullerian duct factor (persistence of the mullerian ducts) (McLachlan, 1981; Schardein, 1985; Steinberger and Lloyd, 1985). DES also causes epididymal cysts, hypotrophic testes, and infertility in males. Some males have reduced ejaculate volume with reduced numbers of motile sperm, and may also experience difficulty in urination. In men, abnormalities of prostatic function normally increase dramatically with age, an effect that might be accelerated by prenatal exposure to DES.

Progestins   In addition to estrogens and DES, a number of progestins also alter human male reproductive differentiation. These compounds include dimethisterone, hydroxyprogesterone, medroxyprogesterone, norethindrone, and progesterone. Effects reportedly include hypospadias, ambiguous genitalia, and occasional testicular atrophy (Schardein, 1985). Similar effects have been obtained in male rodents and monkeys.

Prenatal exposure to estrogens, DES, and progestins can alter sexual differentiation in the human fetal male by blocking the effects of endogenous testosterone. Effects include hypospadias and underdevelopment of the reproductive tract and the testes and infertility. DES treatment also induces a number of pathological conditions in human males that may contribute to an increased infertility rate over that seen in unexposed males during aging.

Effects on Sexual Differentiation in Male Rodents

In male rodents, a number of studies have shown that xenobiotic chemicals have the potential to alter sexual differentiation of the duct system and the CNS following gonadal differentiation. Some of the chemicals are hormonally active, whereas others inhibit the action, synthesis, or metabolism of endogenous hormones that are essential for this process to progress normally.

Androgens   Wilson and Wilson (1943) first demonstrated that neonatal injections of testosterone adversely affected sexual differentiation in the male rodent. Treated males had small testes with hypospermatogenesis and reduced accessory sex gland and epididymal weights, effects that have been attributed to a substantial decrease in the 5 α reductase activity in the prostate and epididymis of adult rats (Baranao et al., 1981). Male rats exposed to another androgen, androstenedione, during pre- and/or neonatal development showed normal patterns of sexual behavior and the accessory sex organs were normal, but testes weights were reduced (Gilroy and Ward, 1978).

Antiandrogens   Antiandrogens, progestins, or maternal stress late in gestation all antagonize the effects of endogenous testosterone in the fetal male rat. Prenatal administration of the antiandrogen flutamide demasculinized the sexual behavior and genitalia of the male rat (Clemens, Gladue, and Coniglio, 1978). The treated males had difficulty achieving intromission, most likely because of the profound morphological changes seen in the genitalia. Similar effects on the genitalia are obtained with prenatal treatment with another antiandrogen, cyproterone acetate. Male rats treated perinatally to cyproterone acetate had the phenotypic appearance of normal females. They did not have a penis or scrotum, although the hypothalamus, in contrast, was not demasculinized (Dohler et al., 1986). Fetal exposure to spironolactone (40 mg/kg/day, Days 13–21, orally), an aldosterone antagonist with antiandrogenic properties, also demasculinized male rats (Hecker, Hasan, and Neumann, 1980). Lower doses (10–20 mg/kg/day, Days 14–20, subcutaneously) led to persistent endocrine dysfunctions (Jaussan, Lemarchand, and Gomez, 1985). The treated males had decreased ventral prostate and seminal vesicle weights, and basal serum and pituitary prolactin levels were 50 percent of control values. In contrast, luteinizing hormone, follicle-stimulating hormone, testosterone, and DHT levels were normal in the treated males. Anand and Van Thiel (1982) claimed that exposing rats in utero and postnatally to cimetidine, which has weak antiandrogen activity, demasculinized the male pups and reduced their sexual performance as adults, but Walker, Bott, and Bond (1987) were unable to replicate these effects. The chemical fenarimol belongs to a class of fungicides that acts by inhibiting ergosterol biosynthesis in fungi (Hirsch et al., 1986). Lifetime treatment with this compound causes a dose-related decrease in fertility in the rat. Hirsch et al. found that fenarimol inhibited aromatase activity in the brain of the neonatal male rat, which prevented the conversion of testosterone to estradiol. They proposed that treated males were incapable of displaying male sex behaviors because masculinization of the CNS did not occur in the absence of estradiol.

Progestins A number of studies have investigated the effects of progesterone on sex differentiation in the male rodent. Neonatal injections of progesterone induced slight changes in the development and function of the adrenal gland and the testis in the rat (Tapanainen, Penttinen, and Huhtaniemi, 1979). Neonatal progesterone injection also interfered with behavioral masculinization (Hull, 1981). Behavioral alterations may result from a lowering of fetal testicular testosterone synthesis (Pointis et al., 1984), thus producing effects similar to the antiandrogens and spironolactone. It has been proposed that the maternal progesterone treatment might impair fetal testosterone synthesis by inhibiting 3-beta-hydroxysteroid dehydrogenase. Male cynomolgus monkeys exposed in utero to medroxyprogesterone acetate had a short penis, hypospadias, and small adrenals (Prahalada et al., 1985).

Prenatal Stress In a number of studies, pregnant rats have been stressed during the period of sexual differentiation. The male offspring showed aberrant sexual behavior in adulthood, shortened anogenital distance at birth, and reduced testicular and adrenal weights as a consequence of the corticosteroids secreted by the stressed mother (Dahlof, Hard, and Larsson, 1977). Treatment of pregnant rats with hydrocortisone (1.5 or 3.0 mg per rat) from Day 14 after conception until birth also resulted in shortened anogenital distance and lowered testis weight in male offspring (Dahlof, Hard, and Larsson, 1978). Rhees and Flemming (1981) found that the copulatory behavior of male offspring from dams subjected to environmental stress (immobilization, illumination, and heat), or injection of adrenocorticotropic hormone (ACTH) (20 IU/day, intramuscularly) was severely impaired. In a similar study, Stylianopoulou (1983) found that males born to dams treated with ACTH (8 IU/day, subcutaneously) during the last third of gestation showed a decreased ability to perform sexually (42 percent failed to mate compared with 3 percent of the control males).

Estrogens Effects seen in male animals exposed in utero or neonatally to estrogens are consistent with some of those in humans. Male mice given DES perinatally develop epididymal cysts; hypospadias; phallic hypoplasia; inhibition of the growth and descent of the testes;

and underdevelopment or absence of the vas deferens, epididymis, and seminal vesicles (McLachlan, 1981). Similar effects are obtained using other potent estrogens like estradiol and RU 2858 (Vannier and Raynaud, 1980). However, the demasculinizing potential of weakly estrogenic xenobiotics like DDT, chlordecone, zearalenone, and methoxychlor has received little attention. A single injection of chlordecone to neonatal hamsters reduced testes and epididymal weights, but sexual behavior was normal and epididymal cysts were not present (Gray, 1982). Although it has been demonstrated that DDT and methoxychlor feminize the gonads and reproductive tracts of male birds (Fry and Toone, 1981), similar effects have not been consistently noted in rodents. Gellert, Heinrichs, and Swerdloff (1974) found that male rats treated as neonates with methoxychlor or DDT had normal reproductive organ weights and motile sperm as adults. Fertility was unaffected in the treated male offspring and no epididymal cysts were reported (Gellert and Wilson, 1979). In contrast, when methoxychlor was administered to the dam, rather than injected directly into the pup, the males had slightly smaller testes, epididymides, and lower sperm counts than did the controls (L. E. Gray, unpublished data). A single neonatal injection of the estrogenic mycotoxin zearalenone masculinized the behavior of female hamsters, whereas sex behavior and reproductive organ weights of the males were not affected (Gray, Ferrell, and Ostby, 1985a).

Antiestrogens A number of investigators have found that antiestrogens can profoundly affect sexual differentiation of the brain of the male rodent. Neonatal administration of the antiestrogen tamoxifen demasculinized the sexually dimorphic nucleus of the preoptic area of the hypothalamus such that it was smaller in size, and hence resembled that of the female rat (Dohler et al., 1984). Perinatal treatment with this compound also drastically inhibited testicular development because the testes were aspermatozoic (Dohler et al., 1986).

Drugs Some compounds that lack steroidal activity have also been shown to alter sex differentiation in the male rodent. Reproductive dysfunction was noted in male rats following prenatal exposure to phenobarbital (Gupta, Shapiro, and Sumner, 1980). Anogenital distance was shorter, and fertility, seminal vesicle weights, serum testosterone, and luteinizing hormone levels were all reduced. Clemens, Popham and Ruppert (1979) reported that neonatal injections of pentobarbital induced sexual behavior deficits in intact and castrated (testosterone supplemented) adult male rats. Tetrahydrocannabinol, the principal psychoactive component of marijuana, was found to alter the hypothalamic–pituitary–gonadal axis and sexual behavior in male mice exposed in utero (Dalterio and Bartke, 1979). Postnatal exposure to cannabinoids also decreased fertility in mice (Dalterio et al., 1982) and rats (Ahluwalia, Rajguru, and Nolan, 1985).

The injection of high doses of monosodium glutamate induces age-specific reproductive effects. Treatment during the late neonatal/early infantile period causes cell death in the arcuate nucleus of the hypothalamus. Male and female mice (Pizzi, Barnhart, and Fanslow, 1977), rats (Bakke et al., 1978), and hamsters (Lamperti and Baldwin, 1982) exposed to monosodium glutamate in this manner suffer endocrine dysfunction and are infertile. The hypothalamic regulation of the release of follicle-stimulating and luteinizing hormones are altered, and thyroid function and growth hormone secretion are abnormal as well.

Infertility also develops after neonatal dermal application of the topical antiseptic hexachlorophene (Gellert et al., 1978). Eleven-month-old male rats exposed as neonates to hexachlorophene were infertile even though testis weights and serum testosterone levels were normal, and motile sperm were present. During an observation of their sexual behavior, it was apparent that the treated males mounted a receptive female but could not ejaculate. Prostatic cysts were also present at necropsy. The authors suggested that this effect was due to a disruption of the organization of the CNS circuits regulating mating behavior.

Recent evidence suggests that the stimulation of the arachidonic acid–prostaglandin pathway is involved in the action of testosterone on the external genitalia (Gupta, 1989). Arachidonic acid administered during embryonic development masculinized the genitalia of females whereas the administration of aspirin, indomethacin, and cortisone, which inhibit the arachidonic acid cascade, inhibited the masculine differentiation of the external genitalia in males. Gupta (1989) also found that prostaglandin (PG) levels were elevated twofold in females exposed to testosterone and an antiandrogen decreased prostaglandin levels in male fetuses. The author proposed that prostaglandins play a critical role in the masculinizing action of fetal testosterone.

Compounds that Induce Liver Function   Changes in liver function during sex differentiation can adversely affect this process by altering the internal hormonal milieu. For example, postnatal administration of polychlorinated biphenyls during the neonatal and juvenile periods can cause a hypoandrogenic condition by inducing the hepatic microsomal enzymes (Sager, 1983). When tested as adults, these males had reduced reproductive capacity and smaller sex accessory gland weights.

Similarly, McCormack, Arneric, and Hook (1979) reported that perinatal polybrominated biphenyls increased steroid catabolism in the male rat, reducing the effectiveness of exogenously administered steroid hormones.

Nitrofen   Ongoing research in our own laboratory indicates that prenatal exposure to the herbicide nitrofen induces anomalous development of the para- and mesonephric duct derivatives in the male hamster via mechanisms that have not yet been determined. Early gestational treatment causes uterus unicornis and occasional ipsilateral renal agenesis in the female, and unilateral agenesis of the vas deferens and/or epididymis and seminal vesicular agenesis in the male. Male hamsters exposed to nitrofen later in gestation displayed lower levels of mounting behavior, reduced fertility, and a high incidence of spermatic granulomas in the epididymis (Gray, Ferrell, and Ostby, 1985b).

In mammals testicular testosterone directs the differentiation of the sex ducts while its metabolite DHT masculinizes the external genitalia. Progestins inhibit masculinization in humans and rodents in a similar fashion. In rodents a number of treatments such as antiandrogens, prenatal stress, polychlorinated biphenyls also inhibit the masculinization of the male. DES is a transplacental carcinogen in rodents and also antagonizes the masculinizing effects of endogenous testosterone on the reproductive system.

Effects on Germ Cells in Male Rodents

The abnormalities of reproductive development discussed in this section have included alterations of sex differentiation that result in abnormal development of the male phenotype. In contrast, treatments that directly affect the germ cells do not usually affect sexual differentiation, and reproductive development proceeds normally until puberty (Hatier, Grigon, and Touati, 1982; Merchant, 1975). For this reason the consequences of toxicant-induced germ cell depletion differ greatly from the previously described alterations of sex differentiation.

In the developing male, the stem cells, referred to as the primordial germ cells, are mitotically active prior to gonadal differentiation, and this activity peaks when these cells reach the indifferent gonad. This prenatal period of mitotic activity lasts for 4 days in the mouse and 80 days in human males. Gonadal differentiation begins on prenatal Day 13 in the mouse and Day 35 in human males, after which the mitotic activity of the stem cells, (now referred to as gonocytes), drops to near zero until the initiation of spermatogenesis. This period of mitotic arrest lasts for only 7 days in the mouse as opposed to 10 years in human males. With the onset of spermatogenesis (postnatal Day 3 in mice and at 10 years of age in human males) the stem cells (now referred to as a stem spermatogonia) resume mitotic activity.

Radiation   It has been clearly demonstrated that the mitotically inactive gonocyte is the most sensitive to the acute effects of irradiation. However, because more stem cells are generated than are needed and many of them normally degenerate in the rodent shortly after birth, it is necessary to kill more than half of the gonocytes before sperm production is reduced in the adult (see Erickson, 1985, for a review). In contrast to the germ cells, the Sertoli cells of the testis are preferentially affected by irradiation on postnatal Days 6–13 following birth.

Chemicals   The consequences of prenatal exposure to a single dose of an alkylating agent, busulfan, are similar to the effects of prenatal irradiation, but in this case the mitotically active stem cells are more sensitive than the resting gonocytes (Hemsworth and Jackson, 1962). The prenatal animal is particularly at risk because doses of busulfan and dimethylbenzanthracene that have no effect on adults will sterilize the prenatal mouse (Erickson, 1981). Work in our laboratory indicates that prenatal administration of some of the benzidine-based diazo dyes (congo red and chlorazol black E) produce effects on the testes similar to those described for busulfan (Gray et al., 1983; Ostby and Gray, 1986), although the prenatal period of vulnerability includes only the pregonadal stage.

In contrast to most chemicals, prenatal dibromochloropropane (DBCP) treatment profoundly affects both germ cell numbers and hormone dependent sex differentiation. A recent report on the effects of fetal exposure to DBCP on adult male reproductive function described rather novel effects in that both sex differentiation and the germ cells were affected. Males whose dams were treated in Days 14–19 of gestation had a 90 percent reduction in testis weight, androgen levels were decreased, the sexually dimorphic nucleus of the preoptic area was reduced in size, and, although none of them displayed mounting behavior, they all showed female sex behavior (lordosis). The most novel effect was the complete absence of seminiferous tubules in many of the males (Warren, Ahmad, and Rudeen, 1988).

The studies presented in the preceding discussion on the effects on germ cells in male rodents demonstrate that prenatal treatment with radiation or the alkylating agent busulfan can reduce sperm production later in life and may even sterilize the male. Prenatal treatment with

DBCP altered both germ cell numbers and sex differentiation of the male offspring.

Conclusion

The studies presented in this review indicate that perinatal exposure of the fetal or neonatal rodent to a toxicant can adversely affect reproductive development, reduce fertility, and accelerate reproductive senescence. In rodents and humans exposure to DES, estrogens, androgens, and progestins during critical developmental periods produces morphological and pathological alterations of the reproductive tract of males and females. DES treatment causes cancer, infertility, and serious morphological abnormalities of the reproductive tract in all species examined.

In female rodents, support was found for the hypothesis that developmental events that occur during perinatal life can "program" the early onset of reproductive senescence. Treatments that deplete oocytes in utero, such as ionizing radiation, procarbazine, the diazo dye congo red, and thymectomy, accelerate reproductive aging and the onset of anestrus. Studies using rats, mice, and hamsters have also found that perinatal exposure to treatments can alter neuroendocrine and hypothalamic sex differentiation. In the female rat such alterations result in abnormal sex behavior and PVC and also accelerate reproductive senescence (via DAS). Some of these treatments include estrogens, antiestrogens, DES, androgens, and estrogenic pesticides.

Although DAS is well established in rodents, the extrapolation of such effects to humans is unclear because the DAS has not been detected in masculinized female monkeys and during aging only rats and mice develop PVC. Although hormones may not induce PVC and DAS, there is indirect evidence for the role of steroids in CNS sex differentiation in human and nonhuman primates. Androgens masculinize some sex behaviors and aggressive play in monkeys and similar sex dimorphisms exist for homologous behaviors in humans. Recently, morphological sex dimorphisms have been reported in the human CNS, one of which resembles the sexually dimorphic nucleus of the preoptic area in the brain of the rat. In addition, one human study has reported that women exposed to DES in utero have altered sex behaviors.

In male rodents, potent estrogens, such as estradiol and RU 2858; antiestrogens; antiandrogens; and progestins alter morphological sex differentiation and cause infertility. In addition, antiestrogens cause infertility by inhibiting CNS development with respect to the regulation of masculine sex behavior. Antiestrogens, testosterone, and progestins all dramatically affect sex differentiation and reduced fertility. Other compounds that are weak estrogens, or somehow antagonize the action of testosterone, may not cause infertility, but often reproductive organ weights are reduced.

In rodents treatments that deplete oocyte levels in females also reduce testicular sperm levels in males. The limited data available indicate that most of the males have a normal reproductive life span. However, few studies have followed the breeding of perinatally treated males long enough to adequately test this hypothesis.

In conclusion, the basic events of reproductive development are similar in all mammalian species, although subtle but important differences exist. Perinatally induced alterations of this process, seen in studies using rodents, should be of concern because similar alterations may occur in humans.

References

Ahluwalia, B. S., Rajguru, S. U., and Nolan, G. H. 1985. The effect of tetrahydrocannabinol in utero exposure on rat offspring fertility and ventral prostate gland morphology. *Journal of Andrology* 6:386–391.

Anand, S., and Van Thiel, D. H. 1982. Prenatal and neonatal exposure to cimetidine results in gonadal and sexual dysfunction in adult males. *Science* 218:493–494.

Arai, Y., and Gorski, R. A. 1968. Protection against neural organizing effect of exogenous androgen in the neonatal female rat. *Endocrinology* 82:1005–1009.

Baker, T. G. 1985. Effects of ionizing radiation on mammalian oogenesis: A model for chemical effects. In Dixon, R. L. (Ed.), *Reproductive Toxicology*. New York, Raven Press, pp. 21–34.

Baker, T. G., and Neal, P. 1977. Action of ionizing radiations on the mammalian ovary. In Zuckerman, S., and Weir, B. J. (Eds.), *The Ovary* (Vol. 3). New York, Academic Press, pp. 1–58.

Bakke, J. L., Lawrence, N., Bennett, J., Robinson, S., and Bowers, C. Y. 1978. Late endocrine effects of administering monosodium glutamate to neonatal rats. *Neuroendocrinology* 26:220–228.

Baranao, J. L. S., Chemes, H. E., Tesone, M., Chiauzzi, V. A., Scacchi, P., Calvo, J. C., Faigon, M. R., Moguilevsky, J. A., Charreau, E. H., and Calandra, R. S. 1981. Effects of androgen treatment of the neonate on rat testis and sex accessory organs. *Biology of Reproduction* 25:851–858.

Barraclough, C. A., and Wise, P. M. 1982. The role of catecholamines in the regulation of pituitary luteinizing hormone and follicle stimulating hormone secretion. *Endocrine Reviews* 3:99–119.

Bern, H. A., Mills, K. T., and Jones, L. A. 1983. Critical period for neonatal estrogen exposure in occurrence of mammary gland abnormalities in adult mice. *Proceedings of the Society for Experimental Biology and Medicine* 172:239–242.

Chamness, G. C., Bannayan, G. A., Landry, L. A., Jr., Sheridan, P. J., and McGuire, W. L. 1979. Abnormal reproductive development in rats after neonatally administered antiestrogen (tamoxifen). *Biology of Reproduction* 21:1087–1090.

Clark, J. H., and McCormack, S. 1977. Clomid or nafoxidine administered to neonatal rats causes reproductive tract abnormalities. *Science* 197:164–165.

Clemens, L. G., Gladue, B. A., and Coniglio, L. P. 1978. Prenatal endogenous androgenic influences on masculine sexual behavior and genital morphology in male and female rats. *Hormones and Behavior* 10:40–53.

Clemens, L. G., Popham, T. V., and Ruppert, P. H. 1979. Neonatal treatment of hamsters with barbiturate alters adult sexual behavior. *Developmental Psychobiology* 12:49–59.

Cooper, R. L., Goldman, J. M., and Rehnberg, G. L. 1986. Neuroendocrine control of reproductive function in the aging female rodent. *Journal of the American Geriatrics Society* 34:735–751.

Dahlof, L. G., Hard, E., and Larsson, K. 1977. Influence of maternal stress on the development of the fetal genital system. *Physiology and Behavior* 20:192–195.

Dahlof, L. G., Hard, E., and Larsson, K. 1978. Sexual differentiation of off-spring of mothers treated with cortisone during pregnancy. *Physiology and Behavior* 21:673–674.

Dalterio, S., Badr, F., Bartke, A., and Mayfield, D. 1982. Cannabinoids in male mice: Effects on fertility and spermatogenesis. *Science* 216:315–316.

Dalterio, S., and Bartke, A. 1979. Perinatal exposure to cannabinoids alters male reproductive functions in mice. *Science* 205:1420–1422.

Dohler, K. D., Coquelin, A., Davies, F., Hines, M., Shryne, J. E., Sickmoller, P. N., Jarzab, B., and Gorski, R. A. 1986. Pre- and postnatal influence of an estrogen antagonist on differentiation of the sexually dimorphic nucleus of the preoptic area of male and female rats. *Neuroendocrinology* 42:443–448.

Dohler, K. D., Srivastava, S. S., Shryne, J. E., Jarzab, B., Sipos, A., and Gorski, R. A. 1984. Differentiation of the sexually dimorphic nucleus in the preoptic area of the rat brain is inhibited by postnatal treatment with an estrogen antagonist. *Neuroendocrinology* 38:297–301.

Ehrhardt, A. A., and Meyer-Bahlburg, F. L. 1981. Effects of prenatal hormones on gender-related behavior. *Science* 211:1312–1318.

Ennis, B. W., and Davies, J. 1982. Reproductive tract abnormalities in rats treated neonatally with DES. *American Journal of Anatomy* 164:145–154.

Erickson, B. H. 1981. Comparison of germ-cell response to polycyclic aromatic hydrocarbons in the mouse, rat and guinea pig. In Mahlum, D. D., Gray, R. H., and Felix, W. D., (Eds.), *Coal Conversion and the Environment*. Springfield, VA, NTIS, pp. 410–418.

Erickson, B. H. 1985. Effects of ionizing radiation on mammalian spermatogenesis: A model for chemical effects. In Dixon, R. L. (Ed.), *Reproductive Toxicology*. New York, Raven Press, pp. 35–46.

Forsberg, J. G. 1985. Treatment with different antiestrogens in the neonatal period and effects in the cervicovaginal epithelium and ovaries of adult mice: A comparison to estrogen-induced changes. *Biology of Reproduction* 32:427–441.

Fry, D. M., and Toone, T. K. 1981. DDT-induced feminization of gull embryos. *Science* 213(21):922–924.

Gellert, R. J. 1978. Kepone, Mirex, Dieldrin and Aldrin: Estrogenic activity and the induction of persistent vaginal estrus and anovulation in rats following neonatal treatment. *Environmental Research* 16:131–138.

Gellert, R. J., Heinrichs, W. L., and Swerdloff, R. 1974. Effects of neonatally-administered DDT homologs on reproductive function in male and female rats. *Neuroendocrinology* 16:84–94.

Gellert, R. J., Wallace, C. A., Wiesmeier, E. M., and Shuman, R. A. 1978. Topical exposure of neonates to hexachlorophene: Long-standing effects on mating behavior and prostatic development in rats. *Toxicology and Applied Pharmacology* 43:339–349.

Gellert, R. J., and Wilson, C. 1979. Reproductive function in rats exposed prenatally to pesticides and polychlorinated biphenyls (PCB). *Environmental Research* 18:437–443.

Gerall, A. A., Dunlap, J. L., and Sonntag, W. E. 1980. Reproduction in aging, normal and neonatally androgenized female rats. *Journal of Comparative and Physiological Psychology* 94:556–563.

Gilroy, A. F., and Ward, I. L. 1978. Effects of perinatal andostenedione on sexual behavior differentiation in male rats. *Behavioral Biology* 23:243–248.

Gorski, R. A. 1963. Modification of ovulatory mechanisms by postnatal administration of estrogen to the rat. *American Journal of Physiology* 205:842–844.

Goy, R. W. 1978. Development of play and mounting behavior in female rhesus virilized prenatally with esters of testosterone or dihydrotestosterone. In Chivers, D. J., and Herbert, J. (Eds.), *Recent Advances in Primatology*. New York, Academic Press, 449–462.

Goy, R., and McEwen, B. 1980. *Sexual Differentiation of the Brain*. Cambridge, MA, MIT Press.

Gray, L. E., Jr. 1982. Neonatal chlordecone exposure alters behavioral sex differentiation in female hamsters. *Neurotoxicology* 3(2):67–80.

Gray, L. E., Jr., Ferrell, J., and Ostby, J. 1985a. Prenatal exposure to nitrofen causes anomolous development of para- and mesonephric duct derivatives in the hamster. *The Toxicologist* 5:183.

Gray, L. E., Jr., Ferrell, J. M., and Ostby, J. S. 1985b. Alteration of behavioral sex differentiation by exposure to estrogenic compounds during a critical neonatal period: Effects of zearalenone, methoxychlor, and estradiol in hamsters. *Toxicology and Applied Pharmacology* 80(1):127–136.

Gray, L. E., Jr., Kavlock, R. J., Ostby, J., and Ferrell, J. 1983. The teratogenic effects of congo red on the reproductive system of the male mouse. *Teratology* 27:46A.

Gray, L. E., Jr., Ostby, J., Ferrell, J., Rehnberg, G., Linder, R., Cooper, R., Goldman, J., Slott, V., and Laskey, J. 1989. A dose–response analysis of methoxychlor-induced alterations of reproductive development and function in the rat. *Fundamental and Applied Toxicology* (12):92–108.

Gupta, C. 1989. The role of prostaglandins in masculine differentiation: Modulation of prostaglandin levels in the differentiating genital tract of the fetal mouse. *Endocrinology* 124:129–133.

Gupta, C., Shapiro, B. H., and Sumner, J. Y. 1980. Reproductive dysfunction in male rats following prenatal exposure to phenobarbital. *Pediatric Pharmacology* 1:55–62.

Hatier, R., Grigon, G., and Touati, F. 1982. Ultrastructural study of seminiferous tubules in the rat after prenatal irradiation. *Anatomy and Embryology* 165:425–435.

Hecker, A., Hasan, S. H., and Neumann, F. 1980. Disturbances of sexual differentiation of rat foetuses following spironolactone treatment. *Acta Endocrinologica* 95:540–545.

Heinrichs, W. L., Gellert, R. J., Bakke, J. L., and Lawrence, N. L. 1971. DDT administered to neonatal rats induces persistent estrus syndrome. *Science* 173:642–643.

Hemsworth, B. N., and Jackson, H. 1962. Effects of busulphan on the foetal gland. *Nature* 195:816–817.

Henry, E. C., and Miller, R. K. 1986. The antiestrogen LY117018 is estrogenic in the fetal rat. *Teratology* 34:59–63.

Hirsch, K. S., Adams, E. R., Hoffman, D. G., Markham, J. K., and Owen, N. V. 1986. Studies to elucidate the mechanism of fenarimol-induced infertility in the male rat. *Toxicology and Applied Pharmacology* 86:391–399.

Holzhausen, C., Murphy, S., and Birke, L. I. A. 1984. Neonatal exposure to a progestin via milk alters subsequent LH cyclicity in the female rat. *Journal of Endocrinology* 100:149–154.

Hull, E. M. 1981. Effects of neonatal exposure to progesterone on sexual behavior of male and female rats. *Physiology and Behavior* 26:401–405.

Huseby, R. A., and Thurlow, S. 1982. Effects of prenatal exposure of mice to "low-dose" diethylstilbestrol and the development of adenomyosis associated with the evidence of hyperprolactinemia. *American Journal of Obstetrics and Gynecology* 144:939–949.

Hutchings, D. E. 1978. Behavioral teratology: Embryopathic and behavioral effects of drugs during pregnancy. In Gottlieb, G. (Ed.), *Studies on the Development of Behavior and the Nervous System* (Vol. 4). New York, Academic Press, pp. 7–34.

Jaussan, V., Lemarchand-Beraud, T., and Gomez, F. 1985. Modifications of the gonadal function in the adult rat after fetal exposure to spironolactone. *Biology of Reproduction* 32:1051–1061.

Kincl, F. A., and Dorfman, R. I. 1962. Influence of progestational agents on the genetic female foetus of orally treated pregnant rats. *Acta Endocinologica* 41:274–279.

Kumagai, S., and Shimizu, T. 1982. Neonatal exposure to zearalenone causes persistent anovulatory estrus in the rat. *Archives of Toxicology* 50:270–286.

Lamperti, A. A., and Baldwin, D. M. 1982. Pituitary responsiveness to LHRH stimulation in hamsters treated neonatally with monosodium glutamate. *Neuroendocrinology* 34:169–174.

Leranth, C. S., Sequra, L. M. G., Palkovits, M., MacLusky, N. J., Shanaburough, M., and Naftolin, F. 1985. The LH-RH containing neuronal network in the preoptic area of the rat: Demonstration of LH-RH containing nerve terminals in synaptic contact with LH-RH neurons. *Brain Research* 345:332–336.

Luttge, W. G., and Whalen, R. E. 1970. Dihydrotestosterone, androstenedione, testosterone: Comparative effectiveness in masculinizing and defeminizing reproductive systems in male and female rats. *Hormones and Behavior* 1:265–281.

Mattison, D. R. 1985. Clinical manifestations of ovarian toxicity. In Dixon, R. L. (Ed.), *Reproductive Toxicology*. New York, Raven Press, pp. 109–130.

McCormack, K. M., Arneric, S. P., and Hook, J. B. 1979. Action of exogenously administered steroid hormones following perinatal exposure to polybrominated biphenyls. *Journal of Toxicology and Environmental Health* 5:1085–1094.

McEwen, B. S. 1980. Gonadal steroid and brain development. *Biology of Reproduction* 22:43–48.

McLachlan, J. A. 1981. Rodent models for perinatal exposure to diethylstilbestrol and their relation to human disease in the male. In Herbst, A. L., and Bern, H. A. (Eds.), *Developmental Effects of Diethylstilbestrol in Pregnancy*. New York, Thieme-Stratton, pp. 148–157.

McLachlan, J. A., and Dixon, R. L. 1973. Reduced fertility in female mice exposed prenatally to procarbazine (abstract). *Federation Proceedings* 32:745.

McLachlan, J. A., Newbold, R. R., Shah, H. C., Hogan, M. D., and Dixon, R. L. 1982. Reduced fertility in female mice exposed transplacentally to diethylstilbestrol (DES). *Fertility and Sterility* 38:364–371.

Mennin, S. P., and Gorski, R. A. 1975. Effects of ovarian steroids on plasma LH in normal and persistent estrous adult female rats. *Endocrinology* 6:486–491.

Merchant, H. 1975. Rat gonadal and ovarian organogenesis with and without germ cells: An untrastructural study. *Developmental Biology* 44:1–21.

Meyer-Bahlburg, H. F. L., Ehrhardt, A. A., Feldman, J. F., Rosen, L. R., Veridiano, N. P., and Zimmerman, I. 1985. Sexual activity level and sexual functioning in women prenatally exposed to diethylstilbestrol. *Psychosomatic Medicine* 47:497–511.

Meyer-Bahlburg, H. F. L., Ehrhardt, A. A., Rosen, L. R., Feldman, J. F., Veridiano, N. P., Zimmerman, I., and McEwen, B. S. 1984. Psychosexual milestones in women prenatally exposed to diethylstilbestrol. *Hormones and Behavior* 18:359–366.

Michael, S. D. 1983. Interactions of the thymus and the ovary. In Greenwald, G. S., and Terranova, P. F. (Eds.), *Factors Regulating Ovarian Function*. New York, Raven Press, pp. 445–463.

Newbold, R. R., Tyrey, S., Haney, A. F., and McLachlan, J. A. 1983. Developmentally arrested oviduct: A structural and functional defect in mice following prenatal exposure to diethylstilbestrol. *Teratology* 27:417–426.

Ostby, J. S., and Gray, L. E., Jr. 1986. The teratogenic effects of two benzidine based dyes on the testes of the mouse. *The Toxicologist* 6(1):91.

Pizzi, W. J., Barnhart, J. E., and Fanslow, D. J. 1977. Monosodium glutamate administration to the newborn reduces reproductive ability in female and male mice. *Science* 196:452–453.

Pointis, G., Latreille, M. T., Richard, M. O., Athis, P. D., and Cedard, P. D. 1984. Effect of maternal progesterone exposure on fetal testosterone in mice. *Biology of the Neonate* 45:203–208.

Pomerantz, S. M., Roy, M. M., Thornton, J. E., and Goy, R. W. 1985. Expression of adult female patterns of sexual behavior by male, female and pseudohermaphroditic female rhesus monkeys. *Biology of Reproduction* 33: 878–889.

Prahalada, S., Carroad, E., Cukierski, M., and Hendrick, A. G. 1985. Embryotoxicity of a single dose of medroxyprogesterone acetate (MPA) and maternal serum MPA concentrations in cynomolgus monkeys (*Macaca fascicularis*). *Teratology* 32:421–432.

Rhees, R. W., and Fleming, D. E. 1981. Effects of malnutrition, maternal stress or ACTH injections during pregnancy on sexual behavior of male offspring. *Physiology and Behavior* 27:879–882.

Rice, J. M. 1981. Effects of prenatal exposure to chemical carcinogens and methods for their detection. In Kimmel, C. A., and Buelke-Sam, J. (Eds.), *Developmental Toxicology*. New York, Raven Press, pp. 191–207.

Sager, D. B. 1983. Effect of postnatal exposure to polychlorinated biphenyls on adult male reproductive function. *Environmental Research* 31:76–94.

Schardein, J. L. 1985. *Drug and Chemical Toxicology: Vol. 2. Chemically Induced Birth Defects*. New York, Marcel Dekker.

Schmidt, G., Fowler, W. C., Talbert, L. M., and Edelman, D. A. 1980. Reproductive history of women exposed to diethylstilbestrol in utero. *Fertility and Sterility* 33:21–24.

Steinberger, E., and Lloyd, J. A. 1985. Chemicals affecting the development of reproductive capacity. In Dixon, R. L. (Ed.), *Reproductive Toxicology*. New York, Raven Press, pp. 1–20.

Stylianopoulou, F. 1983. Effect of maternal adrenocorticotropin injections on the differentiation of sexual behavior of the offspring. *Hormones and Behavior* 17:324–331.

Swaab, D. F., and Fliers, E. A. 1985. Sexually dimorphic nucleus in the human brain. *Science* 228:1112–1114.

Swanson, H. H., and van der Werfften Bosch, J. J. 1964. The early androgen syndrome: Differences in response to prenatal and postnatal administration of various doses of testosterone propinate in female and male rats. *Acta Endocrinologica* 47:37–50.

Tapanainen, J., Penttinen, J., and Huhtaniemi, I. 1979. Effect of progesterone treatment on the development and function of neonatal rat adrenals and testes. *Biology of the Neonate* 36:290–297.

Vannier, B., and Raynaud, J. P. 1980. Long-term effects of prenatal oestrogen treatment on genital morphology and reproductive function in the rat. *Journal of Reproduction and Fertility* 59:43–49.

Vathy, I. U., Etgen, A. M., and Barfield, R. J. 1985. Effects of prenatal exposure to morphine on the development of sexual behavior in rats. *Pharmacology, Biochemistry and Behavior* 22:227–232.

vom Saal, F. S., and Finch, C. E. 1988. Reproductive senescence: Phenomena and mechanisms in mammals and selected vertebrates. In Knobil, E., Niell, J., Ewing, L., Greenwald, G., Markert, C., and Ptaff, D. (Eds.), *The Physiology of Reproduction*. New York, Raven Press, pp. 2323–2413.

Walker, T. F., Bott, J. H., and Bond, B. C. 1987. Cimetidine does not demasculinize male rat offspring exposed in utero. *Fundamental and Applied Toxicology* 8:118–197.

Warren, D. W., Ahmad, N., and Rudeen, P. K. 1988. The effects of fetal exposure to 1,2-dibromo-3-chloropropane on adult male reproductive function. *Biology of Reproduction* 39:707–716.

Wilson, J. G., and Wilson, H. C. 1943. Reproductive capacity in adult rats treated prepubertally with androgenic hormone. *Endocrinology* 33:353–350.

10

The Influence of Age
on Neurotoxicity

Richard F. Walker, Ph.D.

Bruce Fishman, Ph.D.

It is well known that pharmacological and toxicological responses of the nervous system to drugs and chemicals may vary dramatically among individuals depending on their health, sex, endocrine status, and so forth. In addition, the degree to which chemically induced injury occurs is influenced by developmental state. Typically, the greatest damage is inflicted by exposure to toxic substances during early development and again during senescence. In general, vulnerability to neurotoxicants during development coincides with large increases in macromolecular synthesis, neurotransmitter concentrations, and enzymes (Crapper, Krishnan, and Quittkat, 1976; Himwich and Peterson, 1959; Lainer, Dunn, and van Hartesveldt, 1976; Van den Berg, 1974). Cells in the developing nervous system undergoing mitosis as well as those that are proliferating show particular sensitivity to toxic insult (Jacobson, 1978). Axonal proliferation and dendritic arborization usually associated with the aforementioned neurochemical changes are not synchronized in time throughout the brain (Rodier, 1977). Thus, the sequelae resulting from exposure to the same toxicant at different stages of nervous system development may be different. Furthermore, the age-related differences may be qualitative or quantitative. For example, clonidine has been reported to increase or decrease locomotor activity or catalepsy (Nomura and Segawa, 1979; Reinstein and Isaacson, 1977, 1981) and the effects of amphetamine on locomotor activity vary complexly with age (Bauer, 1980; Bauer and Duncan, 1975; Campbell, Lytle, and Fibiger, 1969; Lainer and Isaacson, 1977). Moreover, differential deficits in regional brain growth have been induced by postnatal alcohol treatment (Pierce and West, 1987) while the neu-

rotoxic action of methylmercury was both regionally and receptor subtype selective, depending on the maturational profile of each brain
region (Bartolone et al. 1987).

Unlike the literature that deals with developing organisms, there are
relatively few studies that focus on the responses of aging organisms
to neurotoxicants. However, despite the paucity of comparisons of
neurotoxic responses in young and old subjects, the available data
seem to suggest that the major differences are quantitative rather than
qualitative. Generally, older individuals are more susceptible to toxic
compounds, and this vulnerability results in more profound disturbances with longer duration than those seen in younger individuals.
Presumably, the quantitative differences occur as a consequence of
maladaptive changes in cellular metabolism and degenerative changes
in anatomy that together compromise the nervous system's ability to
sustain function following injury. Thus, in the young animal neurotoxicity is associated with neuronal proliferation and increased neurochemical activity, whereas in the aging animal neurotoxicity is generally linked more to metabolic errors and loss of plasticity than to
cellular proliferation. These generalizations suggest that different
mechanisms underlie vulnerability to neurotoxicants in young and old
individuals. Comparisons of these age-related vulnerability factors are
made below.

Factors Underlying Age-Related Neurotoxicity

A generally accepted notion concerning vulnerability to toxic insult is
that biological systems in change have a greater potential for injury
than those with well-established anatomical connections and homeostatic mechanisms in place. Thus, in contrast to any other stage of life,
exposure of an organism to a teratogen during organogenesis will have
the greatest potential to produce malformations. The same assumption
can be applied to the nervous system and its differential responses
to toxic substances at different stages of life. Once the physiologic/
biochemical "plateau" of maturity is reached, behavioral and neurological functions operate with rather broad limits. Through homeostatic processes acting within these limits, function can be maintained
despite perturbations caused by physical injury or exposure to toxic
substances. Thus, the nervous system possesses a "functional reserve" within which injury can be incurred without affecting performance. However, perturbing factors sometimes reduce the functional
limits within which the nervous system operates so that the ability to
compensate to subsequent exposures is compromised. Because the
capacity to compensate, or "plasticity potential," of the nervous sys-

tem is finite, persistent or repeated neurotoxicant exposure will at some point cause sufficient injury to exceed the functional reserve, and impairments will be recognized as deteriorating performance.

The greatest functional reserve exists in the young adult, whereas, with age, the finite capacity of the nervous system for compensatory response to neurotoxic insult is reduced. Determinants of the limits of compensation or functional reserve seem to be structural redundancy and tolerance (Norton, 1982).

Structural redundancy in association with an ability for remodeling of neuronal connections (reactive synapatogenesis; see next section) allows processes to continue within normal limits despite the destruction of a limited number of cells. Cell death resulting from physical or chemical brain damage will obviously reduce that redundancy and thereby narrow the window for compensation of neurotoxic insults. Similar effects on functional reserve are assumed to occur during aging as the result of spontaneous cell death. For example, McNeill, Koek, and Haycock (1986) recorded the loss of specific subpopulations of nigrostriatal neurons in mice during aging. Furthermore, a 27 percent decrease in synapses of the molecular layer of the dentate gyrus was observed in 25-month-old rats compared with 3-month-old rats. Cell loss has been noted in humans at autopsy, especially in those with senile dementia, in whom cholinergic neurons in the basal nucleus of Meynert were only about 20 percent of those found in controls (McGeer, McGeer, and Suzuki, 1977). The toxicological implication of age-related cell death is that the resulting decrease in structural redundancy increases vulnerability.

Although the neurobiological substrate for tolerance is not completely understood, it can be conceptualized, at least in part, as the ability of links in the chain of neurochemical communication to accommodate changes in the frequency or amplitude of signaling. For example, the density of postsnyaptic receptors and/or their affinity for chemical transmitters released from presynaptic sites can modulate the intensity of signaling within a neuronal circuit. Thus, for perturbations producing quantitative changes in neurochemical signaling, compensatory changes in the number of receptors for the affected neurotransmitter (B_{max}) or those affecting its binding affinity (Kd) could sustain normal communicative functions for distortions within finite limits. Such changes have utility for evaluating neurotoxicity because compensatory changes in receptor populations have been reported following exposure to a diverse array of toxic compounds (DeHaven and Mailman, 1983).

Basically, compensatory changes in postsynaptic receptors alter neuronal functions in at least two ways. First, sensitization occurs when perturbations increase postsynaptic receptors or enhance their affinities for their endogenous ligands. Under these conditions, subsequent signals involving the up-regulated circuit are potentiated.

Potentiation of neurotoxicity following reduced structural redundancy during senescence presumably results from loss of synaptic contacts and subsequent up-regulation or sensitization of existing postsynaptic sites. This phenomenon may account for the fact that tardive dyskinesia is more common in older individuals (Crane, 1973) and those with preexisting brain damage (Edwards, 1970) than in younger individuals. The sensitivity of the aged patient is contrasted to that of the younger patient in that relatively low doses of neuroleptic over surprisingly brief periods may produce the typical buccolingual and masticatory movements associated with tardive dyskinesia in the former. Furthermore, the movements often persist in the elderly long after drug treatment has been discontinued, underscoring not only a reduced capacity to resist drug-induced changes in brain function, but a deterioration of mechanisms for restoring normal function once it is disturbed. The similarities between brain-damaged individuals and aged individuals with regard to their increased sensitivity to tardive dyskinesia suggest that neuronal death during senescence underlies the loss of plasticity and increased vulnerability to toxic insult. In support of this assumption is the observation that a rare idiosyncratic drug reaction to dopamine antagonists such as haloperidol and fluphenazine occurs in elderly patients. The condition, called *neuroleptic malignant syndrome* (Caroff, 1980; Morris, McCormick, and Reinarz, 1980), is characterized by stupor, muscular rigidity, fever, and catatonia. Apparently, these Parkinsonlike symptoms resulting from the dopamine antagonists are exacerbated by a preexisting deficit in dopaminergic neurotransmission associated with senescent loss of nigrostriatal neurons.

Another compensatory postsynaptic change is the reciprocal of potentiation in which receptor number and/or affinity is reduced. The resulting condition is called *tolerance*. In contrast to the generally held notion that all processes slow or degrade with aging, certain ones increase and for some functions produce tolerance. For example, enhanced turnover/accumulation of serotonin with aging (Simpkins et al., 1977) can result in down-regulation of its receptors and thus produce tolerance to compounds whose toxic effects are manifest through the action of serotonin. On the other hand, exposure to certain drugs that affect behavior through serotoninergic stimulation, such as m-chlorophenylpiperazine (MCPP), may be prolonged if the drug's metabolism is prolonged as well (Freo et al., 1988). Furthermore, the age-related increase in monoamine oxidase B (MAO B), an enzyme associated with serotonin metabolism, may play an important role in the age-dependent effects of toxicants that employ this enzyme for their bioactivation (Finnegan et al., 1988).

The differential sensitivities resulting from compensatory changes in postsynaptic receptors produce shifts in dose–response curves for neurotoxicants to the left or right, for sensitization and tolerance, respectively. It would seem that tolerance resulting from receptor down-regulation provides the greatest survival benefit because it increases the amount of toxic substance needed to elicit an effect. However, under some circumstances, receptor down-regulation is accompanied by increased activity of enzymes responsible for the synthesis or degradation of certain neurotransmitters. Under such conditions neurotoxicity may be enhanced. As previously noted, MAO B activity increases with age (Shih, 1979), causing toxicants that employ this enzyme for their bioactivation to be more potent in old than in young individuals.

Reactive Synaptogenesis as a Modulator of Neurotoxicity

Evidence that the developing nervous system is more susceptible to injury than the mature nervous system derives from studies in which pregnant animals have been exposed to a variety of agents such as 5-azacytidine (Rodier and Reynolds, 1977), methylmercury (Chang and Annau, 1984), and X-irradiation (Altman and Anderson, 1972). In these, as well as human tragedies such as the Minamata episode in Japan involving methylmercury ingestion, asymptomatic mothers gave birth to severely retarded offspring. These data support the somewhat obvious conclusion that a system in change is more vulnerable to perturbation than one that is stable and has well-established anatomical connections and homeostatic mechanisms in place. Thus, for these reasons, the developing nervous system as well as the aging nervous system, as previously discussed, is expected to be less resistant to injury than the young adult nervous system. However, in seeming compensation for the greater sensitivity of developing organisms to neurotoxicants, their nervous systems are endowed with remarkable "plasticity" that in some cases can compensate at least in part for functional deficit(s) produced by exposure to a neurotoxicant. An example of this adaptive process is seen in modification of mossy fiber synaptic connections following viral destruction of the cerebellar granule cells (Llinas, Hillman, and Precht, 1973). However, just because regenerative capacity is great in young animals, they are not in all cases less vulnerable to toxicity. On the contrary, exposure to methylmercury early in life leads to mental retardation, whereas adults are less sensitive to these effects. The reason for this difference is that exposure to methylmercury before normal circuitry is established prevents its ever being established, whereas in the adult brain, where circuits are well established, functional reserve is greater. Once neuronal circuitry is established, the nervous system can compensate for experimental lesions by stimulating the undamaged neuronal inputs to the destroyed area to sprout and form new synaptic connections in place of those that were lost (Cotman, Nieto-Sampedro, and Harris, 1981). Through this "sprouting" process or reactive synaptogenesis (Cotman and Lynch, 1976), the circuitry of the brain is remodeled following damage. Examination of sprouting in young adult animals revealed that the process of growth follows very strict temporal parameters, proceeding with great specificity, and in some cases restoring some degree of function. Recovery or retention of normal function in these animals after central nervous system (CNS) damage is associated with lesion-induced growth (Dieringer and Precht, 1977; Goldberger and Murray, 1974; Loesche and Steward, 1977; Murray and Goldberger, 1974; Scheff and Cotman, 1977; Steward, Loesch, and Horten, 1977). If establishment of new synaptic connections is able to replace those destroyed experimentally, as with electrolytic lesions or neurotoxicants, and thereby restore function at least to some degree, then reactive synaptogenesis may be regarded as a compensatory mechanism to oppose functional insults.

Although the aging nervous system retains the potential to compensate for injury, its ability is reduced compared with that of the young nervous system. Rather than being proliferative as in the young, neurochemical and anatomical changes in the aging nervous system are generally maladaptive and regressive (Bondareff and Geinisman, 1976), respectively. Several reports of CNS changes associated with aging indicate that in addition to frank loss of neurons, dendritic branches are lost, reducing the numbers of synapses present. In addition, with aging, the capacity for compensatory regenerative changes characteristic of young organisms is lost to a great extent (Cotman and Scheff, 1979; Scheff, Anderson, and DeKosky, 1984). Thus, the diminished capacity of aged animals to support axon sprouting and hence to adequately reinnervate a massively denervated zone may underlie, at least in part, reduced compensatory potential. If, as previously proposed, reactive synaptogenesis is a compensatory mechanism to oppose functional insults, then deficits in reactive synaptogenesis that are associated with aging may have functional significance (Steward, 1982). Presumably, the loss of neural connections and cell death that occur during the aging process compromise sprouting in the nervous system.

A reduction in the ability of neurons to "sprout" during aging may have obvious detrimental ramifications in terms of aged animals' ability to resist the functional decay following neurotoxicant exposure. Experimental evidence for age-related cognitive deficits has been documented in carefully controlled studies in many species including rats, monkeys, and humans (Bartus and McNaughton, 1980; Birren and Shaie, 1977; Campbell, Krauter, and Wallace, 1980; Doty, 1966; Elias and Elias, 1976; Gold and McGaugh, 1975; Goodrick, 1972; Rigter, Martinex, and Crabbe, 1980) and can be explained, at least in part, by the brain's progressive loss of its ability to remodel through reactive synaptogenesis.

Age-Related Metabolic Products and Vulnerability to Neurotoxicants

Age-associated reductions in nervous system enzymes such as choline acetyltransferase, glutamic acid decarboxylase, and tyrosine hydroxylase have been observed in humans at postmortem examination (McGeer and McGeer, 1976). In addition, accumulation of lipofuscin, an intracellular lipid pigment, is one of the most early recognized metabolic changes in the aging brain, with the potential to reduce neuronal plasticity and cell viability and thus increase sensitivity to neurotoxicants. Several investigators have expressed the opinion that extensive intracellular accumulation of lipofuscin during aging may cause functional diminution of cellular activity, distort cell geometry, and contribute to the regression of neuronal dendrites (Brizze et al., 1983; Samorajski, Ordy, and Keefe, 1965; Zeman, 1971). Evidence for a negative role of lipofuscin on neuronal morphology derives from the fact that the pigment accumulates selectively in cell processes of certain pyramidal neurons filling giant fusiform expansions adjacent to their perikarya (Braak, 1979). Accumulation of lipofuscin in the immediate vicinity of the axon, which presumably leads to cell death, has been observed in the circumscribed parts of apical dendrites of pyramidal neurons of the subiculum (Braak, 1972). Thus, the distinctive regression of aging dendritic fields (Scheibel, Lindsay, and Tomiyasu, 1975, 1976; Scheibel and Scheibel, 1975) could result from excessive accumulation of lipofuscin (Braak, 1979). The significance of lipofuscin accumulation in dendrites is that their subsequent death would reduce functional reserve, as discussed above, and increase sensitivity to neurotoxicants during aging. Prior to death, the involved neurons have regressing rather than expanding dendritic fields, which would be consistent wtih progressive loss of plasticity through decay of the potential for reactive synaptogenesis. Impairments in short-term memory, posture, movement and motor performance, and visual acuity have been correlated with lipofuscin accumulation (Brizzee et al., 1983). The functional nature of the correlation in several cases has been strengthened by the fact that improvements in confusional states, disturbances in concentration and memory, and learning deficits have resolved following pharmacological reduction of neuronal lipofuscin (Nandy, 1978; Riga and Riga, 1974).

Increased Vulnerability to Neurotoxicants
as a Result of Reduced Functional Reserve

It is intuitively obvious that performance in nervous systems with great functional reserves is less likely to be affected by exposure to a neurotoxicant than is performance in nervous systems with small functional reserves. Thus, through age-related processes of cell attrition, reduced reactive synaptogenesis, lipofuscin accumulation and others mentioned above, functional reserve progressively declines and the nervous system becomes more vulnerable to the action of neurotoxicants. An example of this potentiative effect of age on neurotoxicity was previously mentioned whereby tardive dyskinesia occurred more often in old than young individuals (Crane, 1973). In addition, neuroleptic malignant syndrome (Caroff, 1980; Morris, McCormick, and Reinarz, 1980), a rare idiosyncratic reaction to dopamine antagonists, occurred in elderly, not young, patients.

The dopaminergic extrapyramidal circuits controlling motor movements have been the subject of many experimental and clinical studies, providing perhaps one of the best functional units in which to study neurotoxicity in aged patients. Essentially, nigrostriatal neurons are lost as a normal correlate of aging, and although these losses may not be expressed in the majority of individuals as movement disorders, they clearly reduce the functional capacity of the nervous system, making it more vulnerable to neurotoxicants. Several examples of the hypothetical relationship between functional reserve and aging of the nigrostrial dopamine system have been reported, especially with regard to acceleration or simulation of "age-associated" movement disorders by neurotoxicants such as 1-methyl-4-phenyl-1,2,5,6-tetrahydropyridine (MPTP). In primates MPTP causes Parkinsonlike symptoms affecting movement, whereas in rodents these symptoms were not observed after MPTP treatment of young adults. However, it was recently reported that in contrast to 3-month-old mice, 21-month-old mice suffered marked physical symptoms of motor dysfunction following MPTP treatment. The differential effects of MPTP in young and old mice suggest that the senescent decline in functional reserve made the aged mice more vulnerable to MPTP, resulting in motor dysfunction only in that group (Gupta, 1988).

Although the age-related effects of MPTP, ethanol, and other toxic substances may be explained by diminished redundancy in neuronal circuits following cell death, mechanisms involving other than cell attrition could also explain age potentiation of certain neurotoxicants. One alternative is metabolic perturbations that either reduce metabolism of toxic compounds or increase the production of toxic metabolites. An example of reduced metabolism as a mechanism for increased neurotoxicity involved MCPP, a preferential serotonin-1b receptor agonist (Freo et al., 1988). Rotorod performance was maximally impaired 15 min after MCPP administration to young (3 months) and old (24 months) Fischer rats. However, by 90 min after MCPP exposure, normal motor function was regained by the young rats, whereas the 24-month-old rats remained maximally affected. These differences in performance were accompanied by retention of nearly twice the concentration of MCPP in the brains of the old rats compared with the young rats. The results demonstrate an age-related reduction in functional reserve of the rat brain to serotoninergic stimulation that may be due to metabolic decrements.

In contrast to the example above, neurotoxicity may be potentiated in aged animals by metabolic changes that increase production of toxic metabolites. For example, MAO B activity increases during aging, and this change may play an important role in the age-dependent effects of toxicants that employ MAO B for their bioactivation. Thus, the toxicity of DSP-4, a noradrenergic neurotoxicant, was reduced by the MAO B inhibitors pargyline and deprenyl, suggesting that DSP-4 is metabolized by MAO B to a toxic entity (Gibson, 1987). These findings suggest that age-associated potentiation of neurotoxicity for some compounds is related to increased rather than decreased metabolic activity.

Other examples of compounds whose neurotoxicity may be greater in aged individuals because of their effects on systems known to progressively degrade with time include carbon disulfide (CS_2), acrylamide, chlordecone (kepone), lead, and others. These few have been selected because they all affect catecholamine systems whose perturbations during senescence are well documented in experimental as well as clinical literature. CS_2 is an organic solvent with a variety of industrial applications that produces neurobehavioral dysfunctions (Wood, 1981). The mechanism of CS_2 toxicity seems to be inhibition of dopamine-b-hydroxylase, the enzyme that converts dopamine to norepinephrine (McKenna and DiStefano, 1977). Tilson et al. (1979) reported that chronic exposure to CS_2 made rats less sensitive to the effects of amphetamine on spontaneous motor activity and acoustic startle. Because norepinephrine metabolism declines with age, the spectrum of physiological effects regulated by this catecholamine would be expected to suffer greater disturbance by exposure to CS_2 or to pesticides such as methylbromide that reduce brain catecholamines (Honma, Miyagawa, and Sato, 1987) in old individuals than in young ones. Similarly, the commonly used vinyl monomer acrylamide produces "central-peripheral dying-back axonopathy" and associated dopamine-dependent neuromotor impairments that are similar to certain age-related neuropathologies (Spencer and Schaumburg, 1975).

Unlike catecholamines, serotonin metabolism is increased during aging (Simpkins et al., 1977). The implications of this change with regard to potentiated neurotoxicity in elderly individuals derive from the fact that chlordecone (kepone) and the related organochlorine pesticide dichloro-diphenyl-trichloroethane (DDT) produce tremor. That these effects are related to serotonin is indicated by the fact that the serotoninergic antagonist pizotifen (Gerhart, Hong, and Tilson, 1983; Gerhart et al., 1982) or the serotonin synthesis inhibitor p-chlorophenylalanine suppressed the pesticide-induced tremor (Hrdina et al., 1973; Peters et al., 1972). Thus, changes in catecholamine/indolamine "balance" occurring spontaneously during aging have been shown to compromise function in and of themselves. When these deficits are compounded by exposure to certain substances, their neurotoxicities are potentiated.

It is unclear whether changes in cell number or metabolic alterations as referenced above account for the age-related increase in epilepsy (Hauser and Kurland, 1975), but such change in nervous system excitability has the potential to exacerbate the proconvulsant action of certain pesticides. For example, Stark, Albertson, and Joy (1988) reported that treatment of rats with γ-hexachlorocyclohexane (lindane) produced a dose-dependent increase in brain excitability that facilitated the acquisition and retention of amygdaloid seizures. Considering that the clinical data indicate that the increase in brain excitability during aging involves seizures with focal onset (Hauser and Kurland, 1975), lindane may be expected to be more epileptogenic in occupationally or accidentally exposed older individuals than in young ones.

On the basis of the aforementioned studies, it may be generally concluded that the potential for neurotoxicity is enhanced in elderly patients by subtle degenerative changes that in and of themselves may not be expressed as dysfunction, especially in the resting state. However, it is well known that performance deficits in aged individuals are best demonstrated under stressful conditions, where an inadequate "functional reserve" will produce dysfunction at stress levels easily

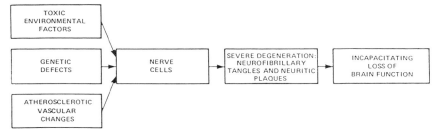

Figure 10.1. The acceleration by neurotoxic substances of senescence in the nervous system. In the presence of predisposing factors, toxic compounds may promote neurodegenerative changes that are associated with advanced age. Repeated exposure or exposure followed by age-related degenerative changes leads ultimately to incapacitating loss of brain function. *Source:* Reprinted with permission from Miquel et al., 1983. Copyright 1983 Raven Press.

tolerated by younger individuals. As in the case of stress, toxic compounds can perturb neural substrates of behavior within limits at which performance can be sustained without overt evidence of toxicity. However, when the limits of that reserve are exceeded, the performance deficits appear. The results of many studies suggest that anatomic and metabolic shrinkage of the functional reserve results in potentiation of neurotoxicity as a correlate of advancing age.

Acceleration of Senescence through Reduced Functional Reserve as a Result of Exposure to Neurotoxicants

As discussed in the preceding section, responses to neurotoxicants may be generally potentiated in older individuals by the progressive reduction of their functional reserve through senescence. The reciprocal has also been reported: Exposure to neurotoxicants can accelerate the onset of age-type diseases, presumably by mimicking the neurodegenerative events that occur spontaneously in some individuals during senescence. Thus, the importance of recognizing pathological changes occurring in normal animals as they age is that similar changes may be pathognomonic of neurotoxicity.

In the presence of vascular changes and/or genetic predisposition, neurotoxic substances could cause degenerative changes in CNS cytoarchitecture that rapidly produce incapacitating loss of brain function. For example, the relationships diagrammed in Figure 10.1 suggest that toxic environmental factors such as aluminum could contribute in the susceptible individual, to development of senile dementia of the Alz-

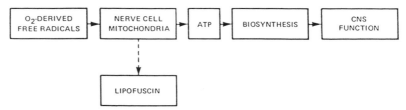

Figure 10.2. The negative effect of metabolic products on the function of the central nervous system (CNS). During age, spontaneous formation of free radicals and accumulation of lipofuscin cause neuronal degeneration. These processes can be accelerated by neurotoxic substances and thereby cause premature senescence of the nervous system. *Abbreviation:* ATP, adenosine triphosphate. *Source:* Reprinted with permission from Miquel et al., 1983. Copyright 1983 Raven Press.

heimer type (see Terry, 1980; Wisniewski and Terry, 1973). A mechanism of neurotoxicant–lipofuscin cooperativity leading to decremental changes in neuronal function is also proposed (see Figure 10.2). The model assumes that under the influence of certain neurotoxicants, oxygen-derived free radicals affecting nerve cell mitochondria could enhance the accumulation of lipofuscin pigment, thereby causing the regressive changes in neuronal morphology and nervous system function cited above. For example, compounds such as ethanol that enhance lipid peroxidation may increase the accumulation of maladaptive intracellular pigments such as lipofuscin and enhance the generation of free radicals (Jou et al., 1988).

During recent years, much of the research done on aging has focused on diseases that are associated with elderly people. These have been studied with the hope of understanding not only the mechanisms that bring about these aberrations but also how they are linked to aging. Alzheimer's disease, a progressive senile dementia, is one such example. The most characteristic mental deficits associated with the disorder are memory loss, speech impairment, and confusion (Slaby and Wyatt, 1974). Neuropathological correlates of Alzheimer's disease consist of cortical atrophy and a high density of neurofibrillary tangles in the cerebral cortex (Perry and Perry, 1982). Consistent with the functional deficits and neuropathology, the postmortem cerebral cortices of Alzheimer's patients normally exhibit decreased choline acetyltransferase activity (Bowen et al., 1976) and acetylcholinesterase activity (Davies and Maloney, 1976). The enzymes are associated with synthesis and degradation of acetylcholine, respectively. The relevance of these symptoms to neurotoxicity derives from the fact that higher than normal concentrations of aluminum were present in brain regions where the neurofibrillary degeneration was most severe (Crapper, Krishnan, and Quittkat, 1976). The aluminum levels were twice those in normal patients, and the metal was associated with chromatin. In contrast, patients who died as the result of dialysis encephalopathy had brain aluminum concentrations 10–20 times greater than normal, but aluminum concentration was not excessively associated with chromatin, as in Alzheimer's patients (Crapper et al., 1978). This difference suggests that aluminum in the Alzheimer's patients gradually increased in brain concentration and bound to DNA. This association may have led to faulty synthesis of any number of proteins critical to the proper functioning of neurons. Thus, for some segment of the population with Alzheimer's disease, aluminum may have slowly increased, gradually becoming toxic by causing cell death and exhausting neuronal redundancy.

Manganese is another metal that causes age-type neuropathology. However, unlike aluminum, it is associated with extrapyramidal disorders, characterized by intention tremor (see Donaldson, 1987). In monkeys, the neurological symptoms of choreathetoid movements, rigidity, and tremor occurred after 18 months of exposure to manganese. These clinical signs in association with severe lesions of the globus pallidus and subthalamic nucleus resembled Parkinson's disease and suggested a possible link between environmental exposure and occurrence of the disease in aging individuals. However, a more popularized chemical that causes premature expression of age-like Parkinson symptoms is the meperidine analog MPTP. Several people exhibited severe symptoms resembling those of Parkinson's disease after exposure to the illicit drug (Langston et al., 1983). Furthermore, the affected individuals responded to therapeutic doses of L-DOPA, a dopamine precursor. Thus, MPTP produced a neurodegenerative condition usually associated with advanced age and thereby accelerated nervous system aging as part of its spectrum of neurotoxicity.

Examples of naturally occurring neurotoxic agents that simulate nervous system senescence have been reported in certain island populations. For example, the Chamorro peoples of the Mariana Islands, specifically Guam and Rota, exhibited a high incidence of amyotrophic lateral sclerosis, parkinsonism, and Alzheimer's-like dementia that was recently linked to their diet. The Chamorros' diet consists in part of a flour made from the seeds of *Cycas circinalis* (Garruto and Yase, 1986). In an experimental study, when one component of that seed, B-n-methylamino-1-alanine (BMAA), a compound similar in structure to excitotoxic amino acids, was fed to macaques, they exhibited signs of motor neuron, extrapyramidal, and behavioral dysfunction (Spencer et al., 1987). The relevance of the dietary cycad-derived flour to the neurodegenerative symptoms is indicated by the fact that with the increasing influence of Western culture and foods on Guam and the concomitant reduction in use of native foods, the frequency of the neurodegenerative disorders has declined. This correlation is a good example of how a neurotoxic agent available in the environment can accelerate nervous system aging in a population.

A case similar to that occurring in Guam is lathyrism, a motor neuron disorder characterized by spastic paraparesis (Gebre-Ab et al., 1978). The neurodegenerative disorder was produced by ingestion of the chick-pea, *Lathyrus sativus*. Recent studies showed that B-n-oxalylamino-L-alanine (BOAA), a component of the chick-pea, had an excitatory effect on CNS neurons in cynomolgus macaques (Spencer et al., 1987). The animals exhibited fine tremor, myoclonic jerks, and hindlimb abnormalities consistent with the symptoms seen in humans after chronic ingestion of the chick-pea.

It seems that several motor neuron disorders are associated with appearance of endogenous, excitotoxic glutamate agonist-type molecules. One such molecule, 2,3-pyridine dicarboxylic acid (quinolinic acid), has been isolated from brains of humans, rabbits, rats, and guinea pigs (Moroni et al., 1984) and has been shown to excite CNS neurons when applied iontophoretically (Perkins and Stone, 1983). An interesting correlate of these observations is the fact that brain concentrations of quinolinic acid increase with age (Moroni et al., 1984), suggesting that the presence of quinolinic acid may result in the spontaneous onset of neurodegenerative conditions that are mimicked by environmental neurotoxicants such as BMAA or BOAA.

Conclusion

Certain generalizations describe the relationship between aging and neurotoxicity. First, neurotoxicants perturb function more profoundly in old than in young animals. A possible explanation of this effect is that the functional reserve of the aging nervous system is low. In short, cellular attrition and declining dendritic arborization attenuate redundancy and the potential for reactive synaptogenesis in aging neural circuits. In addition to having numerically fewer elements to sustain function and support regeneration, maladaptive changes in neuronal metabolism may also fail to provide adequate materials for repair, and in some cases even facilitate neurotoxicity by accelerating the biotransformation of benign substances to those with toxic properties. For example, differences in recovery from exposure to carbon monoxide sufficient to produce coma and respiratory failure were evident when exposure occurred early, rather than later in life (Reiter, 1977). The hyperactivity that is a functional reflection of carbon monoxide neurotoxicity disappeared by 3 months of age when rats were exposed as juveniles, whereas the hyperactivity was irreversible when exposure occurred in old rats (Culver and Norton, 1976). These differences reflect the greater plasticity of the juvenile rats to reinnervate dendritic fields after extensive cell death caused by exposure to carbon monoxide.

The second generalization is that exposure to neurotoxicants may accelerate aging of the nervous system, specifically by reducing functional reserve. For example, the toxicity of Mirex was not observed immediately upon exposure in rats, but became expressed during aging (Reiter, 1977). This observation indicated that immediately after exposure to Mirex, compensation occurred; however, the disruptive influence of the neurotoxicant involved cell death that narrowed the window for compensation to future insults. Subsequent cell death occurring naturally during the aging process then caused functional deterioration because redundancy and the potential for plasticity had been reduced by the earlier encounter with Mirex. Similar examples of delayed neurotoxicity that are expressed as a concomitant of senescence have been reported for nicotine and amphetamine. Exposure to these substances perinatally had no effect until 1–3 years later, when consumatory behavior, activity, and taste preference changed abnormally and tremors appeared (Martin and Martin, 1981; Martin et al., 1979, 1983). In summary, the relationship of neurotoxic substances to senescence is that (a) old animals are generally more sensitive because the neurotoxicants exacerbate preexisting degenerative changes associated with the aging process, or (b) neurotoxic substances accelerate nervous system senescence by reducing functional reserve. On the basis of these assumptions, certain predictions can be made concerning the potency of substances that are known to produce neurobehavioral changes in exposed populations.

References

Altman, J., and Anderson, W. J. 1972. Experimental reorganization of the cerebellar cortex. I. Morphological effects of elimination of microneurons with prolonged x-irradiation started at birth. *Journal of Comparative Neurology* 146:355–406.

Bartolone, J. V., Kavlock, R. J., Cowdery, T., Orband-Miller, L., and Slotkin, T. A. 1987. Development of adrenergic receptor binding sites in brain regions of the neonatal rat: Effects of prenatal or postnatal exposure to methylmercury. *Neurotoxicology* 8:1–14.

Bartus, C. A., and McNaughton, B. L. 1980. Spatial memory and hippocampal synaptic plasticity in senescent and middle-aged rats. In Stein, D. G. (Ed.), *Psychobiology of Aging: Problems and Perspectives*. Amsterdam, Elsevier-North Holland, pp. 253–272.

Bauer, R. 1980. The effects of l-,d-, and parahydroxy-amphetamine on locomotor activity and wall-climbing in rats of different ages. *Pharmacology Biochemistry and Behavior* 13:155–165.

Bauer, R., and Duncan, D. 1975. Differential effects of D-amphetamine in mature and immature rats. *Physiological Psychology* 10:312–316.

Birren, J. W., and Shaie, K. W. 1977. *Handbook of Psychology of Aging*. New York, Van Nostrand.

Bondareff, W., and Geinisman, Y. 1976. Loss of synapses in the dentate gyrus of the senescent rat. *American Journal of Anatomy* 145:129–136.

Bowen, D. M., Smith, C. B., White, P., and Davison, A. N. 1976. Neurotransmitter related enzymes and indices of hypoxia in senile dementia and other abiotrophies. *Brain* 99:459–496.

Braak, H. 1972. Zur pigmentarchitektonik der grobhinrinde des menschen. I. Regio entrohinalis. *Zeitschrift für Zelforschung* 127:407–438.

Braak, H. 1979. Spindle-shaped appendages of IIIab-pyramids filled with lipofuscin. A striking pathological change of the senescent human isocortex. *Acta Neuropathologica* 46:197–202.

Brizzee, K. R., Samorajski, T., Brizzee, D. L., Ordy, J. M., Dunlap, W., and Smith, R. 1983. Age pigments and cell loss in the mammalian nervous system: Functional implications. In Cervos-Navarro, J., and Sarkander, H. I. (Eds.), *Brain Aging: Neuropathology and Neuropharmacology*. New York, Raven Press, pp. 211–229.

Campbell, B. A., Krauter, E. E., and Wallace, J. W. 1980. Animal models of aging: Sensory-motor and cognitive function in aged rats. In Stein, D. G. (Ed.), *Psychobiology of Aging: Problems and Perspectives*. Amsterdam, Elsevier-North Holland, pp. 201–206.

Campbell, B. A., Lytle, L. D., and Fibiger, H. C. 1969. Ontogeny of adrenergic arousal and cholinergic inhibitory mechanisms in the rat. *Science* 166:635–636.

Caroff, S. N. 1980. The neuroleptic malignant syndrome. *Journal of Clinical Psychiatry* 41:79–83.

Chang, L. W., and Annau, Z. 1984. Developmental neuropathology and behavioral teratology of methylmercury. In Yanai, J. (Ed.), *Neurobehavioral Teratology*. Amsterdam, Elsevier, pp. 405–432.

Cotman, C. W., and Lynch, G. S. 1976. Reactive synaptogenesis in the adult nervous system: The effects of partial deafferentation on new synapse formation. In Barondes, S. (Ed.), *Neuronal Recognition*. New York, Plenum Press, pp. 69–108.

Cotman, C. W., Nieto-Sampedro, M., and Harris, E. Q. 1981. Synapse replacement in the adult nervous system of vertebrates. *Physiological Reviews* 61:684–784.

Cotman, C. W., and Scheff, S. W. 1979. Synaptic growth in aged animals. In Cherkin, A., Finch, C. W., Kharasch, N., Makinodan, T., Scott, F. L., and

Strehler, B. L. (Eds.), *Aging, Physiology and Cell Biology of Aging*. New York, Raven Press, pp. 109–120.

Crane, G. 1973. Persistent dyskinesia. *British Journal of Psychiatry* 122: 395–399.

Crapper, D. R., Krishnan, S. S., and Quittkat, S. 1976. Aluminum, neurofibrillary degeneration and Alzheimer's disease. *Brain* 99:67–80.

Crapper, D. R., Quittkat, S., Krishnan, S. S., Dalton, A. J., and Deboni, U. 1978. Intranuclear aluminum content in Alzheimer's disease, dialysis encephalopathy and experimental aluminum encephalopathy. *Acta Neuropathologica* 50:19–24.

Culver, B., and Norton, S. 1976. Juvenile hyperactivity in rats after acute exposure to carbon monoxide. *Experimental Neurology* 50:80–98.

Davies, P., and Maloney, A. J. F. 1976. Selective loss of central cholinergic neurons in Alzheimer's disease. *Lancet* 2:1403.

DeHaven, D. L., and Mailman, R. B. 1983. The use of radioligand binding techniques in neurotoxicology. *Reviews in Biochemical Toxicology* 5:193–238.

Dieringer, N., and Precht, W. 1977. Modification of synaptic input following unilateral labyrinthectomy. *Nature* 269:431–433.

Donaldson, J. 1987. The physiopathologic significance of manganese in brain: Its relation to schizophrenia and neurodegenerative disorders. *Neurotoxicology* 8:451–462.

Doty, B. A. 1966. Age differences in avoidance conditioning as a function of distribution of trials and task difficulty. *General Psychology* 109:249–854.

Edwards, H. 1970. The significance of brain damage in persistent oral dyskinesia. *British Journal of Psychiatry* 116:271–278.

Elias, P. K., and Elias, M. F. 1976. Effects of aging on learning ability: Contributions from the animal literature. *Experimental Aging Research* 2:165–186.

Finnegan, K. T., DeLanney, L. E., Irwin, I., Ricaurte, G. A., Langston, J. W. 1988. The NE depleting effects of DSP-4 are not MAO-A dependent and do not increase with age (abstract). *Society for Neuroscience* 14:774.

Freo, U., Soncrant, T. T., Wozniak, K. M., Larson, D. M., and Rapoporty, S. I. 1988. Age-related differences in behavioral and cerebral metabolic responses to MCPP in the rat (abstract). *Society for Neuroscience* 14:1010.

Garruto, R. M., and Yase, Y. 1986. Neurodegenerative disorders of the Western Pacific: The search for mechanisms of pathogenesis. *Trends in Neurosciences* 9:368–374.

Gebre-Ab, T., Wolde, G. Z., Maffi, M., Ahmed, Z., Ayele, T., and Fanta, H. 1978. Neurol athyrism. A review and a report of an epidemic. *Ethiopian Medical Journal* 16:1–11.

Gerhart, J. M., Hong, J. S., and Tilson, H. A. 1983. Studies on the possible sites of chlordecone-induced tremor in rats. *Toxicology and Applied Pharmacology* 70:382–389.

Gerhart, J. M., Hong, J. S., Uphouse, L. L., and Tilson, H. A. 1982. Chlordecone-induced tremor: Quantification and pharmacological analysis. *Toxicology and Applied Pharmacology* 66:234–243.

Gibson, C. J. 1987. Inhibition of MAO, but not MAO A, blocks DSP-4 toxicity on central NE neurons. *European Journal of Pharmacology* 141: 135–138.

Gold, P. E., and McGaugh, J. L. 1975. Changes in learning and memory during aging. In Ordy, J. M., and Brizzee, K. R. (Eds.), *Neurobiology of Aging.* New York, Plenum Press, pp. 145–158.

Goldberger, M. E., and Murray, M. 1974. Restitution of function and collateral sprouting in the cat spinal cord: The deafferented animal. *Journal of Comparative Neurology* 158:37–54.

Goodrick, C. L. 1972. Learning by mature young and aged Wistar albino rats as a function of task complexity. *Journal of Gerontology* 27:353–357.

Gupta, M. 1988. Dopaminergic neurons in the substantia nigra in MPTP lesioned young and aged mice (abstract). *Society for Neuroscience* 14:12118.

Hauser, W. A., and Kurland, L. T. 1975. The epidemiology of epilepsy in Rochester, Minnesota, 1935 through 1967. *Epilepsia* 16:1–12.

Himwich, W. A., and Peterson, J. C. 1959. Correlation of chemical maturation of the brain in various species with neurologic behavior. In Masserman, J. (Ed.), *Biological Psychiatry.* New York, Grune & Stratton, pp. 67–85.

Honma, T., Miyagawa, M., and Sato, M. 1987. Methyl bromide alters catecholamine and metabolite concentrations in rat brain. *Neurotoxicology and Teratology* 9:369–375.

Hrdina, D. D., Singhal, R. L., Peters, D. A., and Ling, G. M. 1973. Some neurochemical alterations during acute DDT poisoning. *Toxicology and Applied Pharmacology* 25:276–288.

Jacobson, M. 1978. *Developmental Neurobiology.* New York, Plenum Press.

Jou, T.-C., Liu, S.-M, Ahmad, F. F., Cowan, D. L., and Sun, A. Y. (1988). Effect of lipid peroxidation on glucose transport in astrocytes: Potentiation by ethanol (abstract). *Society for Neuroscience* 14:1008.

Lainer, L. P., Dunn, A. J., and van Hartesveldt, C. 1976. Development of neurotransmitters and their function in brain. *Reviews of Neuroscience* 2:195–256.

Lainer, L. P., and Isaacson, R. L. 1977. Early developmental changes in the locomotor responses to amphetamine and their relation to hippocampal function. *Brain Research* 126:567–575.

Langston, J. W., Ballard, P., Tetrud, J. W., and Irwin, I. 1983. Chronic parkinsonism in humans due to a product of meperidine-analog synthesis. *Science* 219:979–980.

Llinas, R., Hillman, D. E., and Precht, W. 1973. Neuronal circuit reorganization in mammalian agranular cerebellar cortex. *Journal of Neurobiology* 4:469–494.

Loesche, J., and Steward, O. 1977. Behavioral correlates of denervation and re-innervation of the hippocampal formation of the rat: Recovery of alteration performance following unilateral entorhinal cortex lesions. *Brain Research Bulletin* 2:31–39.

Martin, J. C., and Martin, D. C. 1981. Voluntary activity in the aging rat as a function of maternal drug exposure. *Neurobehavioral Toxicology and Teratology* 3:261–264.

Martin, J. C., Martin, D. C., Gisman, G., and Day-Pfeiffer, H. 1983. Saccharin preferences in food-deprived aging rats are altered as a function of perinatal drug exposure. *Physiology and Behavior* 30:853–858.

Martin, J. C., Martin, D. C., Radow, B., and Day, H. E. 1979. Life span and pathology in offspring following nicotine and methamphetamine exposure. *Experimental Aging Research* 5:509–522.

McGeer, P. L., and McGeer, E. G. 1976. Enzymes associated with the metabolism of catecholamines, acetylcholine and GABA in human controls and patients with Parkinson's disease and Huntington's disease. *Journal of Neurochemistry* 26:65–76.

McGeer, P. L., McGeer, E. G., and Suzuki, J. S. 1977. Aging and extrapyramidal function. *Archives of Neurology* 34:33–35.

McKenna, M. J., and DiStefano, V. 1977. Carbon disulfide. II. A proposed mechanism for the action of carbon disulfide on dopamine B-hydroxylase. *Journal of Pharmacology and Experimental Therapeutics* 202:253–266.

McNeill, T. H., Koek, L. L., and Haycock, J. W. 1986. Age-correlated changes in dopaminergic nigrostriatal perikarya of the C57BL/6NNia mouse. *Mechanisms of Ageing and Development* 24:293–307.

Miquel, J., Johnson, J. E., and Cervos-Navarro, J. 1983. Comparison of CNS aging in humans and experimental animals. In Cervos-Navarro, J., and Sarkander, H.-I. (Eds.), *Brain Aging: Neuropathology and Neuropharmacology*. New York, Raven Press, pp. 231–258.

Moroni, F., Lombardi, G., Moneti, G., and Aldinio, C. 1984. The excitotoxin quinolinic acid is present in the brain of several mammals and its cortical content increases during the aging process. *Neuroscience Letters* 47:51–55.

Morris, H. H., McCormick, W. F., and Reinarz, J. A. 1980. Neuroleptic malignant syndrome. *Archives of Neurology* 37:462–465.

Murray, M., and Goldberger, M. E. 1974. Restitution of function of collateral sprouting in the cat spinal cord: The partially hemisected animal. *Journal of Comparative Neurology* 158:19–36.

Nandy, K. 1978. Centrophenoxine effects on aging mammalian brain. *Journal of the American Geriatrics Society* 26:74–81.

Nomura, Y., and Segawa T. 1979. The effects of alpha-adrenergic antagonists and metianide on clonidine-induced locomotor stimulation in the infant rat. *British Journal of Pharmacology* 66:531–535.

Norton, S. 1982. Methods in behavioral toxicology. In Hayes, A. W. (Ed.), *Principles and Methods of Toxicology*. New York, Plenum Press, pp. 353–373.

Perkins, M. N., and Stone. T. W. 1983. Pharmacology and regional variations of quinolinic acid-evoked excitations in the rat central nervous system. *Journal of Pharmacology and Experimental Therapeutics* 226:551–557.

Perry, R., and Perry, E. K. 1982. Neuropathology of the brain in old age and psychiatric disease. In Levy, R., and Post, F. (Eds.), *Psychiatry of Late Life*. Oxford, England, Blackwell, pp. 301–335.

Peters, D. A. A., Hrdina, P. D., Singhal, R. L., and Ling, G. M. 1972. The role of brain serotonin in DDT-induced hyperpyrexia. *Journal of Neurochemistry* 19:1131–1136.

Pierce, D. R., and West, J. R. 1987. Differential deficits in regional brain growth induced by postnatal alcohol. *Neurotoxicology and Teratology* 9:129–141.

Reinstein, D. K., and Isaacson, R. L. 1977. Clonidine sensitivity in the developing rat. *Brain Research* 135:378–382.

Reinstein, D. K., and Isaacson, R. L. 1981. Behavioral and temperature changes induced by clonidine in the developing rat. *Neuroscience Letters* 26:251–257.

Reiter, L. W. 1977. Behavioral toxicology: Effects of early postnatal exposure to neurotoxins on development of locomotor activity in the rat. *Journal of Occupational Medicine* 19:201–204.

Riga, S., and Riga, D. 1974. Effects of centrophenoxine on the lipofuscin pigment in the nervous system of old rats. *Brain Research* 72:265–275.

Rigter, H., Martinex, J. L., and Crabbe, J. C. 1980. Forgetting and other behavioral manifestations of aging. In Stein, D. G. (Ed.), *Psychobiology of Aging; Problems and Perspectives*. New York, Plenum Press, pp. 161–176.

Rodier, P. M. 1977. Correlations between prenatally-induced alterations in CNS cell populations and postnatal function. *Teratology* 16:235–246.

Rodier, P. M., and Reynolds, S. S. 1977. Morphological correlates of behavioral abnormalities in experimental congenital brain damage. *Experimental Neurology* 57:81–93.

Samorajski, T., Ordy, J. M., and Keefe, J. R. 1965. The fine structure of lipofuscin age pigment in the nervous system of aged mice. *Journal of Cell Biology* 26:779–795.

Scheff, S. W., Anderson, K., and DeKosky, S. T. 1984. Morphological aspects of brain damage in aging. In Scheff, S. (Ed.), *Aging and Recovery of Function*. New York, Plenum Press, pp. 57–85.

Scheff, S. W., and Cotman, C. W. 1977. Recovery of spontaneous alternation following lesions of the entorhinal cortex in adult rats: Possible correlation to axon sprouting. *Behavioral Biology* 21:286–293.

Scheibel, M. E., Lindsay, R. D., and Tomiyasu, U. 1975. Progressive dendrite changes in aging human cortex. *Experimental Neurology* 47:392–403.

Scheibel, M. E., Lindsay, R. D., and Tomiyasu, U. 1976. Progressive dendritic changes in the aging human limbic system. *Experimental Neurology* 53: 420–430.

Scheibel, M. E., and Scheibel, A. B. 1975. Structural changes in the aging brain. In Harman, D., and Ordy, J. M. (Eds.), *Aging* (Vol. 1). New York, Raven Press, pp. 67–95.

Shih, J. C. 1979. Monoamine oxidase in aging human brain. In Singer, T. P., vonKorff, R. W., and Murphy, D. L. (Eds.), *Monoamine Oxidase: Structure, Function and Altered Functions*. New York, Academic Press, pp. 413–421.

Simpkins, J. W., Mueller, G. P., Juang, H. H., and Meites, J. 1977. Evidence for depressed catecholamine and enhanced serotonin metabolism in aging rats. *Endocrinology* 100:1672–1678.

Slaby, A. E., and Wyatt, R. J. 1974. *Dementia in the Presenium*. Springfield, IL, Charles C Thomas.

Spencer, P. S., Nunn, P. B., Hugon, J., Ludolph, A. C., Ross, S. M., Roy,

D. N., and Robertson, R. C. 1987. Guam amyotrophic lateral sclerosis–parkinsonism–dementia linked to a plant excitant neurotoxin. *Science* 237: 465–564.

Spencer, P. S., and Schaumburg, H. H. 1975. Nervous system degeneration produced by acrylamide monomer. *Environmental Health Perspectives* 11:129–133.

Stark, L. G., Albertson, T. E., and Joy, R. M. 1988. Proconvulsant and anticonvulsant properties of isomers of hexachlorocyclohexane in amygdaloid-kindled rats (abstract). *Society for Neuroscience* 14:1197.

Steward, O. 1982. Assessing the functional significance of lesion-induced neuronal plasticity. *International Reviews of Neurobiology* 23:197–253.

Steward, O., Loesch, J., and Horten, W. C. 1977. Behavioral correlation of denervation and reinnervation of the hippocampal formation of the rat: Open field activity and cue utilization following bilateral entorhinal cortex lesions. *Brain Research Bulletin* 2:41–48.

Terry, R. D. 1980. Some biological aspects of the aging brain. *Mechanisms of Ageing and Development* 14:191–201.

Tilson, H. A., Cabe, P. A., Ellinwood, E. H., and Gonzalez, L. P. 1979. Effects of carbon disulfide on motor function and responsiveness to D-amphetamine in rats. *Neurobehavioral Toxicology* 1:57–63.

Van den Berg, C. J. 1974. Enzymes in the developing brain. In Himwich, W. (Ed.), *Biochemistry of the Developing Brain*. New York, Marcel Dekker, pp. 150–199.

Wisniewski, H. M., and Terry, R. D. 1973. Morphology of the aging brain, human and animal. In Ford, D. H. (Ed.), *Neurobiological Aspects of Maturation and Aging*. Amsterdam, Elsevier, pp. 167–186.

Wood, R. W. 1981. Neurobehavioral toxicity of carbon disulfide. *Neurobehavioral Toxicology and Teratology* 3:397–405.

Zeman, W. 1971. The neuronal ceroid-lipofuscinosis Batten-Vogt syndrome. A model for human aging? *Advances in Gerontological Research* 3:147–169.

11

Electrophysiological Measures in Neurotoxicology

Thomas J. Harbin, Ph.D

The contamination of the environment by toxic substances is a serious problem and is increasing at an alarming rate. The development of new chemicals for industrial, agricultural, and other uses is accelerating dramatically. In addition, the volume of toxic substances released into the air, earth, and water is increasing as the world population grows and as industrial processes and chemical-dependent agricultural practices are introduced into new geographical areas. The development of institutions, legislation, and procedures to protect the environment is lagging well behind the pace of contamination, and coordinated procedures for the registration, testing, distribution, and use of new substances have yet to be formalized in most parts of the world. Similarly, procedures for the treatment of hazardous substances, clean-up of existing areas of contamination, and identification of the sources of contamination are inconsistent and infrequently applied.

Although exposure to environmental toxicants is undesirable for anyone, there are groups for whom certain substances pose a particular hazard. For example, carbon monoxide exposure is especially hazardous to people with coronary artery disease, those with pulmonary disease, and others sensitive to disruption of oxygen intake and metabolism. Developing fetuses and small children are susceptible to a wide range of toxicants, because of the rapid anatomical and physiological changes occurring at this age. Formal and informal testing guidelines now place special emphasis on these groups and others.

The elderly population is a large and identifiable group of persons who may be especially vulnerable to environmental pollutants. Since the beginning of the 20th century, the number of individuals age 65 years or older has increased rapidly: from 3 million persons, or 3 percent of the U.S. population, in 1900 to 25 million, or 11 percent of the population, in 1980. This "graying of America," due to increased fertility rates, increased infant survival rates, and significant improvements in nutrition and health (e.g., the development of vaccines and antibiotics), is expected to continue for the next several decades. By 2025, it is likely that 20 percent of the U.S. population will be 65 years of age or older.

In aged individuals there is an increasing vulnerability to all stressors, including those imposed by the environment. Age-associated changes in anatomy and physiological function place the elderly individual at risk for a variety of medical problems, exemplified by the disproportionately large percentage of older individuals with chronic diseases. The same changes undoubtedly render elderly people susceptible to neurotoxic insult following either acute or chronic exposure to hazardous substances in the environment. Compounding this problem are those substances that pose no greater hazard for healthy older people than for younger persons but that may interact with age-related diseases. The danger of carbon monoxide exposure for patients with coronary heart disease illustrates this concern.

In addition to physiological changes, there are many social factors that increase the risks of toxicological insult to elderly people. Elderly people tend to be located in areas that receive relatively high concentrations of pollutants, because they are more likely to live in older neighborhoods that are closer to industrial centers. In recent years, the average age of farmers has been increasing, and agricultural chemicals are a significant source of environmental pollution. In addition, the current population of elderly persons is less educated than younger cohorts, which means that they are more likely to have worked in hazardous labor situations and to have spent more time in such occupations. These factors render the elderly more susceptible to toxic substances that have delayed effects (e.g., asbestos) or require an extended history of exposure to produce their effects (e.g., coal dust), even though the effects may not be related to age per se.

Despite the overwhelming need for information regarding the interaction between age and the neurophysiological effects of environmental substances, virtually no research has been conducted on this topic. Though the importance of age as a factor in toxicology has long been acknowledged for young organisms, it has yet to be realized that the rapid physiological and psychological changes occurring in elderly persons may also be crucial to consider from a toxicological perspective. The understanding that environmental contamination poses significant hazards for the health of elderly persons has developed slowly, and only recently has the public begun to voice their concerns. However, the elderly are low in political influence, making it difficult for them to have their concerns addressed.

Although there is virtually no information about age differences in the kinetics or dynamics of toxic substances, a small body of pharmacological research suggests that elderly people are likely to be especially vulnerable to neurotoxic substances. Crooks, O'Malley, and Stevenson (1976) reported that there are several physiological changes with age that are problematic for pyschotropic drug therapy and may exacerbate the effects of neurophysiological toxicants. For example, there seem to be consistent age differences in drug metabolism, resulting in prolonged plasma half-lives for most psychotropic drugs. In addition, renal and hepatic function is less efficient in elderly individuals, resulting in slower drug clearance. As a result, adverse reactions to virtually all drugs (likely including toxic compounds) increases with age (Klein, et al., 1976).

Israili (1979) also noted that there are changes with age that may complicate the effects of psychoactive drugs, changes that are also relevant to toxicology. For example, renal anatomical and physiological changes include thickening of membranes, impaired permeability, and decreased blood flow leading to decreased clearance and increased half-life. In addition, liver blood flow decreases, as does production of metabolizing enzymes, leading to decreased metabolism of drugs and increased half-life. There are also changes in blood plasma, especially decreased concentration of protein, leading to a higher level of free drug in the bloodstream. Finally, there is a decrease in the ratio of muscle to fat with age, leading to changes in the distribution and elimination of drugs. One result of these changes is an increased presence of most drugs in elderly individuals coupled with a greater susceptibility to neurotoxic side effects (see Petrie and Ban, 1983, for a review). This suggests that elderly people will also prove to be more susceptible to neurophysiological insult due to environmental toxicants.

Electrophysiological Measures for Neurotoxicological Assessment

There is a pressing need in human neurotoxicology for a reliable, portable, and noninvasive measure of neurotoxic insult. The electrophysiological activity of the brain can potentially provide such a measure. It has been known for some time that the electroencephalogram (EEG) serves as a crude index of the integrity of the central nervous system. Disturbances in the EEG have proved useful in the diagnosis and localization of tumors, epileptic foci, and cerebrovascular abnormalities.

However, the global EEG is not a particularly sensitive index of the neurobehavioral status of the organism. Although there are changes in the EEG that roughly correspond to changes in behavioral state (e.g., decreases in frequency and increases in amplitude accompanying decreases in alertness, such as during sleep or hypoxia), the changes are not unique to specific aspects of cognitive or physiological functioning. In addition, the correspondence between the EEG and nervous system status is very general and is usually informative only in cases of severe brain impairment. However, recent technological advances involved in recording and analyzing electrophysiological response systems have allowed much more detailed exploration of the relationships among cognitive activity, physiological integrity, and the electrical activity of the brain.

Evoked potentials (EP) are changes in the EEG in response to discrete sensory events. These responses are of small amplitude (1–20 μV) and are difficult to detect in the ongoing EEG, which has a much greater amplitude (10–100 μV). However, when multiple samples of the EEG are recorded in response to a stimulus and these samples are then averaged, any EEG activity that is not time-locked to the stimulus approaches zero amplitude, and the response to the eliciting stimulus is more easily distinguished. (For interested readers, a detailed discussion of the procedures for recording EPs has been provided by Vaughn, 1974.)

The positive and negative deflections in the EP, commonly referred to as *components,* are responsive to different aspects of the eliciting stimulus. Components occurring within 80 msec after stimulus onset (relevant latencies differ somewhat by species) are largely a function of relatively simple aspects of the stimulus, such as intensity; are largest when recorded over the relevant areas of sensory cortex; and are relatively insensitive to information processing by the subject (Hillyard and Kutas, 1983). These are often referred to as *exogenous* components of the EP, because of their sensitivity to factors outside the organism, primarily characteristics of the sensory environment.

Components with latencies longer than 80 msec have proved to be a function of more complex cognitive activities. These components are referred to as *endogenous* components because they are not solely a function of the characteristics of the stimulus. Rather, they seem to reflect cognitive processing initiated by the stimulus. The endogenous components of the EP depend on a number of factors, including the task that must be performed by the subject, the direction of the subject's attention, the probability that a particular stimulus will occur, the information value of the eliciting stimulus, and the instructions given to the subject. Endogenous components are similar in waveform and scalp topography regardless of the physical characteristics or sensory modality of stimulation.

EPs are among the oldest tools available to the neurophysiologist and were among the first methods to assess neurotoxicological damage. For example, Xintaras et al. (1966) reported changes in EPs due to carbon monoxide exposure. By selecting certain recording sites and stimulus parameters, increasingly sophisticated evaluations can be made of specific populations of neurons within a sensory system as well as more complex evaluations of sensory information processing.

The exogenous components of the EP have received far more attention in toxicology than the more complicated endogenous components. Somatosensory EPs have proved to be a versatile tool in neurotoxicology (see Dyer, 1987a, for a review). The precise anatomical knowledge of the somatosensory system, coupled with its accessibility in the periphery and somatotopic organization in the brain, permits detailed evaluation by EP techniques. For example, stimulation of a distal receptor such as a finger (usually by a low-amperage electric shock) produces a series of action potentials through the peripheral and spinal portions of the system. These are typically recorded with surface electrodes at preganglionic and spinal locations. Brainstem and cortical potentials (representing cumulated postsynaptic potentials rather than action potentials) are also recorded at cervical and lateral scalp locations. This procedure permits evaluation of conduction velocity at several points in the system from receptor to somatosensory cortex. Somatosensory EPs have proved sensitive to damage from a variety of neurotoxicants, including lead, n-hexane, carbon monoxide, and inorganic mercury (Otto, 1986).

Auditory EPs derived from cortical structures have not been extensively used or investigated in toxicology. However, the "far-field" or brainstem auditory EP is, from an anatomical and physiological perspective, better understood than virtually any other electrophysiological response. This EP, recorded from virtually anywhere on the scalp, is characterized by six commonly measured components occurring within 8–10 msec after stimulation of the ear by a click or tone pip. The components of the brainstem response are thought to originate in the series of nuclei ascending the auditory system. Although the exact origins of each wave are not known, relative changes in the amplitudes and latencies of the waves have been shown to be a sensitive index of the site of neurotoxic insult (Dyer, 1985). The brainstem response is altered by exposure to trimethyltin, triethyltin, chlordimeform (Dyer, 1985), methylmercury (Dyer, 1987b), lead, and toluene (Otto et al., 1988).

Visual EPs have probably received the greatest emphasis in toxicology. They have proved to be a sensitive index of visual system damage and are altered by a wide range of toxicants, including acrylamide, amitraz, cadmium, carbon disulfide, carbon monoxide, chlordimeform, dichloro-diphenyl-trichloroethane (DDT), deltamethrin, lead, manganese, methylmercury, methylpiridines, organic mercury, parathion, hexane, sulfolane, toluene, triethyltin, trimethyltin, and xylene (Otto et al., 1988). Visual EPs are a flexible tool in that different parameters of stimulation can be used to assess different aspects of visual system integrity. For example, flash EPs, elicited by brief, intense light flashes, can be obtained in both humans and other animals, permitting valuable cross-species comparisons. Precise fixation and acuity are not required, facilitating the development of animal models as well as assessment in humans who are unable or unwilling to control their vision precisely. Although this measure has been used widely in neurotoxicological assessment, it is not a diagnostically sensitive procedure. The flash stimulates all retinal cells and a wide range of cortical neurons as well, and differentiation of various sites of visual system damage is not possible (Dyer, 1985).

Visual EPs can also be elicited by patterns of light and dark (usually checkerboards) that suddenly reverse, with light areas becoming dark and dark areas switching to light. Such pattern reversal EPs selectively stimulate the foveal region of the retina (Dyer, 1985). By varying the size of the pattern elements, information regarding visual acuity can be obtained. There are some disadvantages to the use of pattern reversal stimulation. The primary drawback is the requirement that the animal fixate a visual stimulus. This makes assessment in humans who are unable or unwilling to cooperate difficult to accomplish and assessment in animals problematic. Thus cross-species comparisons, which are essential for neurotoxicological assessment, are difficult to make.

These techniques represent the most heavily researched electrophysiological measures for neurotoxicological assessment of sensory systems. There are other methods that, in the future, may prove useful in this regard. For example, single-cell recording, EPs elicited with visual sine-wave gratings, and EPs generated by the initiation of voluntary movements are receiving considerable attention from basic researchers and will receive increasing attention in toxicology.

Age Differences in the Effects of Neurotoxicants on Electrophysiological Measures

Before discussing potential age differences in the effects of neurotoxicants on these measures, it is fruitful to briefly review what is known about the effects of age. In addition, interactions between age and other causes of decreased neurophysiological integrity (e.g., age-related diseases of the nervous system) may provide hypotheses to be explored in the neurotoxicology of aging. In general, the elderly EEG is characterized by slowing (Marsh and Thompson, 1977). This slowing is manifest in two primary ways. First, there is an increase in the percentage of time (during the awake state) in which low-frequency activity (1–7 Hz) is evident. It is still speculative, however, whether this is a product of maturation per se or age-related central nervous system pathology, such as vascular disease or Alzheimer's disease. The second type of slowing is a decrease in the frequency of alpha activity. The mean frequency for young adults is 10–11 Hz, compared with 8–9 Hz in elderly persons.

EPs are also known to change in old age. For example, the latencies of various components of the brainstem auditory EP increase with age. By examining latency differences within various portions of the response, Harkins and Lenhardt (1980) concluded that changes in co-chlear, and possibly medullary, portions of the auditory system are responsible for the differences, as opposed to more superior, cortical areas. The changes noted include a reduced amplitude and increased latencies among early portions of the EP. This illustrates the potential utility of this response in localizing auditory system damage. Somatosensory EPs are generally characterized by increased latencies and decreased amplitudes of most components with age (Marsh and Thompson, 1977). However, clinical or neurotoxicological applications must take into account the fact that the conduction velocity of peripheral nerves slows with age (Marsh and Thompson, 1977). Visual EPs seem to change very little with age for components with latencies less than 100 msec. Beyond this range, latencies tend to increase while amplitudes may decrease in the elderly. Though this has been found for the flash EP (Schenkenberg, 1970), there has been very little, if any, research on adult age differences in the pattern reversal EP.

The application of EPs to assess potential neurotoxic insult in the elderly patient will require knowledge of the normative changes with age. A further complication is likely to be the effects of age-related disease processes. For example, Wave V of the brainstem response has been shown to increase in latency and decrease in amplitude in Alzheimer's disease (Harkins and Lenhardt, 1980). Although striking differences in the early and middle portions of visual EPs have not been attributed to dementing illnesses, there are reliable changes in late portions of the response, as discussed below. With a few exceptions, the gerontological and neurotoxicological literatures in electrophysiology have not overlapped. Age-comparative neurotoxicological studies of humans are clearly needed before the measures will be useful in the screening of elderly individuals exposed to toxicants. Perhaps more important in the near future is the development of animal models of electrophysiological aging, in order to allow screening of various substances for their toxic effects on senescent organisms. In one of the first age-comparative electrophysiological studies of a suspected neurotoxicant, Groll-Knapp et al. (1982) measured click EPs during sleep in young and elderly subjects exposed to carbon monoxide. They reported generally increased amplitudes after exposure, especially for earlier components. There were no pronounced age differences in the effects of the carbon monoxide.

In addition to the exogenous components of the EP, there are longer latency components that are less sensitive to the characteristics of the stimulus and more influenced by cognitive activity initiated by the stimulus. The contingent negative variation (CNV) is a negative shift in the electrical activity of the brain that lasts for several seconds and occurs in conjunction with certain sensory, motor, and cognitive activities. For example, during a reaction-time task in which a warning signal precedes a stimulus signaling the necessity of a motor response, a CNV develops between the warning signal and the "go" signal. The CNV is often correlated with various aspects of cognitive responses and is considered by some to be an index of attention and arousal (Tecce, 1972). The magnitude of this negative shift has been found to decrease with age and to be sensitive to neurotoxicants and other drugs. According to Otto (1983), the amplitude of the CNV is increased by amphetamines and caffeine and reduced by depressants, tranquilizers, and anxiolytics. The CNV is also altered by exposure to carbon monoxide, but the effects have not been consistent. A reliable relationship has been found between CNV amplitude and blood lead levels in children (Otto, 1983).

There is a component of the EP that is a positive deflection occurring at a latency of 300–800 msec. This late positive component (LPC; also referred to as P300 or P3), is maximal over central and parietal areas of the scalp and was originally detected in response to low-probability stimuli (Sutton, Braren, and Zubin, 1965). The amplitude of the LPC is a function of stimulus probability as well as the significance, or information value, of the stimulus (Johnson, 1986). The latency of the LPC is thought to be a reflection of the timing of various cognitive processes (Duncan-Johnson and Donchin, 1977). In general, the latency of the LPC increases in response to increases in task difficulty or complexity. For example, in a tone discrimination task, LPC latency typically increases as the tones become more similar (i.e., discrimination between them becomes more difficult; Squires et al., 1977). When deciding whether a probe item is a member of a previously presented set of items, LPC latency to the probe has been found to increase with increases is set size (Marsh, 1975). The LPC has recently been shown to be sensitive to various forms of neurophysiological insult. LPC latency is prolonged in Alzheimer's disease, in cerebrovascular disease (Squires et al., 1980), in Parkinson's disease (Brown, Marsh, and LaRue, 1983), after neurological surgery and traumatic insult (Squires et al., 1980), in hyperkinetic children (Prichep, Sutton, and Hakerem, 1976), and in mentally retarded individuals (Galbraith et al., 1979). LPC amplitude is reduced in Alzheimer's disease, cerebrovascular disease (Squires et al., 1980), and schizophrenia (Roth et al., 1980).

As noted by Rebert (1983) and Harbin (1985), few toxicological studies of the LPC have been conducted. Teo and Ferguson (1985) reported a significantly greater LPC latency in workers exposed to high doses of organophosphate pesticides. Alterations in the LPC have also been reported subsequent to subanesthetic doses of enflurane (Adam and Collins, 1979). Harbin et al. (1987) investigated the effects of low-level carbon monoxide exposure on the LPC in young and elderly men. Results indicated no effects of carbon monoxide on either the amplitude or latency of the LPC in either group. Young subjects in this study absorbed more of the gas than did the elderly subjects. This may be the result of a paradoxically advantageous decline in respiratory function with age.

Electrophysiological measures have been studied quite extensively in the context of monitoring the effects of anesthesia and the health of brain structures during surgical procedures (Grundy, 1982). However, extrapolation to toxicology is problematic for at least two reasons. First, the emphases of anesthesia and toxicology are somewhat different. Anesthesiologists want information on the patient's response to the somatosensory stimulation of surgery and are therefore interested in correlates between electrophysiological response and "depth of anesthesia." Toxicologists are more interested in the health of various structures as indicated by their electrophysiological activity. One prominent area of overlap is represented by the anesthesiologists monitoring of EPs during surgery for the purpose of ascertaining the adequacy of blood flow, proper retraction of brain structures, and so forth (Grundy, 1982), which corresponds to the evaluation of the health of brain structures by neurotoxicologists. However, the emphasis of this chapter is on alteration in EPs due to chemical insult; other uses of EPs, such as localizing specific structures, monitoring the adequacy of spinal column function during spinal surgery, and ascertaining the health of auditory system structures during brainstem and related surgery are reviewed elsewhere (e.g., Grundy, 1982).

The differences in emphasis lead to differences in the information obtained by the two disciplines. In anesthesiology, the EEG and EPs are evaluated for their gross normality. Toxicologists desire information regarding abnormalities in more discrete components and frequency characteristics of the measures. The global EEG has not proved to be particularly useful as an index of brain status in anesthesiology. As in toxicology (e.g., Dyer, 1987b), anesthesiologists have found that the EEG is much less sensitive to the effects of drugs than other measures (Levy, Grundy, and Smith, 1984). Most agents have little effect on the EEG until anesthetic levels are reached. According to Levy, Grundy, and Smith (1984), narcotics initially produce an increase in overall frequency and then result in a greater prominence in high-voltage, low-frequency activity. Barbiturates and halogenated compounds result in slight increases in high-frequency activity, followed by decreases in frequency and increased voltage at higher doses. The appearance of slow wave activity usually coincides with loss of consciousness (Clark and Rosner, 1973). Continued increases in dose result in "suppression bursts," or episodic reductions in voltage, to the point that the EEG is virtually flat.

Although EPs can provide more detailed information regarding the functioning of discrete portions of the brain, they are not particularly sensitive to anesthetics. This conclusion must be tempered by the recognition that very little work has been done on this topic. The brainstem EP seems to be reduced in amplitude during anesthesia (Grundy, 1983). Uhl et al. (1980) reported that the latency of the P1 component of the flash EP was increased by halothane, though amplitude was not affected. Similarly, Adam and Collins (1979) reported increased latencies of several components of visual EPs, including the late positive component, at low doses of enflurane. However, as noted by Grundy (1982), the effects of anesthetics on EPs are not well researched. The effects seem to depend on the particular anesthetic, modality of stimulation, recording site, and secondary effects of the anesthetic such as hypo- or hyperthermia.

In summary, the effect of anesthetics on the EEG seems to be primarily an increase in high-voltage, low-frequency activity. As with neurotoxicants, however, the EEG is not particularly sensitive to the effects of the drugs. This corroborates the conclusion of toxicologists that, at present, the EEG is not a useful index of central nervous system integrity, and the contribution of EPs in anesthesiology and toxicology is an open question. It also appears that differences in recording techniques and emphases between the fields are sufficiently great as to make it difficult for researchers to learn from one another. Further work in areas common to both disciplines (e.g., the neurophysiology of the EEG and EPs) will render fruitful collaboration more likely. Finally, as is evident from the preceding discussion, there is little or no research on the effects of anesthetics on the brain's electrical activity from an adult developmental perspective.

More complete knowledge is needed regarding changes with age in the kinetics and dynamics of neurophysiological toxicants. Many age-related diseases have deleterious effects on neurophysiological integrity, most notably Alzheimer's disease. Because at present there is no treatment for this disease, afflicted individuals receive mainly custodial treatment. It is frequently the case that elderly individuals who present symptoms of neurological dysfunction are believed to be suffering from Alzheimer's disease when, in fact, a different condition is causing the symptoms. Thus, a toxicant-induced neurobehavioral disorder must be accurately distinguished from normal age changes and chronic disease if elderly patients are to receive the appropriate treatment.

At this point, EEG and EPs make only small contributions to the applied assessment of neurotoxicological insult. Although they are useful in limited circumstances, there are a number of areas in which further development and refinement are required. Norms for the amplitudes and latencies of various components are needed. These norms should be compiled for different ages and genders at the very least (see Grundy, 1982). If EPs are to be useful in the differentiation of toxicant-induced changes and other disease processes, norms for the different disease conditions are also needed. Similarly, basic knowledge of CNV amplitude and morphology as well as the frequency–power spectrum of the EEG, again by age and gender, must be obtained. One of the advantages of EPs is the cross-species comparability of many aspects of the measures. Further work in comparative neurotoxicology from an adult developmental framework is necessary.

Currently, very little is known about toxicant-induced changes in EPs and the nature of the underlying anatomical or physiological damage. Although alterations in the EP now serve as indicators that *something* is amiss, toxicologists must rely on other measures to elucidate the nature of the damage. Small exceptions to this are the brainstem EP and the pattern reversal EP, which can provide some information regarding the nature of the damage. Basic research describing the origins of various aspects of the brain's electrical activity is warranted.

Otto (1983) evaluated the utility of various aspects of the EP as neurotoxicity screens and concluded that their use is sufficiently promising to warrant further development. The potential for electrophysiological measures to be especially useful from an adult developmental perspective is considerable. Other measures, especially behavioral methods, may suffer from age-related differences in such factors as compliance, attitudes toward testing, and cautiousness. The EEG and EPs are impervious to these and many other potential confounds that may be related to age. It is difficult to intentionally alter these measures, in contrast to others that can be "faked." Electrophysiological measures are easily quantified, encouraging precise use and sensitive evaluation of potential toxicant-induced changes at all ages.

With the exception of the developing fetus and young children, there is probably no larger group in the United States who can be considered more susceptible to the effects of environmental toxicants than elderly people. The virtual absence of research in this area is disturbing. In view of the increased risk of neurophysiological problems in elderly people, and the enormous cost both in monetary terms and in terms of human suffering, it is to be hoped that this state of affairs will soon be rectified.

References

Adam, N., and Collins, C. I. 1979. Alteration by enflurane of electrophysiological correlates of search in short-term memory. *Anesthesiology* 50:93–97.

Brown, W. S., Marsh, J. T., and LaRue, A. 1983. Exponential electrophysiological aging: P3 latency. *Electroencephalography and Clinical Neurophysiology* 55:277–285.

Clark, D. L., and Rosner, B. S. 1973. Neurophysiologic effects of general anesthetics: I. The electroencephalogram and sensory evoked responses in man. *Anesthesiology* 38:564–582.

Crooks, J., O'Malley, K., and Stevenson, I. H. 1976. Pharmacokinetics in the elderly. *Clinical Pharmacokinetics* 1:280–296.

Duncan-Johnson, C. C., and Donchin, E. 1977. The P300 component of the event-related brain potential as an index of information processing. *Biological Psychology* 14:1–52.

Dyer, R. S. 1985. The use of sensory evoked potentials in toxicology. *Fundamental and Applied Toxicology* 5:24–40.

Dyer, R. S. 1987a. Somatosensory evoked potentials. In Lowndes, H. H. (Ed.), *Electrophysiology in Neurotoxicology* (Vol. 2). Boca Raton, FL, CRC Press, pp. 1–33.

Dyer, R. S. 1987b. Macrophysiological assessment of organometal neurotoxicity. In Tilsen, H. A., and Sparber, S. B. (Eds.), *Neurotoxicants and Neurobiological Function. Effects of Organoheavy Metals*. New York, John Wiley and Sons, pp. 137–184.

Galbraith, G. C., Squires, N., Altair, D., and Glidden, J. B. 1979. Electrophysiological assessments in mentally retarded individuals: From brainstem to cortex. In Begleiter, H. (Ed.), *Evoked Brain Potentials and Behavior*. New York, Plenum Press, pp. 229–244.

Groll-Knapp, E., Haider, M., Jenker, H., Liebich, H., Neuberger, M., and

Trimmel, M. 1982. Moderate carbon monoxide exposure during sleep: Neuro- and psychophysiological effects in young and elderly people. *Neurobehavioral Toxicology and Teratology* 4:709–716.

Grundy, B. L. 1982. Monitoring of sensory evoked potentials during neurosurgical operations: Methods and applications. *Neurosurgery* 11:556–575.

Grundy, B. L. 1983. Intraoperative monitoring of sensory evoked potentials. *Anesthesiology* 58:72–87.

Harbin, T. J. 1985. The late positive component of the evoked cortical potential: Application to neurotoxicity testing. *Neurobehavioral Toxicology and Teratology* 7:339–344.

Harbin, T. J., Benignus, V. A., Muller, K. M., and Barton, C. N. 1988. The effects of low-level carbon monoxide exposure upon visually evoked potentials in young and elderly men. *Neurotoxicology and Teratology* 1:93–100.

Harkins, S. W., and Lenhardt, M. 1980. Brainstem auditory evoked potentials in the elderly. In Poon, L. W. (Ed.), *Aging in the 1980s: Psychological Issues*. Washington, DC, American Psychological Association, pp. 101–114.

Hillyard, S. A., and Kutas, M. 1983. Electrophysiology of cognitive processing. *Annual Review of Psychology* 34:33–61.

Israili, Z. H. 1979. Age-related change in the pharmacokinetics of some psychotropic drugs in its clinical implications. In Nandy, K. (Ed.), *Geriatric Psychopharmacology*. New York, Elsevier, pp. 31–62.

Johnson, R., Jr. 1986. A triarchic model of P300 amplitude. *Psychophysiology* 23:367–384.

Klein, U., Klein, M., Sturm, H., Rothenbuhler, M., Huber, R., Stucki, P., Gikalov, I., and Keller, M. 1976. The frequency of adverse drug reactions as dependent upon age, sex and duration of hospitalization. *International Journal of Clinical Pharmacology and Biopharmacy* 13:187–195.

Levy, W. J., Grundy, B. L., and Smith, N. T. 1984. Monitoring the electroencephalogram and evoked potentials during anesthesia. In Saidman, L. J., and Smith, N. T. (Eds.), *Monitoring in Anesthesia*. Boston, Butterworth, pp. 227–267.

Marsh, G. R. 1975. Age differences in evoked potential correlates of memory scanning process. *Experimental Aging Research* 1:3–16.

Marsh, G. R., and Thompson, L. W. 1977. Psychophysiology of aging. In Birren, J. E., and Schaie, K. W. (Eds.), *Handbook of the Psychology of Aging*. New York, Van Nostrand Reinhold, pp. 219–248.

Otto, D. 1983. The application of event-related slow brain potentials in occupational medicine. In Gilioli, R., Cassitto, M. G., and Foa, V. (Eds.), *Neurobehavioral Methods in Occupational Health*. New York, Pergamon Press, pp. 71–78.

Otto, D. 1986. The use of sensory evoked potentials in neurotoxicity testing of workers. *Seminars in Occupational Medicine* 1:175–183.

Otto, D., Hudnell, K., Boyes, W., Janssen, R., and Dyer, R. S. 1988. Electrophysiological measures of visual and auditory function as indices of neurotoxicity. *Toxicology* 49:205–218.

Petrie, W. M., and Ban, T. A. 1983. Drugs and the aged. In Burrows, G. D., and Werry, J. S. (Eds.), *Advances in Human Psychopharmacology* (Vol. 3). Greenwhich, CT, JAI Press, pp. 187–210.

Prichep, L. S., Sutton, S., and Hakerem, G. 1976. Evoked potentials in hyperkinetic and normal children under certainty and uncertainty: A placebo and methylphenidate study. *Psychophysiology* 13:419–428.

Rebert, C. S. 1983. Multisensory evoked potentials in experimental and applied neurotoxicology. *Neurobehavioral Toxicology and Teratology* 5:659–672.

Roth, W. T., Horvath, T. B., Pfefferbaum, A., and Kopell, B. S. 1980. Event-related potentials in schizophrenics. *Electroencephalography and Clinical Neurophysiology* 48:127–139.

Schenkenberg, T. 1970. Visual, auditory, and somatosensory evoked responses of normal subjects from childhood to senescence. Unpublished doctoral dissertation, University of Utah.

Squires, K. C., Chippendale, K. C., Wrege, K. S., Goodin, D. S., and Starr, A. 1980. Electrophysiological assessment of mental function in aging and dementia. In Poon, L. W. (Ed.), *Aging in the 1980s: Psychological Issues.* Washington, DC, American Psychological Association, pp. 125–134.

Squires, N. K., Donchin, E., Squires, K. C., and Grossberg, S. 1977. Bisensory stimulation: Inferring decision-related process from the P300 component. *Journal of Experimental Psychology: Human Perception* 3:299–315.

Sutton, S., Braren, M., and Zubin, J. 1965. Evoked potential correlates of stimulus uncertainty. *Science* 150:1187–1188.

Tecce, J. J. 1972. Contingent negative variation (CNV) and psychological processes in man. *Psychological Bulletin* 77:73–108.

Teo, R. K. C., and Ferguson, D. A. 1985. The effects of organophosphate pesticide exposure on event-related potentials (ERPs) in pest control operators. In *Neurobehavioral Methods in Occupational and Environmental Health.* Copenhagen, World Health Organization, pp. 163–167.

Uhl, R. R., Squires, K. C., Bruce, D. L., and Starr, A. 1980. Effect of halothane anesthesia on the human cortical visual evoked response. *Anesthesiology* 53:273–276.

Vaughn, H. G. 1974. The analysis of scalp-recorded brain potentials. In Thompson, R. F., and Patterson, M. M. (Eds.), *Bioelectric Recording Techniques, Part B.* New York, Academic Press, pp. 158–207.

Xintaras, C., Johnson, B. L., Ulrich, C. E., Terrill, R. E., and Sobecki, M. F. 1966. Application of the evoked response technique in air pollution toxicology. *Toxicology and Applied Pharmacology* 8:77–87.

12

Neuropsychological Toxicology
and Aging

Frederick A. Schmitt, Ph.D.
John D. Ranseen, Ph.D.

Neuropsychological toxicology involves the study of the effects of exposure to toxic substances on human behavior, cognition, and emotion. This field has evolved recently from behavioral toxicology, which has primarily employed animal models in research to analyze exposure to toxicants. Hartman (1987a) expressed the importance of a separate discipline of neuropsychological toxicology, because the traditional approach of animal research cannot easily be generalized to the effects in humans of exposure to toxicants, which involve changes in emotionality and higher cognitive functions. Perhaps the first study in this area was that of Hanninen (1971), who employed psychological methods to examine workers exposed to carbon disulfide. Subsequently, numerous investigations have evaluated the effects of naturally or industrially produced central nervous system (CNS) toxicants on neuropsychological functioning in children and adults.

The objective assessment of neurotoxicity is currently the primary contribution of neuropsychological investigation (e.g., White, 1986). As noted by Lezak (1984, p. 28), "neuropsychological assessment probably offers the most sensitive means of examining the effects of toxic exposure, of monitoring for industrial safety, and of understanding the complaints and psychosocial problems of persons exposed to these toxins." Neuropsychological assessment provides a variety of techniques to examine change in behavior, emotion, and cognition. It is hoped that this form of evaluation will contribute to a better understanding of the nature and course of exposure to different toxic substances, facilitate the care and treatment of exposed patients, and possibly assist in monitoring industrial safety.

As the field of neuropsychological toxicology has matured it has become evident, however, that a variety of problems are encountered in the accurate determination of the effects of exposure to toxic substances. Currently there is no general consensus concerning which tests are most sensitive to exposure effects. In addition, it seems likely that various neuropsychological procedures may not be equally sensitive to different neurotoxicants, particularly because environmental variables such as duration and concentration of exposure are impossible to control and often difficult to delineate both for research and clinical purposes. Prior to any formal evaluation, however, there must be some understanding of the environment in which exposure may have occurred. This can often be quite difficult because exposure often involves retrospective assessment. Finally, the clinician or researcher cannot ignore subject variables such as level of education and additional indices of premorbid functioning including evidence of other risk factors for cognitive impairment. Many of these issues involving neuropsychological performance specifically related to exposure have been extensively discussed in previous reviews (e.g., Baker, White, and Murawski, 1985; Weiss, 1983).

Subject age, both at time of exposure and at time of evaluation, is also a critical variable. Although age has often been considered a possible confounding variable in studies of neurotoxic effects, there has been relatively little systematic study of the relationship of age to the effects of CNS toxicants. Nevertheless, it is evident that interpretation of the behavioral effects seen with exposure to toxicants must consider the individual's age. In addition, research suggests that a variety of diseases associated with aging may be the end result of chronic exposure to a toxicant. This chapter highlights some of the typical behavioral changes associated with exposure to metals, organic solvents, and pesticides while stressing age as an important variable often neglected in the study of neuropsychological toxicology. Methodological approaches to the study of neuropsychological toxicology examining the impact of age on these procedures are examined.

Evaluation of Exposure to Toxicants

Evaluation of the patient with suspected exposure to a toxicant is complex and involves medical, pharmacological, and physiological assessment as well as neurological and neuropsychological evaluation. A thorough history is also necessary, particularly to ascertain the nature of the environment in which this exposure occurred. McGuigan (1983) provided a summary of identifying signs and symptoms resulting from exposure and discussed medical management of the poisoned patient. Information concerning the acute care aspects of medical evaluation and management can be found in comprehensive reviews by Baker, White, and Murawski (1985) and Rumack and Lovejoy (1986). Generally, the neurological examination is oriented toward assessment of objective signs of structural central (CNS) and peripheral nervous system (PNS) involvement. Documentation of chronic sequelae of toxic exposure, estimation of recovery and prognosis, and identification of potential psychosocial aspects of treatment also rely on thorough neuropsychological evaluation (e.g., Strub and Black, 1981).

The neuropsychological evaluation has increasingly been recognized by physicians as an adjunct to the clinical examination because it is well established that exposure to a toxicant often leads to significant subjective complaints of emotional and cognitive difficulties in the absence of objective medical or neurological signs. Thus, the neuropsychological examination can be used to understand the nature and severity of cognitive and motor changes that imply subtle structural impairment in the CNS and PNS (Feldman, 1987; White and Feldman, 1987). Performance on these noninvasive psychological tests has increasingly proved to be an important index of toxic exposure because behavior is "the final common pathway for all neural and non-neural activity" and, as such, "represents an integrated response to an environmental stimulus or insult" (Cranmer and Goad, 1983, p. 97).

The clinical picture of generic exposure usually includes subtle psychiatric problems that can be viewed as a "neurasthenic syndrome" involving numerous emotional and somatic complaints such as fatigue, nervousness, dizziness, and depression (Baker and Letz, 1986; Juntunen, 1978; Juntunen et al., 1982). A variety of standard psychological tests such as the Minnesota Multiphasic Personality Inventory, Beck Depression Inventory, and Profile of Mood States can be used to objectify such complaints. Perhaps of greater importance to the neuropsychologist is the delineation of typical cognitive deficits seen following exposure, such as decreased attention and concentration, slowed reaction time and psychomotor ability, and poor memory and learning (Lezak, 1984; Ryan, Morrow, and Hodgson, 1988). There are a large number of cognitive measures that can potentially be used to assess suspected impairment following exposure. Unfortunately, there are numerous issues involving test sensitivity and selection, availability of appropriate normative data, and validity of interpretation of subtle deficits that render neuropsychological evaluation a difficult enterprise (Smith, 1985).

In general, tests used to monitor neuropsychological change associated with exposure to a toxicant have relied on standard clinical instruments and/or cognitive psychological methodologies. Many of these tests have been administered in the traditional pencil-and-paper format, although the advent of computers has led to an interest in the development of microcomputer-assisted test batteries. Descriptions of computer-based evaluation systems can be found by referring to individual test batteries (e.g., Baker et al., 1985; Baker and Letz, 1986; Branconnier, 1985; Eckerman et al., 1985). Usually these computer test batteries contain variants of standardized clinical neuropsychological assessments as well as newer measures of reaction time, vigilance, and memory scanning that may be the most sensitive to early toxic exposure. Other comprehensive clinical batteries previously used to monitor neurotoxic effects have been described by Baker et al. (1983) and more recently by Ryan et al. (1987).

In sum, there are a variety of neuropsychological tests from which to choose, and it is not always clear which of these tests will best detect neuropsychological deficits in an efficient manner. In general, all of these batteries advocate assessment of the usual variety of cognitive domains including intellectual functioning, psychomotor and visuospatial ability, attentional and memory skills, and language as well as examination of specific motor functions and psychiatric complaints as are typically seen in individuals exposed to toxicants. Although choice of test battery should consider the availability of appropriate normative data for the population under consideration, such data are surprisingly lacking for many standard tests (Dodrill, 1988). This is particularly true for older adults. A notable exception is the Pittsburgh Occupational Exposures Test Battery (Ryan et al., 1987), which is based on standard clinical neuropsychological procedures and provides excellent age-scaled norms.

Interpretation of neuropsychological tests is difficult in older populations, not only because of the lack of appropriate norms, but because of the inherent problem of differentiating subtle, and perhaps subclinical, neurotoxic effects associated with exposure from decline associated with normal or accelerated aging. Further, these test batteries have been used as measures of neurobehavioral functioning across groups of individuals who exhibit a wide range in age and differing exposure histories. Thus, group differences that appear on cognitive tests may not necessarily generalize to individual assessment to guide clinical practice. Individual analyses of neurotoxic effects are further compounded by indirect factors. For instance, symptoms such as change in motivation and arousal, which have reportedly been associated with exposure to a toxicant, might greatly affect the evaluative process of both computerized and standard tests. Finally, many test batteries do not take into account the possibility that subjects who actually complete evaluations may represent a very selective group of workers who have survived in the workplace. Therefore, this population may have an exposure history that is quite different from that of individuals who actually left the workplace possibly as a result of impairment secondary to exposure. In sum, there are many unresolved issues associated with the detection of neuropsychologic deficits secondary to toxic exposure, and in an older adult population these difficulties are exacerbated.

Exposure to Toxic Substances and Age-Associated Disease

Exposure to toxic substances has not only been compared with age-related dementing conditions evident in the studies discussed previously, but has also been implicated as a causal factor in the onset of such disorders. The two most commonly diagnosed organic brain syndromes in the elderly are delirium and dementia (Trzepacz, Teague, and Lipowski, 1985), and both of these problems have been linked to various forms of exposure. Delirium involves an abrupt onset of global cognitive–behavioral disruption and is much more common in older than younger adults (Mesulam and Geschwind, 1976; Morse and Litin, 1969). Although it is well accepted that toxic exposure can result in delirium (e.g., Albert, 1981), most studies have examined delirium as a toxic–metabolic disturbance associated with the postoperative period (e.g., Mesulam and Geschwind, 1976) or with other physical factors including drug intoxication, cardiovascular disorders, infection, and neurological illness (Libow, 1977; Sloane, 1980).

A few studies have attempted to link environmental and industrial exposure to a toxicant with increased risk of general organic brain syndromes (OBS) rather than to a specific disease process. For example, Rasmussen, Olson, and Lauritsen (1985) reported a case control study among nursing home applicants with a history of exposure to an occupational solvent. This study revealed that workers applying for nursing home admission, who had been exposed to solvents, appeared to have an increased risk of developing encephalopathy. Although their data did not show a statistically significant difference in the risk of having developed some form of OBS between workers with and without exposure, workers with a history of solvent exposure exhibited approximately five times the risk of psychosis, which is suggestive of a delirium, and twice the risk of dementia and cerebrovascular disease compared with the nonexposed applicants.

Recently, interest has been expressed concerning the possibility that toxic exposure not only may be related to a brief and transient disruption in behavioral functioning but may also be a mechanism related to chronic progressive dementing conditions. For instance,

Gresham et al. (1986) provided some data suggesting that amyotrophic lateral sclerosis could be linked to occupational exposure to heavy metals. Also, the spectrum of parkinsonian symptoms has been associated with both carbon monoxide (Klawans et al., 1982) and cyanide poisoning (Uitti et al., 1985). For a review of possible etiologies of Parkinson's disease, see Duvoisin (1986).

There has also been a particular interest in a potential link between Alzheimer's disease (AD) and aluminum toxicity. It was initially reported that the autopsied brains of AD patients showed elevated aluminum (e.g., Perl and Brody, 1980). Subsequently, however, Markesbery et al. (1981), in comparing the brains of AD patients with older adult controls, found no correlation between the density of aluminum content and the density of neurofibrillary tangles and neuritic plaques. They also found that brain aluminium levels significantly increased as a function of age in both populations. Consequently, it is questionable whether there is an actual correlation between the increased presence of aluminium and AD and there are no data to firmly suggest that exposure to aluminium is causally related to AD. This research, however, has stimulated the search for other environmental substances that may be linked to development of AD. For example, Bianchi, Bittesini, and Brollo (1986) evaluated the brains of 10 workers exposed to asbestos and found that 8 showed senile plaques in the cortex and 7 showed neurofibrillary tangles in the cortex and hippocampus as might be seen with AD. As a result, this suggests a possible link between asbestos and the development of Alzheimer-like changes although, again, much further research would be necessary to examine whether this relationship has any true link to the development of AD.

Although research investigating links between exposure to toxic substances and the development of OBS is valuable, there is little evidence that firmly establishes the association of exposure and specific dementing conditions. These studies serve to highlight the complexity of the relationship among exposure, age, and resultant neuropsychological deficits. Zbinden (1983) and Annau (1983) both argued that behavioral change secondary to exposure may occur without observable physiological abnormality or may precede or lag behind obvious physiologic change. Furthermore, Zbinden (1983) noted that behavioral changes may not always be a consequence of a direct toxic CNS effect but rather may be secondary to other organ lesions. Taking into account the obvious changes in the physiology of older adults (discussed in other chapters in this text), the elderly may be more at risk for exposure to toxicants because of the indirect toxic effects on other organ systems. Consequently these concerns raise the issue of whether an increased risk for neuropsychiatric disease might be manifested long after the patient has been removed from exposure to neurotoxic agents. It is plausible that aging may encompass numerous subacute CNS insults that include exposure to a toxicant as a factor for the development of progressive dementing conditions (e.g., Mortimer, 1980). In reviewing the literature on exposure to toxicants, however, age has generally been used as a matching variable rather than as a summary variable that could moderate the emergence of neuropsychological deficit associated with exposure.

Neuropsychological Effects of Exposure to Toxic Substances

The literature summarizing the behavioral effects of exposure to pollutants and industrial toxicants suggests that individuals typically experience nonspecific psychological complaints such as forgetfulness, headache, dizziness, and insomnia as well as varying types of cognitive disturbances as documented by psychological test instruments. Unfortunately, much of what is known about neuropsychological impairment associated with exposure is based on a wide variety of tests often uncomparable between studies, resulting in conflicting data. With regard to the specific behavioral effects of exposure, a number of excellent reviews can be found in the current literature (Baker, Smith, and Landrigan, 1985; Feldman, Ricks, and Baker, 1980; Grandjean, 1983; Hartman, 1987b, 1988).

The neurotoxic effects of metals have been widely studied, and many reports summarize their neurotoxic effects including emotional and cognitive symptoms (e.g., Weiss, 1983). Perhaps the most widely studied metal has been lead, which has been implicated in reduced intellectual abilities in children (Needleman et al., 1979), slowed reaction time (Hunter et al., 1985) and impairment in other cognitive abilities (e.g., Hansen et al., 1985; Winneke, Hrdina, and Brockhouse, 1982). Lead has also been studied for its effect on CNS functioning in adults. Although psychophysiological measures appear relatively insensitive to low levels of lead exposure (Assennato et al., 1983), a number of studies have demonstrated both cognitive and emotional effects as a result of long-term exposure to lead. For example, Hogstedt et al. (1983) studied 49 workers exposed to lead in secondary lead smelters and battery factories. Compared with a control group of 27 workers from steel wire plants, machine shops, and ammunition plants the workers exposed to lead (average exposure of 18 years) showed significant decrements in reaction time and memory. However, Hogstedt et al. were unable to demonstrate a significant correlation between their exposure measures and the psychologic tests or reported symptoms.

Similar findings have been reported by Jeyaratnam et al. (1986), who studied the neuropsychological performance of 49 workers in Singapore who were exposed to lead while manufacturing polyvinyl chloride (PVC). These workers were compared with a control group matched for education and ethnicity. Performance of the lead workers was significantly poorer on a number of tests including simple reaction time, the Santa Anna Dexterity Test, Trail Making Test Part A, and Digit Symbol Substitution. Subjective symptoms reported by the exposed group revealed significantly more complaints of depression, anxiety, and other somatic complaints including memory and concentration problems than reported by the controls. Once again, however, a relationship between blood lead values and test performance was not demonstrated.

Correlations between psychological performance and biological indicators of lead toxicity have been reported by other researchers, however. Valciukas et al. (1978) studied 90 smelter workers with an average 10-year occupational exposure to lead. They found significant correlations between levels of zinc protoporphyrin (a biological indicator of long-term lead effects) and three of five performance tests administered. These correlations were seen for the Block Design, Digit Symbol Substitution, and Embedded Figures tests, even when these test scores were corrected for age of the exposed worker. The authors reported that this age correction in performance had only a small effect on the relationship between dose response and performance. Finally, Mantere et al. (1984) completed a follow-up study of workers exposed to low levels of lead. These workers were exposed while working at a storage battery factory and were evaluated before exposure and after 1, 2, and 4 years of work. These workers were compared with a group of nonexposed subjects from electrical power and cable manufacturing plants. Their data showed that a learning effect (improved performance with repeated testing) that was obvious among the case controls was not seen for workers exposed to lead in the battery plant. Further, they reported that the lead-exposed workers showed significant impairment after the first 2 years of follow-up in visual intelligence and visuomotor functioning.

Other metals have also been implicated as having neurotoxic effects that influence neuropsychological functioning. Uzzell and Oler (1986) demonstrated mild changes in short-term nonverbal memory and emotional distress in dental auxillary workers with probable chronic low-level exposure to inorganic mercury. Interestingly, these workers did not show changes in general intelligence as measured by the Wechsler Adult Intelligence Scale (WAIS) or in attention, verbal memory, or motor skills. Long-term exposure to mercury vapor has been reported to interfere with verbal intelligence as assessed by the WAIS Similarities subtest as well as a dose–response curve among exposure level, concentration of mercury in the blood, and memory performance (Piikivi et al., 1984). As with lead toxicity, mercury-induced abnormalities seemed to affect a broad variety of neuropsychological functions. Hanninen (1982) suggested that abnormalities due to mercury exposure affect the motor system and result in intellectual impairment, a gradual and progressive deterioration of memory functioning, and emotional disability. Other metals including copper, iron, and manganese have also been described as causing CNS dysfunction as indicated by both neuropsychological and neurological symptoms (e.g., Grandjean, 1983; Hartman, 1988). It is interesting to note, however, that, consistent with other forms of diffuse brain impairment, some of the early symptoms of metal poisoning appear to involve affective changes and complaints of memory disturbance whereas more objective measures of intellectual dysfunction appear with higher levels of exposure (Grandjean, 1983).

As is the case with metals, organic solvents also appear to damage the CNS, resulting in neuropsychological deficits. Juntunen (1978; Juntunen et al., 1982) has described the diagnostic criteria for organic solvent intoxication. These criteria include the quantitative and qualitative assessments of exposure to the neurotoxic solvent and the documentation of CNS and PNS damage. The clinical picture of organic solvent disease would then include the host of subjective "neurasthenic" symptoms and documented dysfunction on neurological examination, electroencephalograph (EEG), electromyograph, and psychologic evaluation. Toluene has been a focus of some studies (Hanninen et al., 1976) as have other organic solvents used by painters (Baker and Seppalainen, 1986). In general, brief exposure to a solvent appears to impair reaction time as well as psychomotor functioning (Gambrale, 1976). Chronic neurotoxic effects of solvents have been reported by a number of authors (e.g., Mikkelsen, 1980; Spencer and Schaumburg, 1985) and are reviewed by Baker, Smith, and Landrigen (1985).

Cherry and colleagues have been instrumental in investigating the neuropsychological effects of occupational exposure to various solvents. In an early study Cherry et al. (1980) examined workers employed in a boat-building factory who were exposed to styrene. Twenty-seven boat builders were compared with a control group similar in education and age. Workers were evaluated for blood styrene concentrations and measures of mood and reaction time during the day. Mood changes were correlated with blood styrene concentrations; reaction time measures varied on the basis of level of blood styrene concentration. Although the exposed workers did not differ from the control group on the Digit Symbol Substitution and Digit Span tests, they did differ in simple reaction time. More detailed analyses revealed that those workers with a high blood styrine level showed very little improvement in reaction time from morning to afternoon test sessions. Individuals with low blood styrine concentrations were comparable to the control group in performance in the afternoon, after having shown slower reaction times in the morning. These data appear consistent with the hypothesis that styrene exposure may affect CNS functioning only at high concentrations.

In a follow-up study, Cherry et al. (1981) evaluated reaction time performance associated with urine mendelic acid levels (a metabolite of styrine) in workers with high styrine exposure as well as workers with lower styrine exposure. Once again, correlations between mendelic acid as an index of styrine exposure and reaction time were significant. These data suggest that the slowing of reaction time may have been the result of acute styrine exposure.

In a study of dockyard workers exposed to toluene and paint solvents, Cherry et al. (1985) evaluated 44 men exposed to paint solvents and 52 men exposed to toluene versus a control group matched to the exposed groups in terms of age and alcohol use. The behavioral measures included tests of vigilance, visual search, motor speed, memory, and reaction time. In an attempt to adjust for premorbid abilities, the National Adult Reading Test was administered to provide an index of premorbid intellectual ability. Although group differences emerged on the various tests, once the data were adjusted for premorbid ability, only the reaction time tests showed decrements for the workers exposed to solvents.

Other studies of solvent-exposed workers have reported similar results. Hane et al. (1977) evaluated 52 house painters with an average exposure of 14.2 years. These painters were compared with an age-matched control group of industrial workers from other industries. Significantly poorer performance on choice reaction time, visual memory, psychomotor coordination, and figure classification tests was found for the painters compared with the control group. Additional behavioral measures including verbal ability, spatial ability, vigilance, learning, and coordination showed no differences between the two groups. Of interest is the fact that there appeared to be no correlation between workers' age and performance on the psychological tests. Years of probable exposure, however, did not correlate with performance on the various psychological measures.

A similar pattern of findings was described by Lindstrom (1980) in his study of 56 workers diagnosed as suffering from organic solvent disease. These workers had a mean exposure duration of approximately 9 years, having used a mixture of paint solvents as well as halogenated and aromatic hydrocarbons. These 56 workers were compared with a group of 98 styrine-exposed workers as well as a nonexposed control group of 43 construction workers. The psychological tests that were administered were derived from the WAIS as well as the Wechsler Memory Scale, symmetry drawing, the Santa Anna Dexterity Test and the MIRA Test (psychomotor ability). Group comparisons revealed similar performance between the styrine-exposed group and the nonexposed control group with the exception of a higher number of reversals on the symmetry drawing test in the styrine-exposed group. On the other hand, patients with diagnosed solvent exposure showed statistically significant lower scores on the WAIS Digit Symbol, Block Design, and Digit Span subtests. In addition, the solvent-exposed group showed poorer performance on symmetry drawing, the Santa Anna Dexterity Test, and the MIRA Test, suggesting poorer visuomotor performance. Poor visuomotor scores also appeared to be related to duration of solvent exposure.

An important aspect of this study is that Lindstrom (1980) also attempted to control for the effect of different mean ages between the three groups. The mean age of each of the groups was 38.8 years for the solvent-exposed workers, 29.5 years for the styrine-exposed workers, and 33.3 years for the control group. An analysis of covariance revealed that only the visual memory test and Santa Anna Dexterity Test correlated with duration of exposure. Once again, these data support some disruption of visuomotor performance as a result of exposure to solvents. A similar pattern of visuomotor dysfunction has also been described for workers exposed to pesticides (e.g., Misra, Nag, and Murti, 1984), suggesting the possibility of frontal and parietal lobe insult for these toxicants.

Other studies of organic solvents appear to corroborate the findings of Cherry et al. (1980, 1981) as well as Lindstrom (1980). Elofsson et al. (1980) reported poorer reaction time, manual dexterity, and short-term memory in car and industrial spray painters. The authors were also able to demonstrate changes in PNS function, EEG, visual evoked potentials, computed tomographic (CT) scans, and ophthomologic examinations based on exposure. In a more recent study, Linz et al. (1986) evaluated 15 industrial painters who showed no consistent deficits on neurologic exam. Nevertheless, typical neurasthenic symptoms of depression, anxiety, and somatization were seen in these industrial painters and differences on psychologic measures emerged when the painters were compared with a control group matched for age, sex and education level. Among the industrial painters, 80 percent had a Halstead-Reitan Impairment Index greater than 0.5 (moderate impairment). As a group they showed deficits on tests of cognitive flexibility, memory, visuospatial skills, reasoning, and attention.

A host of other solvents have been implicated for their effects on the CNS and resulting impairment in neurological and neuropsychological dysfunction. Carbon disulfide has also been studied extensively, with findings indicating a similar pattern of deficits in motor speed and psychomotor performance as well as emotional impairment. The effects of carbon disulfide exposure have also been linked to peripheral neuropathy as evaluated by nerve conduction velocity studies in workers even 10 years after exposure (Corsi et al., 1983).

Other reports have implicated jet fuel, a mixture of various hydrocarbons including benzine and toluene, in epidemiological studies of exposed workers. Knave et al. (1978) reported a higher number of psychiatric symptoms in workers exposed to jet fuel along with deficits in attention, motor speed, and findings suggesting abnormal EEGs and peripheral neuropathy.

More recently a neurological study of solvent vapor abuse has been reported by Hormes, Filley, and Rosenberg (1986), who studied 20 patients with a history of vapor abuse. These patients were studied after at least 4 weeks of abstinence to reduce the effects of acute intoxication. Sixty percent of these patients showed cognitive deficits, and half showed pyramidal and cerebellar findings. Brainstem and cranial nerve findings were found in 25 percent of the sample, and eight of the nine CT scans that were obtained revealed diffuse atrophy. These data suggest that in highly exposed individuals, objective and observable neurological abnormalities may form the basis of the neuropsychological abnormalities seen in exposed patients.

Age as a Moderating Variable

In the majority of studies discussed in this section, age was seen primarily as a potential confounding variable in the evaluation of exposure to a toxicant. It has been suggested by Cherry et al. (1985) that age and measures of exposure to toxicants (usually based on duration of employment) will invariably show a positive correlation. Therefore, age should always be considered as a moderating variable in the interpretation of results from studies of exposure. Furthermore, if uncontrolled, subject age is likely to be a major confound because many of the neuropsychologic tests that are used in toxicology studies are tests that are also sensitive to age-related change in performance. A number of studies and reviews document the fact that many neuropsychological tests show declines with age (e.g., Bornstein, Paniak, and O'Brien,

1987; Heaton, Grant, and Matthews, 1986; Kaszniak, 1987). Consequently, interpretation of subtle neuropsychologic deficits will be extremely difficult in elderly subjects exposed to toxic substances who
may exhibit impairment simply as a function of age. This is further
complicated because normative data concerning performance by older
adults on neuropsychological tests are often unavailable or based on
restricted samples (e.g., Schmitt and Ranseen, 1989).

Gerontological researchers have discussed the nature of age as a
variable in research designs. They argue that many developmental phenomena are time dependent but not age related even though correlations between chronological age and certain time-ordered processes
appear (Schaie and Hertzog, 1985). Other concepts regarding age as a
variable for study have appeared in the gerontological literature but
have not yet been included in research efforts in neuropsychological
toxicology. Furthermore, many studies investigating CNS effects of
toxicants generally employ a limited age range of approximately 18–60
years because of the nature of the work force. Few studies have extended the age range beyond 65 because most researchers attempt to
enroll workers who are being exposed at the workplace who have not
yet retired. The notion of functional age (McFarland, 1953; Stagner,
1985) or primary aging (disease free) versus secondary aging (disease-
related processes; Birren and Cunningham, 1985) might be useful in
defining the effects of exposure to toxic substances in older workers,
particularly after they leave the work environment. Further discussion
of the nature of age as a variable in psychological research can be
found in chapters by Birren and Renner (1977) and other reviews (e.g.,
Baltes and Willis, 1977; Birren and Cunningham, 1985).

Age and Neuropsychological Toxicology

Chronological age usually serves as a matching variable in research
involving workers exposed to toxicants. As mentioned previously, age
might encompass both the degree and duration of exposure experienced by the individual. Age may also reflect generational differences
as indexed by changes in the work environment through the use of
protective measures or changes in the worker's role within the workplace. In addition, behavioral measures used to evaluate CNS function
may be subject to problems with regard to the use of appropriate age
norms. As a result, chronological age may confound interpretation of
suspected decline or test abnormalities. The use of test procedures
that are not appropriately age normed should be avoided; yet it is only
recently that age-appropriate norms have become available for many
widely used clinical procedures. Several studies have attempted to

account for age effects by matching exposed workers with controls on age and other pertinent variables such as sex and education. These studies that have attempted to account for the effects of workers' age have generally shown inconsistent associations between age and outcomes of exposure.

For example, Juntunen et al. (1982) studied 106 patients exposed to solvents using standard neurologic criteria. Eighty of these patients were seen by a neurologist roughly 6 years after their initial evaluation. These patients averaged approximately 11 years of exposure and were divided by neurological criteria into two groups. The first group showed neurologic and psychologic abnormalities; the second group showed no obvious neurologic symptoms, but other abnormalities including psychological and subjective symptoms were evident. The authors noted a significant decline as indexed by patient symptoms at the 6-year follow-up. Sixteen patients, originally without symptoms, developed abnormalities at follow-up. Five patients who had initially been rated as abnormal were unimpaired at follow-up. The symptoms documented in this report included neurasthenia, sensory problems, gait disturbances, as well as cerebellar signs. The authors noted that gait disturbances were worse with higher levels and longer durations of exposure. They did not find any particular age effects in this group of patients, however.

Letz and Baker (1986) used a computer-administered test battery to evaluate painters for early indications of CNS damage. Their group consisted of painters ranging in age from approximately 25 to 65 years. Comparison groups included patients with head trauma and patients exposed to lead. Their continuous performance test (CPT) revealed poorer performance (CPT latency) for the head injury group compared with the painters. Patients exposed to lead also performed worse than the painters even after the authors adjusted for the effects of age. This age adjustment was necessary because many of the computerized tests were sensitive to chronological age.

Using a questionnaire for neurasthenic symptoms, Rasmussen and Sabroe (1986) studied solvent exposure in metal and electronics workers in Denmark. Control groups included semiskilled metal workers, and although the mean age of their sample was approximately 38 years, some subjects over age 60 were included. Although they found the usual neurasthenic symptoms of headache, dizziness, fatigue, forgetfulness, and irritability in the solvent-exposed workers, Rasmussen and Sabroe (1986) were unable to demonstrate group differences associated with exposure once they adjusted for the age of the worker.

In a comprehensive study, Eskelinen et al. (1986) compared 21 patients with organic solvent exposure (average of 10.5 years) with patients who had vertebrobasilar circulation insufficiencies, patients with headache, and patients with a history of closed head injury. They used WAIS subtests as well as subtests from the Wechsler Memory Scale, the Santa Anna Dexterity Test, finger tapping, the MIRA Drawing Test, and symmetry drawing to compare these groups. The patients exposed to organic solvents performed worse than the other three control groups on measures of intelligence and memory. A potential confound emerged, however, in that the patients with vertebrobasilar circulation insufficiency were significantly worse than the solvent-exposed, headache, or closed head injury patients on the psychomotor or visual–graphic measures. Using a discriminate function analysis, Eskelinen et al. were able to best differentiate the four groups' performance on the Block Design test, the Similarities test, Digit Span, visual reproduction, and Santa Anna Dexterity Test. The group differences may have been influenced by the age of the patients; however, whereas the average ages for the solvent-exposed, headache, and head injury groups were equivalent, the vascular group's mean age was more than 10 years older. Consequently, their poor performance on psychomotor and visual graphic tests may well have been accounted for by their being older rather than their medical condition per se.

Another example of the high correlation between workers' age and exposure estimates can be found in a study by Gregersen, Klausen, and Elsnab (1987), who studied solvent-exposed painters in Denmark over a 5-year period. Their study attempted to look at workers with chronic toxic encephalopathy by including patients who quit work because of other organic factors such as head injury, alcohol, transient ischemic attacks, stroke, and so forth. Their group of 21 painters (ages 23–56 years) were evaluated using neuropsychological measures of learning, memory, attention, and abstraction. Patients were evaluated roughly 9 months after exposure (average duration of exposure was approximately 26 years). Compared with the other organic groups, the painters showed a wide variety of neurologic problems including sensory abnormalities (29 percent), motor abnormalities (5 percent), and cerebellar ataxia (5 percent). The authors found that memory was much more impaired than abstraction in the chronic toxic encephalopathy group and that ratings of exposure correlated with the degree of psychological impairment. For example, measures of learning and memory showed a correlation of .61 with exposure, and attention and concentration measures showed a correlation of .57 with exposure. On the other hand, age of the solvent-exposed patients also correlated with the neuropsychological tests, with a correlation coefficient of .48 between age and psychological impairment.

Maizlish et al. (1987) used multiple linear regression models to evaluate 240 subjects with a history of exposure to organic solvents controlling for the moderating variables of age, sex, and alcohol use. They noted neurological abnormalities, predominantly polyneuropathy, in 16 percent of their subjects and found that exposed workers compared with nonexposed controls showed a higher frequency of symptoms that was associated with solvent level. Nevertheless, once they controlled for the effects of moderator variables, including age, sex, and alcohol use, no significant relationship was found between the ratings of poor neurological function and solvent exposure.

Effects of subject age are also apparent in studies comparing neuropsychological tests and physiological measures in the evaluation of chronic toxic encephalopathy. For example, Arlien-Soborg et al. (1982) derived cerebral blood flow indices in nine house painters with a mean exposure of 22 years. These house painters had mild to moderate neuropsychological impairment but showed only minimal or no cerebral atrophy on CT scan. These nine painters were compared with 11 age- and sex-matched volunteers on the blood flow measures. Mean age of the painters was 41 years (range of 24–59 years) and the age range for the volunteers was 30–57 years. Although the results revealed significant differences in cerebral blood flow based on the xenon inhalation technique, cerebral blood flow appeared to be correlated with subject age as well. Even though the painters revealed lower blood flow rates overall, they did not show any hemispheric flow differences, consistent with a diffuse chronic brain syndrome following solvent exposure.

In a more recent study, Orbaek et al. (1987) evaluated 62 patients with organic solvent exposure on neurologic and neuropsychological tasks. Their sample of exposed patients included 32 men between the ages of 33 and 69 (median age of 55 years) with a median exposure to solvents of 26 years. They also used a control group of 40 age- and socioeconomic status-matched men. Comparisons of the neuropsychological tests revealed a wide range of neuropsychological deficits, including visual memory, verbal memory, spatial skills, simple and choice reaction time, mental processing speed, and basic motor functioning. No differences were found between the patients with chronic toxic encephalopathy in the control group on the CT scan measures. Although the CT scan measures appeared to be age dependent, the differences between patients and controls did not increase with increasing subject age. Orbaek et al. adjusted for the age of patients and then looked at correlations between neuropsychological test impairment and the CT scans as well. They were able to find some significant interrelationships between the CT scan measures and such tasks as Block Design and attention. Because these correlations appeared only within the solvent-exposed group, the authors suggested that the deficits seen in psychomotor speed and attention were associated with structural changes in the brains of the patients with chronic toxic encephalopathy.

Two other studies comparing neuropsychological functioning and structural brain measures have been reported. White (1987) addressed the issue of differential diagnosis between toxicant exposure and probable Alzheimer's disease in older workers in which four diagnostic cases were presented. From these cases, as well as a review of the literature, White concluded that several differences in neuropsychological evaluation exist between individuals exposed to solvents and those with Alzheimer's disease. The primary difference that White inferred between these two groups on neuropsychological examination was in the nature of their language disturbance. Alzheimer's disease was viewed as resulting in dysnomia as well as verbal paraphasic errors and accompanying disruptions in reading and writing. The solvent-exposed patient, on the other hand, may show little dysnomia and reading and writing performance within normal limits. The nature of the memory disturbance between the two disorders may also be qualitatively different. In the case of the solvent-exposed encephalopathic patient, retrograde memory problems would date only from the time of exposure and be more extensive and severe than with patients with Alzheimer's disease. A final diagnostic consideration is progression of the neuropsychological deficits associated with each disease. The general pattern of Alzheimer's disease is a steady and progressive decline that may or may not be seen with solvent-exposed patients. Although there is some evidence that solvent-exposed patients can improve in neuropsychological performance once they are removed from exposure (Baker, White, and Murawski, 1985). White argued that a slow and progressive decline in solvent-exposed individuals could be possible if the neurotoxic agent is stored in body tissues and continues to disrupt CNS functioning. Again, these are useful clinical hypotheses based on case studies, but they do not constitute a test of differential neuropsychological functioning in these two groups of cognitively impaired patients.

A more direct comparison of occupational exposure to toxicants and Alzheimer's disease was recently reported by Koss et al. (1988). Eighteen patients with Alzheimer's disease who were assessed for possible occupational exposure to solvents and other environmental toxicants on the basis of their occupational history were studied. Patients with greater than 5 years' exposure according to their history (10 patients) were compared with the nonexposed group (8 patients) using neuropsychological tests and positron emission tomography. Both groups showed neuropsychological impairment consistent with the diagnosis of Alzheimer's disease. Further, both groups showed reduced glucose metabolism, which is commonly associated with Alzheimer's disease. On the other hand, patients with the 5-year history of occupational exposure showed an additional impairment in frontal glucose metabolism. Apparently, patients with this history showed a relative frontal hypometabolism compared with the patients with Alzheimer's disease and no history of potential exposure.

These data are important in the study of neuropsychological toxicology and aging because, as mentioned earlier, no relationship between exposure to neurotoxicants and eventual development of progressive dementia has been documented. These data also point to the possible coexistence of solvent encephalopathy and primary degenerate dementia such as Alzheimer's disease. Data such as those reported by Koss et al. (1988) serve to emphasize the lack of research data in the areas of both long-term toxicant exposure in the workplace as associated with the aging process and possible age-associated sequelae once exposure to neurotoxicants has been eliminated. Koss et al.'s study further emphasizes the diagnostic dilemmas posed by evaluations of older adults with cognitive impairment, particularly given the range of possible exposure not only in the workplace but in day-to-day life, which in the final analysis, can only be looked at retrospectively.

Conclusions and Future Directions

This chapter has raised the issue of age as an important variable within the field of neuropsychological toxicology. This is a very new field with promise to facilitate our understanding of toxic effects on human function, assist in patient evaluation and treatment, and possibly help us better understand the aging process. It is also a field with potentially far-reaching consequences within industry to assist in monitoring safety. It is not inconceivable that conclusions concerning the adverse neuropsychological effects of exposure to toxicants may involve serious legal issues as well. For these reasons, well-designed research will continue to be necessary.

General conclusions indicate that there is little question that exposure to metals, solvents, and pesticides can have serious effects on human behavior, emotion, and cognition that can be documented with neuropsychological procedures. These effects, however, involve a complex spectrum of impairment, the extent of which is likely to depend on variables such as duration and degree of exposure, the exposed subject's biological integrity, and history of premorbid risk factors. It is generally believed that the behavioral dysfunction associated with exposure reflects a process of diffuse CNS impairment. As with other diffuse CNS disorders, such as closed head injury or the toxic effects of alcoholism, the neuropsychological changes that occur are easier to detect and understand when the precipitating event is both acute and relatively severe. This would also appear to be the case for exposure to toxicants. Methodological and clinical problems are encountered, however, in the differentiation of subtle emotional and cognitive impairments, particularly if they are caused by events that are temporally removed from the onset of symptomatology.

These problems confront the researcher and clinician with serious problems in the evaluation of neuropsychological sequelae following exposure to toxicants, especially in elderly patients. Subtle affective and cognitive dysfunction may be virtually impossible to distinguish from the declines that are often associated with normal aging. The elderly patient is also much more likely to be removed in time from the events that might have involved exposure, particularly if this exposure occurred in the workplace and the patient presents for evaluation some time after retirement. The problem of the timing of exposure and evaluation therefore reduces the reliability of diagnostic procedures geared toward documenting exposure to a toxicant and the resultant neuropsychological deficits. Further, some researchers have suggested that there are differences in the neuropsychological profiles between exposure to a toxicant and disorders associated with aging such as Alzheimer's disease (White, 1987), whereas others have suggested toxicant exposure as one possible etiology for Alzheimer's disease (e.g., Mortimer, 1980). Consequently, there are many unresolved issues in the area of neuropsychological toxicology involving elderly patients. Although it has been suggested that prospective studies that assess workers prior to possible exposure would provide a better way to evaluate such concerns (Baker and Letz, 1986), this approach raises other issues associated with repeated evaluation, lengthy follow-up, and potential ethical problems.

As already discussed, there is a desperate need for additional normative data with which to interpret test findings from older adults. Such data would clearly enhance both clinical and research efforts in this field. A related need, which is rarely addressed in the literature, concerns the functional relevance of impaired performance associated with exposure. For instance, it is of theoretical interest that exposure to different types of toxicants results in a statistically significant difference between exposed and nonexposed groups on simple reaction-time tasks (a finding equally typical for normal aging). On the other hand, what is the importance of such a finding in terms of the individual's ability to function on a day-to-day basis? Such questions will be of particular importance as the health professional is asked to address clinical and perhaps legal concerns.

In sum, many questions remain concerning the exact nature and impact of exposure to various neurotoxicants on neuropsychological functions, and these issues become increasingly complex as we consider the additional impact of patient age on these functions. Although "the impact of these environmental phenomenon on aging processes and the aged is not well understood, there are sound biological reasons to assume that the effect of the environment on people changes with age, as does the ability to respond to environmental exposures" (Committee on Chemical Toxicity and Aging, 1987, p. 162). As we begin to understand the CNS mechanisms of toxicants and the relationship between the brain and behavior in neuropsychological toxicology, we will no doubt increase our knowledge regarding the early detection and age-associated changes involved in the disorders associated with environmental exposure to toxicants.

References

Albert, M. A. 1981. Geriatric neuropsychology. *Journal of Consulting and Clinical Psychology* 49:835–850.

Annau, Z. 1983. Screening strategies. In Zbinden, G., Cuomo, V., Racagni, G., and Weiss, B. (Eds.), *Application of Behavioral Pharmacology in Toxicology*. New York, Raven Press, pp. 87–95.

Arlien-Soborg, P., Henriksen, L., Gade, A., Gyldensted, C., and Paulson, O. B. 1982. Cerebral blood flow in chronic toxic encephalopathy in house painters exposed to organic solvents. *Acta Neurologica Scandinavica* 66:34–41.

Assennato, G., Sborgia, G., L'Abbate, N., Paci, C., De Marinis, L., De Marinis, G., Gagliardi, T., Montrone, N., Ambrosi, L., Ferrannini, E., Masi, G., Specchio, L. M., Olivieri, G., LaNeve, A., De Tommaso, M., and Benedetto, G. 1983. Evaluation of neurophysiological tests in monitoring lead exposure. In Zbinden, G., Cuomo, V., Racagni, G., and Weiss, B. (Eds.), *Application of Behavioral Pharmacology in Toxicology*. New York, Raven Press, pp. 345–348.

Baker, E. L., Feldman, R. G., White, R. F., Harley, J. P., Dinse, G. E., and Berkey, C. S. 1983. Monitoring neurotoxins on industry: Development of a neurobehavioral test battery. *Journal of Occupational Medicine* 25:125–130.

Baker, E. L., and Letz, R. 1986. Neurobehavioral testing in monitoring hazardous workplace exposures. *Journal of Occupational Medicine* 28:987–990.

Baker, E. L., Letz, R. E., Fidler, A. T., Shalat, S., Plantamura, D., and Lyndon, M. 1985. A computer-based neurobehavioral evaluation system for occupational and environmental epidemiology: Methodology and validation studies. *Neurobehavioral Toxicology and Teratology* 7:369–377.

Baker, E. L., and Seppalainen, A. M. 1986. Human aspects of solvent neuro-behavioral effects. *Neurotoxicology* 7:43–56.

Baker, E. L., Smith, T. J., and Landrigan, P. J. 1985. The neurotoxicity of industrial solvents: A review of the literature. *American Journal of Industrial Medicine* 8:207–217.

Baker, E. L., White, R. F., and Murawski, B. J. 1985. Clinical evaluation of neurobehavioral effects of occupational exposure to organic solvents and lead. *International Journal of Mental Health* 14:135–158.

Baltes, P. B., and Willis, S. L. 1977. Toward psychological theories of aging and development. In Birren, J. E., and Schaie, K. W. (Eds.), *Handbook of the Psychology of Aging* (1st ed.). New York, Van Nostrand Reinhold, pp. 128–154.

Bianchi, C., Bittesini, L., and Brollo, A. 1986. Asbestos exposure and Alzheimer disease. *Italian Journal of Neurological Sciences* 7:145–151.

Birren, J. E., and Cunningham, W. R. 1985. Research on the psychology of aging: Principals, concepts and theory. In Birren, J. E., and Schaie, K. W. (Eds.), *Handbook of the Psychology of Aging* (2nd ed.). New York, Van Nostrand Reinhold, pp. 3–34.

Birren, J. E., and Renner, V. J. 1977. Research on the psychology of aging: Principles and experimentation. In Birren, J. E., and Schaie, K. W. (Eds.), *Handbook of the Psychology of Aging* (1st ed.). New York, Van Nostrand Reinhold, pp. 3–38.

Bornstein, R. A., Paniak, C., and O'Brien, W. 1987. Preliminary data on classification of normal and brain-damaged elderly subjects. *The Clinical Neuropsychologist* 1:315–323.

Branconnier, R. J. 1985. Dementia in human populations exposed to neuro-toxic agents: A portable microcomputerized dementia screening battery. *Neurobehavioral Toxicology and Teratology* 7:379–386.

Cherry, N., Hutchins, H., Pace, T., and Waldron, H. A. 1985. Neurobehavioral effects of repeated occupational exposure to toluene and paint solvents. *British Journal of Industrial Medicine* 42:291–300.

Cherry, N., Rogers, B., Venables, H., Waldron, H. A., and Wells, G. G. 1981. Acute behavioral effects of styrene exposure: A further analysis. *British Journal of Industrial Medicine* 38:346–350.

Cherry, N., Waldron, H. A., Wells, G. G., Wilkinson, R. T., Wilson, H. K., and Jones, S. 1980. An investigation of the acute behavioral effects of styrene on factory workers. *British Journal of Industrial Medicine* 377:234–240.

Corsi, G., Maestrelli, P., Picotti, G., Manzoni, S., and Negrin, P. 1983. Chronic peripheral neuropathy in workers with previous exposure to carbon disulphide. *British Journal of Industrial Medicine* 40:209–211.

Cranmer, J. S., and Goad, P. T. 1983. Validation of selected behavioral tests for evaluating low-level toxicity. In Zbinden, G., Cuomo, V., Racagni, G., and Weiss, B. (Eds.), *Application of Behavioral Pharmacology in Toxicology*. New York, Raven Press, pp. 97–112.

Dodrill, C. B. 1988. What constitutes normal performance in clinical neuropsychology? Paper presented at the annual meeting of the American Psychological Association, Atlanta, GA.

Duvoisin, R. C. 1986. Etiology of Parkinson's disease: Current concepts. *Clinical Neuropharmacology* 9 (Suppl. 1):S3–S11.

Eckerman, D. A., Carroll, J. B., Fooree, D., Gullion, C. M., Lansman, M., Long, E. R., Waller, M. B., and Wallsten, T. S. 1985. An approach to brief field testing for neurotoxicity. *Neurobehavioral Toxicology and Teratology* 7:387–393.

Elofsson, S., Gamberale, F., Hindmarsh, T., Iregren, A., Isaksson, A., Johnsson, I., Knave, B., Lydahl, E., Mindus, P., Persson, H. E., Philipson, B., Steby, M., Struwe, G., Soderman, E., Wennberg, A., and Welden, L. 1980. Exposure to organic solvents: A cross-sectional epidemiologic investigation on occupationally exposed car and industrial spray painters with special reference to the nervous system. *Scandinavian Journal of Work, Environment and Health* 6:239–273.

Eskelinen, L., Luisto, M., Tenkanen, L., and Mattei, O. 1986. Neuropsychological methods in the differentiation of organic solvent intoxication from certain neurological conditions. *Journal of Clinical and Experimental Neuropsychology* 8:239–256.

Feldman, R. G. 1987. Occupational neurology. *Yale Journal of Biology and Medicine* 60:179–186.

Feldman, R. G., Ricks, N. L., and Baker, E. L. 1980. Neuropsychological effects of industrial toxins: A review. *American Journal of Industrial Medicine* 1:211–227.

Gambrale, F. 1976. Behavioral effects of exposure to solvent vapors: Experimental and field studies. In Horvath, M. (Ed.), *Adverse Effects of Environmental Chemicals and Psychotropic Drugs* (Vol. 2). Amsterdam, Elsevier, pp. 111–113.

Grandjean, P. 1983. Behavioral toxicology of heavy metals. In Zbinden, G., Cuomo, V., Racagni, G., and Weiss, B. (Eds.), *Application of Behavioral Pharmacology in Toxicology*. New York, Raven Press, pp. 331–339.

Gregersen, P., Klausen, H., and Elsnab, C. U. 1987. Chronic toxic encephalopathy in solvent-exposed painters in Denmark 1976–1980: Clinical cases and social consequences after a 5-year follow-up. *American Journal of Industrial Medicine* 11:399–417.

Gresham, L. S., Molgaard, C. A., Golbeck, A. L., and Smith, R. 1986. Amyotrophic lateral sclerosis and occupational heavy metal exposure: A case-control study. *Neuroepidemiology* 5:29–38.

Hane, M., Axelson, O., Blume, J., Hogstedt, C., Sundell, L., and Ydreborg, B. 1977. Psychological function changes among house painters. *Scandinavian Journal of Work, Environment and Health* 3:91–99.

Hanninen, H. 1971. Psychological picture of manifest and latent carbon disulphide poisoning. *British Journal of Industrial Medicine* 28:374–381.

Hanninen, H. 1982. Behavioral effects of occupational exposure to mercury and lead. *Acta Neurologica Scandinavica* 66 (Suppl. 92):167–175.

Hanninen, H., Eskelinen, L., Husman, K., and Nurminen, M. 1976. Behavioral effects of long-term exposure to a mixture of organic solvents. *Scandinavian Journal of Work, Environment and Health* 4:240–255.

Hanninen, H., Nurminen, M., Tolonen, M., and Martelin, T. 1978. Psychological tests as indicators of excessive exposure to carbon disulfide. *Scandinavian Journal of Psychology* 19:163–174.

Hansen, O. N., Trillingsgaard, A., Beese, I., Lyngbye, T., and Grandjean, P. 1985. Neurobehavioral methods in assessment of children with low-level lead exposure. In *Neurobehavioral Methods in Occupational and Environmental Health, Document 3*. Copenhagen, World Health Organization, pp. 183–187.

Hartman, D. E. 1987a. *Neuropsychological Toxicology*. Workshop presented at the annual meeting of the National Academy of Neuropsychologists, Chicago, IL.

Hartman, D. E. 1987b. Neuropsychological toxicology: Identification and assessment of neurotoxic syndromes. *Archives of Clinical Neuropsychology* 2:45–65.

Hartman, D. E. 1988. *Neuropsychological Toxicology: Indentification and Assessment of Neurotoxic Syndromes*. New York, Pergamon Press.

Heaton, R. K., Grant, I., and Matthews, C. G. 1986. Differences in neuropsychological test performance associated with age, education, and sex. In Grant, I., and Adams, K. M. (Eds.), *Neuropsychological Assessment of Neuropsychiatric Disorders*. New York, Oxford University Press, pp. 100–120.

Hogstedt, C., Hane, M., Agrell, A., and Bodin, L. 1983. Neuropsychological test results and symptoms among workers with well-defined long-term exposure to lead. *British Journal of Industrial Medicine* 40:99–105.

Hormes J. T., Filley, C. M., and Rosenberg, N. L. 1986. Neurologic sequelae of chronic solvent vapor abuse. *Neurology* 36:698–702.

Hunter, J., Urbanowicz, M. A., Yule, W., and Landsdown, R. 1985. Automated testing of reaction time and its association with lead in children. *International Archives of Occupational and Environmental Health* 57: 27–34.

Jeyaratnam, J., Boey, K. W., Ong, C. N., Chia, C. B., and Phoon, W. O. 1986. Neuropsychological studies on lead workers in Singapore. *British Journal of Industrial Medicine* 43:626–629.

Juntunen, J. 1978. Neurotoxic syndromes in man. In *Third International Course in Industrial Toxicology*. Helsinki, Institute of Occupational Health, pp. 164–168.

Juntunen, J., Antti-Poika, M., Tola, S., and Partanen, T. 1982. Clinical prognosis of patients with diagnosed chronic solvent intoxication. *Acta Neurologica Scandinavica* 65:488–503.

Kaszniak, A. W. 1987. Neuropsychological consultation to geriatricians: Issues in the assessment of memory complaints. *The Clinical Neuropsychologist* 1:35–46.

Klawans, H. L., Stein, R. W., Tanner, C. M., and Goetz, C. G. 1982. A pure parkinsonian syndrome following acute carbon monoxide intoxication. *Archives of Neurology* 39:302–330.

Knave, B., Olson, B. A., Elofsson, S., Gamberale, F., Isaksson, A., Mindus, P., Persson, H. E., Struwe, G., Wennberg, A., and Westerholm, P. 1978. Long-term exposure to jet fuel. A cross-sectional epidemiologic investigation on nervous system. *Scandinavian Journal of Work, Environment and Health* 4:19–45.

Koss, E., Friedland, R. P., Luxenberg, J. S., and Moore, A. 1988. Occupational exposure to toxins in Alzheimer's disease: Metabolic and behavioral correlates. Presented at the annual meeting of the International Neuropsychological Society, New Orleans, LA.

Letz, R., and Baker, E. L. 1986. Computer-administered neurobehavioral testing in occupational health. *Seminars in Occupational Medicine* 1:197–203.

Lezak, M. D. 1984. Neuropsychological assessment in behavioral toxicology—developing techniques and interpretative issues. *Scandinavian Journal of Work, Environment and Health* 10:25–29.

Libow, L. S. 1977. Senile dementia and pseudosenility: Clinical diagnosis. In Eisdorfer, C., and Friedel, R. O. (Eds.), *Cognitive and Emotional Disturbance in the Elderly*. Chicago, Year Book, pp. 75–88.

Lindstrom, K. 1980. Changes in psychological performance of solvent-poisoned and solvent-exposed workers. *American Journal of Industrial Medicine* 1:69–84.

Linz, D. H., deGarmo, P. L., Morton, W. E., Wiens, A. N., Coull, B. M., and Maricle, R. A. 1986. Organic solvent-induced encephalopathy in industrial painters. *Journal of Occupational Medicine* 28:119–125.

Maizlish, N. A., Fine, L. J., Albers, J. W., Whitehead, L., and Langolf, G. D. 1987. A neurological evaluation of workers exposed to mixtures of organic solvents. *British Journal of Industrial Medicine* 44:14–25.

Mantere, P., Hanninen, H., Hernberg, S., and Luukkonen, R. 1984. A prospective follow-up study on psychological effects on workers exposed to low levels of lead. *Scandinavian Journal of Work, Environment and Health* 10:43–50.

Markesbery, W. R., Ehmann, W. D., Hossain, T. I. M., Alauddin, M., and Goodin, D. T. 1981. Instrumental neutron activation of brain aluminum in Alzheimer's disease and aging. *Annals of Neurology* 10:511–516.

McFarland, R. A. 1953. *Human Factors in Air Transportation: Occupational Health and Safety*. New York, McGraw-Hill.

McGuigan, M. A. 1983. Clinical toxicology. In Hayes, J. A., and Pelikan, E. W. (Eds.), *A Guide to General Toxicology*. New York, Karger, pp. 23–69.

Mesulam, M., and Geschwind, N. 1976. Disordered mental status in the postoperative period. *Urologic Clinics of North America* 3:199–215.

Mikkelsen, S. 1980. A cohort study of disability pension and death among painters with special regard to disabling presenile dementia as an occupational disease. *Scandinavian Journal of Social Medicine* 16(Suppl.):34–43.

Misra, U. K., Nag, D., and Krishna Murti, C. R. 1984. A study of cognitive functions in DDT sprayers. *Industrial Health* 22:199–206.

Morse, R. M., and Litin, E. M. 1969. Postoperative delirium: A study of etiological factors. *American Journal of Psychiatry* 126:388–395.

Mortimer, J. A. 1980. Epidemiological aspects of Alzheimer's disease. In Maletta, G. J., and Pirozzolo, F. J. (Eds.), *The Aging Nervous System*. New York, Praeger Scientific, pp. 307–332.

National Research Council, Committee on Chemical Toxicity and Aging. 1987. *Aging in Today's Environment*. Washington, DC: National Academy Press.

Needleman, H. L., Gunnoe, C., Leviton, A., Reed, R., Peresie, H., Maher, C., and Barret, P. 1979. Deficits in psychologic and classroom performance of children with elevated dentine lead levels. *New England Journal of Medicine* 300:689–695.

Orbaek, P., Lindgren, M., Olivecrona, H., and Haeger-Aronson, B. 1987. Computed tomography and psychometric test performances in patients with solvent induced chronic toxic encephalopathy and healthy controls. *British Journal of Industrial Medicine* 44:175–179.

Perl, D. P., and Brody, A. R. 1980. Alzheimer's disease: X-ray spectrometric evidence of aluminum accumulation in neurofibrillary tangle-bearing neurons. *Science* 208:207–209.

Piikivi, L., Hanninen, H., Martelin, T., and Mantere, P. 1984. Psychological performance and long-term exposure to mercury vapors. *Scandinavian Journal of Work, Environment and Health* 10:35–41.

Rasmussen, H., Olsen, J., and Lauritsen, J. 1985. Risk of encephalopathia among retired solvent-exposed workers: A case-control study among males applying for nursing home accommodation or other types of social support facilities. *Journal of Occupational Medicine* 27:561–566.

Rasmussen, K., and Sabroe, S. 1986. Neuropsychological symptoms among metal workers exposed to halogenated hydrocarbons. *Scandinavian Journal of Social Medicine* 14:161–168.

Rumack, B. H., and Lovejoy, F. H. 1986. Clinical toxicology. In Klaassen, C. D., Amdur, M. O., and Doull, J. (Eds.), *Casarett and Doull's Toxicology: The Basic Science of Poisons* (3rd ed.). New York, Macmillan, pp. 879–901.

Ryan, C. M., Morrow, L. A., Bromett, E. J., and Parkinson, D. K. 1987. Assessment of neuropsychological dysfunction in the workplace: Normative data from the Pittsburgh Occupational Exposures Test Battery. *Journal of Clinical and Experimental Neuropsychology* 9:665–679.

Ryan, C. M., Morrow, L. A., and Hodgson, M. 1988. Cacosmia and neurobehavioral dysfunction associated with occupational exposure to mixtures of organic solvents. *American Journal of Psychiatry* 145:1442–1445.

Schaie, K. W., and Hertzog, C. 1985. Measurement in the psychology of adulthood and aging. In Birren, J. E., and Schaie, K. W. (Eds.), *Handbook of the Psychology of Aging*. New York, Van Nostrand Reinhold, pp. 61–92.

Schmitt, F. A., and Ranseen, J. D. 1989. Neuropsychological assessment of older adults. In Hunt, T., and Lindley, C. (Eds.), *Testing Older Adults*. Austin, TX, Pro-Ed, pp. 51–69.

Sloane, R. B. 1980. Organic brain syndrome. In Birren, J. E., and Sloane, R. B. (Eds.), *Handbook of Mental Health and Aging*. Englewood Cliffs, NJ, Prentice-Hall, pp. 554–590.

Spencer, P. S., and Schaumburg, H. 1985. Organic solvent neurotoxicity: Facts and research needs. *Scandinavian Journal of Work, Environment and Health* 1(Suppl.):53–60.

Smith, P. J. 1985. Behavioral toxicology: Evaluating cognitive functions. *Neurobehavioral Toxicology and Teratology* 7:345–350.

Stagner, R. 1985. Aging in industry. In Birren, J. E., and Schaie, K. W. (Eds.), *Handbook of the Psychology of Aging*. New York, Van Nostrand Reinhold, pp. 789–817.

Strub, R. L., and Black, F. W. 1981. *Organic Brain Syndromes: An Introduction to Neurobehavioral Disorders*. Philadelphia, F. A. Davis.

Trzepacz, P. T., Teague, G. B., and Lipowski, Z. J. 1985. Delirium and other organic mental disorders in a general hospital. *General Hospital* 7:101–106.

Uitti, R. J., Rajput, A. H., Ashenhurst, E. M., and Rozdilsky, B. 1985. Cyanide-induced parkinsonism: A clinicopathologic report. *Neurology* 35: 921–924.

Uzzell, B. P., and Oler, J. 1986. Chronic low-level mercury exposure and neuropsychological functioning. *Journal of Clinical and Experimental Neuropsychology* 8:581–593.

Valciukas, J. A., Lilis, R., Fischbein, A., Selikoff, I. J., Eisinger, J., and Blumberg, W. E. 1978. Central nervous system dysfunction due to lead exposure. *Science* 201:465–467.

Weiss, B. 1983. Behavioral toxicology and environmental health science: Opportunity and challenge for psychology. *American Psychologist* 38: 1174–1187.

White, R. F. 1986. The role of the neuropsychologist in the evaluation of toxic central nervous system disorders. *Seminars in Occupational Medicine* 1:191–196.

White, R. F. 1987. Differential diagnosis of probable Alzheimer's disease and solvent encephalopathy in older workers. *The Clinical Neuropsychologist* 1:153–160.

White, R. F., and Feldman, R. G. 1987. Neuropsychological assessment of toxic encephalopathy. *American Journal of Industrial Medicine* 11:395–398.

Winneke, G., Hrdina, K. G., and Brockhouse, A. 1982. Neuropsychological studies in children with elevated tooth-lead concentrations: A pilot study. *International Archives of Occupational and Environmental Health* 51:169–183.

Zbinden, G. 1983. Definition of adverse behavioral effects. In Zbinden, G., Cuomo, V., Racagni, G., and Weiss, B. (Eds.), *Application of Behavioral Pharmacology in Toxicology*. New York, Raven Press, pp. 1–14.

13

Aging and the Impact
of Environmental Hazards
on Sensory Function

Gail R. Marsh, Ph.D

Vision and hearing are the two senses that have received the lion's share of the research on the effects of aging on sensory systems. This chapter reviews the research on these two senses as well as smell, taste, and the somatosensory senses. Many of the studies have not differentiated between "normal" aging and those changes that have taken place as a result of disease or the accumulated insults acquired from a hazardous environment. I shall attempt to make this differentiation where possible. The number of studies that have addressed issues of sensory function in aging with respect to toxic substances is meager. However, a number of studies have examined aging sensory systems with regard to environmental insult or the accumulated effects of a lifetime of exposure to environmental pollutants or hazards. These are interleaved in the present discussion so that contrasts can be drawn with the relevant normal studies.

It will become apparent in the discussion below that, as our knowledge has grown, an easy division between what is sensory and what is cognitive is no longer possible. We now know that there are multiple feedback loops between higher brain centers and the sensory apparatus that guides our perceptions before we are ever aware of what we are sensing. Thus, changes in the central nervous system (CNS) during aging can alter how we perceive, and changes in the sensory apparatus can alter how the CNS processes the sensory data. Unlike anatomical or physiological changes, when measuring perceptual functions it is often not possible to know at what levels the aging changes have taken place.

To clarify what we know and what remains in question regarding each sensory system, I first describe the most prominent changes in the anatomy and physiology of the sensory system under discussion. The perceptual changes are then described, some of which may be due to anatomical and physiological changes, and some to alterations in the CNS that remain relatively unknown.

For further information and other points of view on aging changes in the special senses, readers are referred to several recent reviews. These reviews include three general references (Birren and Schaie, 1977, 1985; Corso, 1981) and one specifically on vision (Sekuler, Kline, and Dismukes, 1982).

Vision

Anatomical and Physiological Changes with Aging

For humans there is little doubt that vision is considered the cardinal sense, and its loss is considered the most severe. The earliest changes in the eye are in the anterior portion; deterioration in the retina comes later. The important structures in this anterior portion are the cornea, the iris, the crystalline lens, and the chamber enclosed by the cornea and the lens. The cornea, which is the most important refractive element of the eye (performing about two-thirds of the total refraction), flattens a bit but is relatively unchanged with age. It must be kept relatively unhydrated, and special cells on the inner surface pump water out of the cornea into the anterior chamber. These cells are reduced in number with age, which reduces control of hydration in old age, but this is a relatively minor problem.

The most significant changes that occur with age are in the iris and the crystalline lens. The iris, which functions to control the amount of light entering the eye through the pupil, begins to constrict to a relatively more closed position in the elderly person. An individual in his or her 70s receives about one-third the light on the retina as a twenty-year-old (some of this is due to decreased transmission internal to the eye) (Weale, 1961). The iris also becomes less able to react quickly to a change in lighting conditions. However, this is a relatively benign change compared with its more chronic state of constriction. Several theories have been advanced to explain this condition: (1) a relative overbalance of sympathetic to parasympathetic influence, (2) atrophy of the dilator muscles and growing inelasticity of the iris, and (3) chronic partial sleep deprivation in the elderly, which induces constriction, one of the chief signs of sleepiness (Pressman, DePhillipo, and Fry, 1986). The explanations are not mutually exclusive. This loss of light undoubtedly leads to loss of visual abilities under conditions of low illumination.

The iris loses some of its pigmentation with age and is a less effective barrier to light. This light leakage, since it strikes the retina in random fashion, functions as noise superimposed on the focused image.

The cornea and the lens cannot contain capillaries to provide the usual support functions of the vascular system because these vessels would impede light transmission. Thus, another system developed: the flow of a clear fluid, aqueous humor, a blood derivative, through the anterior chamber of the eye. However, nutrients and oxygen must perfuse into the tissue and waste products diffuse out. This is not a problem for the cornea, but it is for the lens.

The lens of the eye derives from ectoderm and continues to display its heritage by growing continuously throughout life. Consequently, the lens is about three times larger in a 70-year-old than in a 20-year-old. The growth of the lens is like an onion with new tissue spreading over the outer surface that forms a lens with its oldest cells in the center. This continuous growth of the lens, without shedding any old cells, leads to several problems.

First, it becomes difficult to provide nutrients to the cells buried deeply in the core of the lens. When the thickness of the lens prevents adequate penetration of nutrients to the core of the lens, those cells begin to turn dark and to deteriorate. Also, these cells lose their nucleus, alter parts of the cytoskeleton, and become insufficient in enzymes necessary for proper metabolism and protection from insults, such as the oxidation of membranes from free radicals. They also are less able to prevent the incorporation of sulfide-linked protein aggregates, found in cataract formation, which scatter light rather than properly refracting it. Thus, the cells near the center of the lens are more susceptible to lasting injury of several kinds (Spector, 1982; Tripathi and Tripathi, 1983).

Second, the lens begins to change from pale yellow to a stronger yellow, which strengthens its filter capacity to reduce the input of shorter wavelengths of light. The pale yellow filters out some ultraviolet light and provides correction of a mild chromatic aberration (Lerman, 1980). The stronger yellow provides better ultraviolet protection, but reduces the ability of the eye to pass purples and blues.

Lastly, the lens becomes resistant to changing shape. It needs to be squeezed to a flatter shape to focus distant objects on the retina and must return to its former oval shape when the compression force is released so that it can focus near objects. The accommodative power of the lens to respond to the control of the ciliary muscle is gradually lost, being initially felt between the ages of 40 and 50. The loss is both static and dynamic: (1) a loss of ability to form a clear image of objects close to the eye and (2) the ability to change focus quickly from near to far objects.

The posterior portion of the eye holds the retina and other supporting membranes at the rear of the chamber. The chamber itself is filled with a gelatinous substance called the *vitreous humor,* which helps hold the retina in place and the eye in the correct shape. With age the vitreous begins to liquify and pockets of fluid develop. This accumulation of fluid usually begins about two-thirds of the distance from the lens to the retina. This fluid accumulation slowly grows and migrates toward the retina, which reduces support for the retina. Further, the fluid and remnants of the vitreous move during rapid accelerations of the eye or head and the pull on the retina can cause injury. It has been suggested that the possibility of injury through eye movements or vibration is much higher in older workers (Balazs and Denlinger, 1982).

The retina and its supporting tissue show several different kinds of changes with age: loss of retinal elements, a decrease in the pigmentation in the retinal pigment epithelium, and evidence of sclerosing of the blood vessels. The most devastating loss to visual function is the loss of elements in the macula, a tightly packed mass of receptive elements at the center of which is the fovea, the point of visual focus on the retina, where the receptors are packed very closely. This is the part of the retina that supports high visual acuity. The retinal elements are cones, elements that are sensitive to color and operate only at high levels of light. These elements begin to show evidence of aging between 40 and 60 years of age, when there is significant loss of cones. If the macular degeneration is accompanied by extensive deterioration of the pigmented epithelium just behind the retina, which supports the parts of the rods and cones that actually transform light into electrical impulses, then blood vessels from the choroid that normally supply the pigmented epithelium may invade the retina. These new vessels are very prone to leakage and quickly lead to a complete loss of macular function.

The role played by the retinal pigmented epithelium in aging has not been fully explored. It is one of the most active tissues of the body and is very sensitive to loss of vascular support. Without this membrane the photoreceptors cannot function, and this loss could induce a progressive chain of deterioration in the retinal elements. The main function of the epithelium is the breakdown and synthesis of the lipid pigments used by the rods and cones to sense light. Free radicals can produce nonmetabolizable lipid compounds that accumulate, causing deterioration of function and consequent loss of elements in the overlying retina (Marmor, 1982).

Phototoxicity from ultraviolet and visible light may also play a role in deterioration of the retina and supporting tissues. These elements have as much exposure as the skin, but without replacement of the exposed cells. Sclerosis of the blood vessels is well known and has been shown to be involved in patchy losses of retinal elements, as already mentioned. Its role in slow loss of individual elements is not as well established.

Diabetic retinopathy is considered to be an acceleration of the normal aging deterioration of the retina. The blood vessels of the retina deteriorate in what is thought to be the usual deterioration of the small vessels seen with diabetes—growth of small vessels followed by sclerosis of the vessels and deterioration of blood flow leading to loss of the cells being supported by those vessels. This type of deterioration in the retina is seen most strongly in persons who have had diabetes a long time. There is 90 percent prevalence of significant deterioration after 20 years, even in young adulthood in those with juvenile onset (Type I).

In addition to senile macular degeneration, there are two other diseases of the eye that are common and are strongly linked to aging: glaucoma and cataract (Greenberg and Branch, 1982; Pitts, 1982). Glaucoma is a condition of increased pressure within the eye. The eye continuously operates at pressures above normal to aid in holding the structure in its proper shape. The formation of aqueous humor from the vascular system allows for the quick flow of this liquid through the eye and then out through small ducts. Pressure builds beyond normal limits when there is excess fluid in the anterior chamber, often because of blockages of the outflow of fluid, and creates no perceptible sensation or pain. Also, ocular pressure is regulated to some degree by the systolic blood pressure. Thus, with the increases of blood pressure often seen in aging, there can be a parallel increase in intraocular pressure leading to glaucoma. Treatment of blood pressure can also concomitantly treat the high-pressure problem of the eye (Bulpitt, Hodes, and Everitt, 1975).

Cataracts, the opacification of the lens, form in two principal ways. One is that the nuclear portion of the lens becomes so dark or opaque or scatters light so badly that transmission of light through the central portion of the lens becomes severely impaired. Because most of central vision must take place through this portion of the lens, the lens is removed and often replaced with a plastic lens insert or wearing of special contact lenses. Surprisingly, surgery to remove cataracts is the fifth most often conducted surgery in the United States. There is some evidence that exposure to ultraviolet light could be an important element in development of cataracts (Hollows and Moran, 1981). However, the data suggest that sufficient exposure to trigger cataract production is unlikely except for those who spent the vast majority of their life outdoors. Even for those persons, if wearing protective lens (or sunglasses) was common practice, the effects of ultraviolet exposure would be insufficient to speed cataract production.

The second process of generating cataracts is linked to diabetes. In this case the lens develops opacity, but it is on the outer edges, where the cells developing the new lens layers are located, rather than at the central core. The outer edge deteriorates when lens cells deteriorate as a result of filling with sorbitol, generated only when blood sugar is at high levels. Cellular metabolism is disrupted and the cells deteriorate. This relatively opaque tissue then slowly moves outward toward the center of the lens in the usual motion of a forming layer.

These two forms of cataract influence sight quite differently. The cortical cataract provides greatest interference under lower light conditions when the pupil is relatively open, thus interfering most with peripheral vision. On the other hand, the nuclear cataract interferes most under bright conditions when the pupil is constricted; under dim conditions, when the pupil is relaxed, some light can enter through the peripheral portion of the lens and peripheral sight can function, as well as provide a modicum of central vision.

There are undoubtedly changes in brain tissue, such as the loss of 50 percent of the primary visual cortex cells by age 70 (Devaney and Johnson, 1980), which underlie some of the changes in visual perception that are described below. Most of the changes in brain tissue that have been discussed in the literature have not been found by direct experimentation carried out on the primary visual system. Thus, we do not know the exact changes in the visual system and instead work by analogy to the changes seen elsewhere in brain tissue.

Perceptual Alteration with Aging

Acuity   Visual acuity (the ability to see fine detail) has always received a great deal of attention, most likely because it is so readily detected. During early childhood objects within a few inches of the face can be brought into focus. However, by middle age objects must often be a foot or more away from the face before they can be brought into focus. As the lens becomes increasingly less able to bring near objects into focus, spectacles with multiple focal lengths are used to bring relatively near objects into focus.

Dynamic acuity is even more heavily altered by age. Dynamic acuity is the ability to maintain clear focus for fine detail on objects that are in motion. With an increasingly less resilient lens, quick changes of focus become very difficult. In addition, for moving objects the eyes must be able to track that object, which is an additional problem. In a study of a very large number of individuals from ages 16–92 years, Burg (1966) found that older individuals could not track rapidly moving objects well and thus were unable to see them clearly. These decreased abilities to track and focus were reflected in the driving abilities of older drivers (Panek et al., 1977).

One element in loss of acuity is loss of light on the retina. When the amount of light entering the eye is reduced, the eye's resolving power is reduced. As noted earlier, the retina of a 70- to 80-year-old receives about one-third the light of a young adult because of decreased pupil aperture and the loss of transmission through lens and vitreous. This is shown maximally by testing under low levels of illumination after an adequate period of adaptation, but it is also seen under well-illuminated conditions.

Another problem, in addition to the loss of signal, is the extent of visual "noise." The older eye produces more stray light on the retina from scattered light from the lens and through the iris. This introduction of stray light is glare. Glare takes several forms: simple addition of stray light, washing out of the image from too much light, and being blinded by persisting images of light that take a long time to fade (as in the response to a flashbulb). Also, the image is often less sharply formed in the older eye. All of these conditions partially disable the visual imaging processes of the eye and CNS.

Acuity also depends on the number of receptive elements in the retina. The number of such elements is reduced, but, as calculated by Weale (1982), the loss of acuity is greater than would be predicted just on the loss of these elements alone. Thus, CNS changes with age contribute substantially to the loss of acuity.

A related aspect of visual acuity is brightness contrast, that is, the ability to note differences in brightness between two adjacent fields. There are little data on changes in this function with aging, but in one study comparing 20- to 30-year-olds with 60- to 70-year-olds, the illumination difference had to be about 2.5 times greater for the older group to perceive the difference (Blackwell and Blackwell, 1971).

Contrast sensitivity, another way of assessing visual acuity, is closely associated with brightness contrast. This method assesses acuity by determining how great the difference in contrast must be between two adjacent areas for the person to perceive the difference. Test stimuli can have sharp border contrasts, such as a checkerboard, or more slowly changing borders, such as sinusoidal gratings (somewhat like waves or ripples seen from above). The spatial distance between the bars, checks, or waves determines the spatial frequency. To use the checkerboard example, as the checks get smaller the spatial frequency increases. With increasing age there is a need for greater contrast at the intermediate and higher spatial frequencies, and little change at the low frequencies (Owsley, Sekuler, and Siemsen, 1983).

Obviously, acuity can be measured in a number of ways. The most familiar, the Snellen chart, measures only the ability to see small objects under high contrast at far distances. The most comprehensive acuity measure is contrast sensitivity, because it covers resolving power of the eye for both small and large objects under a number of illumination and contrast conditions. However, none of the methods used to measure acuity have any good way of translating across methods for comparisons. Further, acuity is influenced by a number of systems in the eye, all of which may age in different ways and at different rates. Thus, acuity is an important measure as a summary of how well the eye functions, but is a slippery measure when one must specify what the measures mean in terms of the aging of various eye functions. In fact, Birren and Williams (1982) pointed out that changes in vision often involve changes in all aspects of eye and brain function, overlapping into what would normally be considered cognitive functions.

Depth Perception   Depth perception is thought to fall off after about age 45 at which time deterioration in function parallels the decline in acuity with age (Bell, Wolf, and Bernholz, 1972; Jani, 1966). This is reasonable, considering that depth cues can be extracted only if the eye is able to clearly resolve the visual field. Because depth perception is believed to involve extensive high-level processing of a number of cues from the visual field, it might be expected on theoretical grounds to be an important function to study in aging, but it has received little attention. Fortunately, having a smaller pupil increases the ability to perceive depth as long as sufficient light reaches the retina to provide adequate acuity.

Field of Vision   The ability to detect a stimulus shrinks from a wide visual field in young adults to a field about two-thirds this size by the age of 75 and drops to about half the original field by age 80–90 (Burg, 1968; Wolf, 1967). The field of vision is tested by various means, using both moving and static targets. The same general tendency has emerged: a small constriction in visual field between ages 40 and 50, and increasingly larger losses in succeeding decades with loss greater in the temporal fields than in the nasal. There is an enlargement of the blind spot that marks the point at which the optic nerve leaves the retina. The mechanism involved in loss of the visual field is not known. The loss of elements can be substantial before the person begins noticing the loss, because the visual system is very accomplished at "filling in'' missing parts of a visualized object. The losses of the visual elements in the peripheral visual field, the rods, may be especially large before they are noticed because many rods feed information to one retinal ganglion cell. This may explain why the large losses that are often noted anatomically are not always reflected in complaints of lost function. It may also be due to the fact that peripheral vision is more automatic and receives less conscious consideration.

Because the peripheral visual field has as one of its chief functions detecting motion, which then allows us to turn our gaze directly to the moving object, those methods of assessing peripheral function that use detection of motion are the most useful. Whether the speed of this motion is critical has not been studied in aging.

Darkness Adaptation and Color Vision   The eye can respond immediately to changes in illumination by altering the size of the iris. It can attain a wider range of sensitivity by altering the level of sensitivity of the retina through photochemical and neural changes. These latter processes take place over a much longer time period, and in two phases. The cones operate over a more restricted range under fairly high levels of illumination. The rods operate only at lower levels of illumination and take much longer to adapt to these lower levels of illumination. The aging eye is less able to alter its sensitivity in response to changing levels of illumination.

Adaptation in elderly individuals is at about the same rate as younger adults, and Weale (1965) showed that the principal cause of these elevated thresholds with age is the deterioration of light transmission in the ocular media. The lens is the major culprit, because older persons with the lens removed surgically showed thresholds very similar to those of young adults when tested with an artificial pupil that kept both old and young subjects with an equal amount of light entering the eye (Gunkel and Gouras, 1963). In reality, of course, the older eye, which has less light entering because of the persisting senile miosis (small pupil), has poorer sensitivity.

The aged eye shows less transmission of the shorter wavelengths (violets and blues) than the long wavelengths (reds) because of the yellowing of the lens. When tested with the shorter wavelengths, the older eye appears far worse than when tested with the younger ones. Also, the older eye works with color distortion resulting from the filtering of the lens, which grows worse with age (Carter, 1982).

Changing Temporal Abilities in the Eye   The older eye has increased persistence (i.e., it holds images longer). The threshold for flicker fusion, whereby a flickering light is speeded until it is seen as a constant light, drops with age, even when pupil size is taken into account. Because photoreceptors can follow flickering light far above the reported thresholds, the limitation must be in the nervous system.

Stimulus persistence has also been shown in other ways. An experiment that allowed a tradeoff between integration of light over time verses increased light intensity (Eriksen, Hamlin, and Breitmeyer, 1970) showed that older persons could integrate over a longer period than young adults. Likewise, an experiment using color showed that older adults fuse separate sequential flashes of red and green light into yellow far more than do young adults (Kline, Ikeda, and Schieber, 1982).

Kline and Schieber (1985) proposed a hypothesis to explain the slowed temporal processing in the visual system with age: a "sustained/transient shift." The visual system has been shown to have two different types of processing channels involving different types of neurons and neuronal activity; these channels were dubbed *sustained* and *transient*. The sustained channel operates from the fovea, responds to sustained images, has high spatial resolution, and can integrate input over a longer period of time. The transient channel operates largely from peripheral retina, responds to moving/pulsing stimuli, has poor spatial resolution, and when triggered tends to elicit an attentional response (usually an eye movement to bring the stimulus on to the fovea for closer examination). Kline and Schieber proposed that the transient system declines faster with age than the sustained channel. Consistent with this, Owsley, Sekuler, and Siemsen (1983) found that threshold for detection of grating patterns was lowered for young adults by motion in the gratings, but hardly changed the thresholds for older adults.

The rate at which visual stimuli are processed has been measured by a method called *backward masking*. In this method a stimulus is presented and then followed after a short interval by a stimulus in the same area of the visual field, which if it follows quickly enough, prevents the subject from perceiving the previously presented target. The subject's task is to report the target stimulus. Masking is more easily achieved in older adults and may reflect several aspects of visual system performance. Target and mask delivered sequentially to the same eye produce masking in the retina. Masking at higher levels can also be shown by delivering the target to one eye and the mask to the other. This masking at higher levels of the nervous system is also more easily achieved in the older adult. This may be due to the slowed processing discussed above. However, it may additionally reflect a lowered signal-

to-noise ratio in the older nervous system that requires a longer processing time to extract the signal (Salthouse, 1980, as quoted by Kline
and Schieber, 1985).

Higher-Level Functions   Older adults have difficulty using unfamiliar
stimuli, report fewer switches in many visual illusions such as the
Necker cube, and seem more ruled by context effects than younger
adults. Elderly persons have been characterized as being more cau-
tious in their reports of perceptions, and this may bias their responses
under some circumstances. However it seems equally likely that difficulties with signal-to-noise ratio may have an equally broad explana-
tory effect. It also seems certain that elderly persons are not able to
use partial information to resolve difficult perceptual problems (Danziger and Salthouse, 1978). The basis of this difficulty is unknown but
surely resides in higher-level functions of the CNS.

Our high-technology culture has some implications for how some of
the above information impinges on the older adult. Driving an automobile after dark is perhaps one of the most difficult assignments for
an older adult. Glare of several types is encountered from oncoming
headlights that blinds the older driver during the encounter and for
some time afterward as the older visual system adapts to the low light
levels. Reading dials on the dashboard requires rapid accommodation
under quite different levels of illumination, and all of this under life-
and-death circumstances. Reading signs under lower levels of illumination is far more difficult for the older person who is suffering from
poorer acuity. Also, the transient/peripheral visual system is chiefly
used in driving a car, not the relatively spared sustained/foveal system.
As a consequence of all these changes, most older drivers stop driving
after dark.

Audition

Anatomical and Physiological Changes with Age

The external ear parts, the pinna and the external auditory canal, do
not contribute to degradations of hearing with aging except for two
factors: buildup of ear wax and collapse of the external canal. The
latter is not common, but does occur occasionally in extreme old age.
The buildup of ear wax because of changes in the skin of the external
canal is a more common finding. It can be easily treated by wax removal.

The middle ear contains the tympanum and ossicles, the means by
which sound is transmitted to the inner ear. Despite some known
changes in both the tympanum and ossicular chain, neither has been

shown to greatly alter the transmission of sound with normal aging. The tympanum grows stiffer with age and likely alters the pattern of response somewhat to different frequencies. Likewise, the ossicular chain often stiffens arthritically with age, but this has not always been associated with hearing loss. However, ossification of the final ossicle in the chain at the entry to the inner ear does induce a loss of input.

The main changes with aging are in the inner ear (cochlea) and the CNS. There are four major changes with age: (1) atrophy of the stria vascularis, (2) loss of elasticity of the basilar membrane, (3) loss of the sensory receptors (hair cells in the organ of Corti), and (4) loss of neurons innervating the organ of Corti.

The atrophy of the stria vascularis produces one of the main sources of deterioration with age, the loss of metabolic support for the inner ear (Schuknecht, 1974). It is accompanied by lower flow of endolymph and a lower standing electrical potential in that portion of the cochlea that transforms sound into nerve impulses. Persons with such atrophy have impaired hearing across all frequencies. They also often show loudness recruitment, which is an enhanced perception of loudness as the intensity of sound is increased. Thus, the person suffering from this problem has a very short range of comfortable intensities and passes quickly from just perceptible loudness to uncomfortably loud sounds over a short range of sound intensity increase.

Loss of elasticity in the basilar membrane impairs the ability of the cochlea to respond precisely to sound (Hansen and Reske-Nielson, 1965). The end of the basilar membrane that is closest to the input of sound at the oval window is most sensitive to high frequencies. The other end is most sensitive to low frequencies. The basilar membrane bends in response to the sound waves as they pass through the cochlea. When the membrane stiffens it bends less and bends over a longer distance. Thus, a smaller stimulus is provided to the receptors and this stimulation is spread over a wider band of receptors. This provides a lower amplitude and less precise signal to the CNS. The effect is strongest for the higher frequencies. The receptors are packed most densely near the oval window, and most frequencies used in speech are crowded into this region. This area of the basilar membrane is the thickest. Thus the combination of crowding of elements and thickness of membrane combine to enhance the loss due to membrane stiffness. Higher frequencies are thereby more dramatically affected.

The organ of Corti is a specialized apparatus that lies along the basilar membrane and contains the sensory receptors, which are of two types—inner and outer hair cells. When the basilar membrane flexes in response to sound, the organ of Corti flexes in a complex motion that provides the hair cells the necessary stimulation to excite the neurons of the 8th nerve. With age the number of hair cells decreases, especially the outer hair cells, which seem to support the detection of low-level input.

Loss of neurons in some cases follows the loss of sensory receptors, but in other cases seems to be based on loss of blood supply or pinching by bone growth on the 8th nerve. The loss is not understood, and some of it may be genetically based. Because there are more neurons devoted to high frequencies, those frequencies are harder hit.

There are some changes in the nuclei of the brain. There is both shrinkage of nuclei and darkening of some areas. However, there are no direct links between any of these changes and specific losses of function.

Perceptual Alteration with Aging

The most notable change with age is the loss of sensitivity, especially for the higher frequencies. The ability to detect sound diminishes with age at all frequencies, but the ability to hear sound from 50 Hz up to 1 KHz remains relatively preserved compared with the increasingly greater losses at the higher frequencies (Lebo and Reddell, 1972; Spoor, 1967). Men show this loss to a somewhat greater extent than do women.

Frequency discrimination also diminishes with age (Jesteadt and Sims, 1975; König, 1957), being somewhat worse for discrimination of lower frequencies. However, the amount of loss is relatively minor.

Masking of stimuli can occur in the auditory system as it can in the visual. Masking can be measured by how loud a band of noise overlapping the stimulus frequency must be to prevent the stimulus's being heard. There can also be temporal masking, in which pulses of noise before or after a stimulus prevent it from being perceived. Elderly individuals have a moderate loss when confronted with masking (Smith and Prather, 1971). The results are consistent with animal models that predict loss of function due to loss of the outer hair cells (Bonding, 1979).

Masking sounds can also be perceived as coming from different or similar locations in space. The ability to spatially locate a stimulus provides another dimension to better differentiate signal from noise. The auditory system uses both time delay and intensity differences between the ears to spatially locate sound sources. Older listeners are less able to use time delay cues to distinguish signal from noise, but they use intensity differences as effectively as young adults do (Herman, Warren, and Wagener, 1977). Younger listeners are better able to use such "stereo" effects to distinguish words from masking noise or speech (Tillman, Carhart, and Nicholls, 1973; Warren, Wagener, and Herman, 1978).

The greatest problem for the elderly person is the perception of speech against a background of noise. This difficulty arises as a result of a number of changes in the auditory system of the older person. Some of those changes have been noted above. In addition, another effect seems to have a powerful role, namely, the inability to rapidly encode speech sounds when they are embedded in other noise. This is essentially a loss of cognitive processing capability. This is most strongly supported by the finding that with increasing age the ability to identify single words against a noisy background is actually better than identifying entire sentences (Jerger and Hayes, 1977). The fact that words used in spoken sentences actually change their sounds depending on surrounding words undoubtedly provides a more difficult and amorphous stimulus to deal with and adds to the difficulty of encoding the stimulus, especially when the peripheral receptors are already producing a distorted or degraded output. The losses found in speech perception under difficult conditions are not well predicted by hearing thresholds or other tests of lower-level functions, most likely because those tests examine only receptor sensitivity and not the more important CNS functions involved in encoding speech.

Noise

The role that noise, or at least excessive exposure to sound, may play in the loss of hearing over a lifetime is not clear. It is clear that high-energy sound, over a relatively short period, can damage the cochlea and produce permanent shifts in hearing thresholds. It has been speculated that the greater impairment seen in men might be due to greater exposure to high levels of sound in the workplace and that industrial workers in Western society might have greater exposure than people in more primitive cultures. One series of studies provided such a contrast by comparing the Mabaan tribesmen of the Sudan with similar-aged groups in the United States (Rosen et al., 1962, 1964a). The Mabaan tribesmen did have better hearing on all measures. However, there were no controls in these studies for such important variables as genetic endowment or diet. For instance, such differences as very low levels of cardiovascular disease among the Mabaan men compared with the high levels of such disease in the United States provide better explanations (Rosen et al., 1964b). Further, the supposition that the desert is a quiet place to live is contradicted by the high levels of sound under such conditions as violent wind storms. It should also be noted that the original studies of auditory function in the United States were done on selected populations that had not had high levels of noise exposure (Corso, 1959; Hinchcliff, 1959).

The usual model for how excessive noise injures the ear is by continuous exposure over a long period of time, such as is found during a lifetime of working under high noise conditions. A lifetime of working at 83- to 85-dB noise exposure can produce some hearing loss, but women show less injury (Szanto and Ionescu, 1983; von Gierke and Johnson, 1976). Corso (1980) argued for differentiating between normal hearing loss due to age and that due to other causes, like excessive noise. The intensity of the noise alters the amount of time necessary before damage takes place. Over 140-dB sound pressure level damage is immediate and permanent and can continue for up to 10 min, after which no further damage can be done. At 130 dB, immediate damage will occur and can continue for up to 1 hr. At 120 dB, some damage can be done immediately, but most is delayed, but continuous exposure up to 72 hr will continue to produce damage. In the range of 90–120 dB some damage will occur if exposure is long enough (Spoendlin, 1976). Below 90 dB laboratory experiments are not practical; long exposure times of workers seem more practical as an assessment tool.

Impulse noise is likely more similar to our natural environment than is continuous noise. However the data on how impulse noise affects hearing have been more difficult to assess and remain controversial. One report shows exposure to intermittent impulse noise will not produce as much damage as continuous noise at the same level (Ward, 1976). But another (Ratloff, 1982) indicates that impulse noise produces damage faster than continuous noise of equal energy.

Antibiotics, Ototoxic Drugs, and Noise   The action of some drugs, aspirin being the most popular, can bring temporary loss of sensitivity. The permanence of the effect is controversial. The cochlea was found to have no increase in vulnerability during aspirin exposure in one study (Hamernik and Henderson, 1976), but a potentiation was found in another (McFadden and Plattsmier, 1983). There is also evidence that such interaction does take place with kanamycin (Marques, Clark, and Hawkins, 1975). This family of aminoglycoside antibiotics are all toxic to the cochlea and will produce damage (Prazma, 1981), and may depend on sound to produce damaging effects.

Smell and Taste

Smell and taste have received insufficient research attention to adequately describe their alteration with aging. The sense of smell has been particularly poorly addressed in older populations. There is general agreement that both taste and smell deteriorate with age, but these decrements are not well documented across age groups and across the various classes of stimuli within these two sense modalities.

One major review of this area (Engen, 1977) concluded that age had little effect on olfactory and gustatory sensitivity and that shifting preferences with age and health might be the greatest factor to be dealt with in aging studies. However, there have been several studies showing large losses in olfactory sensitivity, with men showing greater loss than women, again with health an important factor (Chalke, Dewhurst, and Ward, 1958; Kimbrell and Furchgott, 1963). Taste and smell at suprathreshold levels are quite similar for young and old adults (Bartoshuk et al., 1986).

The number of taste buds seems to be linked to the level of gonadal hormones. Thus, there is a decrease for women starting in the mid-40s while for men it falls about a decade later. For both sexes more than half of the papillae are gone for those over 75 years of age (Arey, Tremaine, and Monzingo, 1936). Using the traditional categories of taste, salty deteriorates most with age, sweet, and sour are just behind, and bitter seems best preserved, but still shows decline in most studies (Byrd and Gertman, 1959; Cooper, Bilash, and Zubek, 1958). Recognition of food by elderly persons is diminished and they use fewer dimensions to describe their sensations (Schiffman, 1977), with the overriding hedonic quality of the sensations being negative. Many factors come into play in assessing taste and smell and many of them have not been assessed or have been poorly controlled. For instance, the mucus content and pH of the saliva, as well as the amount produced, are known to change with age and could seriously alter the perception of taste. Some studies have ignored the factor of dentures, which can cover important portions of the palate, especially for sour and bitter, as well as altering the mouth environment. Improved oral hygiene can improve the taste sensitivity of many older persons.

Somesthesis

Tactile and Temperature Sensitivity

The ability to detect a warm stimulus on the forearm is somewhat less in older persons than in young adults (Clark and Mehl, 1971). However, another study could only detect a difference using the soles of the feet (Kenshalo, 1986). There is little deterioration with age of the systems employed in detecting temperature change at the skin. But perhaps of greater significance is the ability to detect and control internal body temperature. Although older persons are often seen wearing more clothing or seem to prefer warmer environments, this is not related to their perception of the environment, but to how well they are able to maintain their core body temperature. They prefer the same temperature environment as younger persons (Rohles, 1969); they just have a more difficult time controlling their internal temperature. One study in which core body temperature and finger temperature were obtained found a number of older persons near hypothermia (35° C), but they did not report feeling cold; nor were they shivering (Fox et al., 1973).

With age, skin loses elastin and collagen, becoming inelastic and rigid and therefore less deformable (Gilchrest, 1984). The hairy skin relies largely on free nerve endings, whereas the nonhairy (glabrous) skin of the palms and soles relies on a number of special receptors for touch sensation. The number of free nerve endings does not seem to diminish with age, but the specialized receptors show large losses or distorted forms in most cases (e.g., Meissner corpuscles decrease by about 90 percent by late life). Both punctate and vibratory stimulation shows reduced function on hands, feet, and wrist of the elderly person (Kenshalo, 1986). Also, the two-point threshold (distance between two stimulating points before the person feels two instead of one) was larger on both thumb and palm for an older group as compared with a younger group (Axelrod and Cohen, 1961).

Pain is a sensation that has emotional properties, can only be inferred to be present, and is exceptionally open to bias on the part of the responding person. As such only those testing methods that permit bias-free reporting can be considered reliable. Kenshalo (1986) reported no age difference. Other studies have reported that older persons are less able to detect a painful stimulus and women start earlier (Clark and Mehl, 1971; Harkins and Chapman, 1976, 1977). Interestingly, although there was a decrease in detectability, these persons also showed a bias toward not labeling the sensation as pain until it was relatively painful, whereupon they labeled the stimulation as quite painful. A large group of industrial workers, a number of which had been subjected to varying degrees of vibration during their working lives, were tested for pain perception (but not using the bias-free methods mentioned above) on the fingers and forearm (Radzyukevich, 1974, as quoted by Corso, 1981). Those exposed to vibration felt the least pain, and the lack of pain perception seemed linked to the extent of exposure to vibration.

References

Arey, L. B., Tremaine, M. J., and Monzingo, F. L. 1936. The numerical and topographical relations of taste buds to human circumvallate papillae throughout the life span. *Anatomical Record* 64:9–25.

Axelrod, S., and Cohen, L. D. 1961. Senescence and embedded-figure performance in vision and touch. *Perception and Psychophysics* 12:283–288.
Balazs, E. A., and Denlinger, J. L. 1982. Age changes in the vitreus. In Sek-
uler, R., Kline, D., and Dismukes, K. (Eds.), *Aging and Human Visual
Function*. New York, Alan R. Liss, pp. 45–57.
Bartoshuk, L. M., Rifkin, B., Marks, L. E., and Bars, P. 1986. Taste and
aging. *Journal of Gerontology* 41:51–57.
Bell, B., Wolf, E., and Bernholz, C. D. 1972. Depth perception as a function
of age. *Aging and Human Development* 3:77–81.
Birren, J. E., and Schaie, K. W. (Eds.). 1977. *Handbook of the Psychology
of Aging*. New York, Van Nostrand Rheinhold.
Birren, J. E., and Schaie, K. W. (Eds.). 1985. *Handbook of the Psychology
of Aging* (2nd ed.). New York, Van Nostrand Rheinhold.
Birren, J. E., and Williams, M. V. 1982. A perspective on aging and visual
function. In Sekuler, R., Kline, D., and Dismukes, K. (Eds.), *Aging and
Human Visual Function*. New York, Alan R. Liss, pp. 7–19.
Blackwell, O. M., and Blackwell, H. R. 1971. Visual performance data for 156
normal observers of various ages. *Journal of the Illuminating Engineering
Society* 1:3–13.
Bonding, P. 1979. Critical bandwith in presbycusis. *Scandinavian Audiology*
8:205–225.
Bulpitt, C. J., Hodes, C., and Everitt, M. G. 1975. Intraocular pressure and
systematic pressure in the elderly. *British Journal of Ophthalmology* 59:
717–720.
Burg, A. 1966. Visual acuity as measured by dynamic and static tests: A
comparative evaluation. *Journal of Applied Psychology* 50:460–466.
Burg, A. 1968. Lateral visual field as related to age and sex. *Journal of Applied
Psychology* 52:10–15.
Byrd, E., and Gertman, S. 1959. Taste sensitivity in aging persons. *Geriatrics*
14:381–384.
Carter, J. H. 1982. The effects of aging upon selected visual functions: Color
vision, glare sensitivity, field of vision and accommodation. In Sekuler, R.,
Kline, D., and Dismukes, K. (Eds.), *Aging and Human Visual Function*.
Newn York, Alan R. Liss, pp. 121–130.
Chalke, H. D., Dewhurst, J. B., and Ward, C. W. 1958. Loss of sense of smell
in old people. *Public Health* 72:223–230.
Clark, W. C., and Mehl, L. 1971. Thermal pain: A sensory decision analysis
of the effect of age and sex on d', various response criteria, and 50 percent
pain threshold. *Journal of Abnormal Psychology* 78:202–212.
Cooper, R. M., Bilash, M. A., and Zubek, J. P. 1958. The effect of age on
taste sensitivity. *Journal of Gerontology* 14:56–58.
Corso, J. F. 1959. Age and sex differences in pure-tone thresholds. *Journal of
the Acoustic Society of America* 31:498–507.
Corso, J. F. 1980. Age correction factor in noise-induced hearing loss: A
quantitative model. *Audiology* 19:221–232.
Corso, J. F. 1981. *Aging Sensory Systems and Perception*. New York,
Praeger.

Danziger, W. L., and Salthouse, T. A. 1978. Age and the perception of incomplete figures. *Experimental Aging Research* 4:67–80.

Devaney, K. O., and Johnson, H. A. 1980. Neuron loss in the aging visual cortex of man. *Journal of Gerontology* 15:836–841.

Engen, T. 1977. Taste and smell. In Birren, J. E., and Schaie, K. W. (Eds.), *Handbook of the Psychology of Aging*. New York, Van Nostrand Rheinhold, pp. 554–561.

Eriksen, C. W., Hamlin, P. M., and Breitmeyer, B. G. 1970. Temporal factors in perception as related to aging. *Perception and Psychophysics* 7:354–356.

Fox, R. H., Woodward, P. M., Eston-Smith, H. N., Green, M. F., Donnison, D. V., and Wicks, M. H. 1973. Body temperature in the elderly: Anatomical study of physiological, social, and environmental conditions. *British Medical Journal* 1:200–206.

Gilchrest, B. A. 1984. *Skin and Aging Processes*. Boca Raton, FL, CRC Press.

Greenberg, D. A., and Branch, L. G. 1982. A review of methodological issues concerning incidence and prevalence data of visual deterioration in elders. In Sekuler, R., Kline, D., and Dismukes, K. (Eds.), *Aging and Human Visual Function*. New York, Alan R. Liss, pp. 279–296.

Gunkel, R. D., and Gouras. P. 1963. Changes in scotopic visibility thresholds with age. *American Medical Association Archives of Ophthalmology* 69:4–9.

Hollows, F., and Moran, D. 1981. Cataract—the ultraviolet risk factor. *Lancet* 2:1249–1253.

Hamernik, R. P., and Henderson, D. 1976. The potentiation of noise by other ototraumatic agents. In Henderson, D., Hamernik, R. P., Dosanjh, D. S., and Mills, J. H. (Eds.), *Effects of Noise on Hearing*. New York, Raven Press, pp. 291–307.

Hansen, C. C., and Reske-Nielson, E. 1965. Pathological studies in presbycusis. *Archives of Otolaryngology* 82:115–132.

Harkins, S. W., and Chapman, C. R. 1976. Detection and decision factors in pain perception in young and elderly men. *Pain* 2:253–264.

Harkins, S. W., and Chapman, C. R. 1977. The perception of induced dental pain in young and elderly women. *Journal of Gerontology* 32:428–435.

Herman, G. E., Warren, L. R., and Wagener, J. W. 1977. Auditory lateralization: Age-differences in sensitivity to dichotic time and amplitude cues. *Journal of Gerontology* 32:187–191.

Hinchcliff, R. 1959. The threshold of hearing as a function of age. *Acoustica* 9:303–308.

Jani, S. N. 1966. The age factor in stereopsis screening. *American Journal of Optometry and Physiological Optics* 43:653–655.

Jerger, J., and Hayes, D. 1977. Diagnostic speech audiometry. *Archives of Otolaryngology* 103:216–222.

Jesteadt, W., and Sims, S. L. 1975. Decision processes in frequency discrimination. *Journal of the Acoustical Society of America* 57:1161–1168.

Kenshalo, D. R. 1986. Somesthetic sensitivity in young and elderly humans. *Journal of Gerontology* 41:732–742.

Kimbrell, G. McA., and Furchgott, E. 1963. The effect of aging on olfactory threshold. *Journal of Gerontology* 18:364–365.

Kline, D. W., Ikeda, D., and Schieber, F. 1982. Age and temporal resolution in color vision: When do red and green make yellow? *Journal of Gerontology* 37:705–709.

Kline, D. W., and Schieber, F. 1985. Vision and aging. In Birren, J. E., and Schaie, K. W. (Eds.), *Handbook of the Psychology of Aging* (2nd ed.). New York, Van Nostrand Reinhold, pp. 296–331.

König, E. 1957. Pitch discrimination and age. *Acta Oto-Larynologica* 48: 475–489.

Lebo, C. P., and Reddell, R. C. 1972. The presbycusis component in occupational noise-induced hearing loss. *Laryngoscope* 82:1399–1409.

Lerman, S. 1980. *Radiant Energy and the Eye.* New York, Macmillan.

Marmor, M. F. 1982. Aging and the retina. In Sekuler, R., Kline, D., and Dismukes, K. (Eds.), *Aging and Human Visual Function.* New York, Alan R. Liss, pp. 59–78.

Marques, D. M., Clark, C. S., and Hawkins, J. E., Jr. 1975. Potentiation of cochlear injury by noise and ototoxic antibiotics in guinea pigs (abstract). *Journal of the Acoustic Society of America* 57:S60.

McFadden, D., and Plattsmier, H. S. 1983. Aspirin can potentiate the temporary hearing loss induced by noise. *Hearing Research* 9:295–316.

Owsley, C., Sekuler, R., and Siemsen, D. 1983. Contrast sensitivity throughout adulthood. *Vision Research* 23:689–699.

Panek, P. E., Barrett, G. V., Sterns, H. L., and Alexander, R. A. 1977. A review of age changes in perceptual information processing ability with regard to driving. *Experimental Aging Research* 3:387–449.

Pitts, D. G. 1982. The effects of aging on selected visual functions: Dark adaptation, visual acuity, stereopsis, and brightness contrast. In Sekuler, R., Kline, D., and Dismukes, K. (Eds.), *Aging and Human Visual Function.* New York, Alan R. Liss, pp. 131–159.

Prazma, J. 1981. Ototoxicity of aminoglycoside antibiotics. In Brown, R. D., and Daigneault, E. A. (Eds.), *Pharmacology of Hearing.* New York, Wiley, pp. 153–195.

Pressman, M. R., DiPhillipo, M. A., and Fry, J. M. 1986. Senile miosis: The possible contribution of disordered sleep and daytime sleepiness. *Journal of Gerontology* 41:629–634.

Radzyukevich, T. M. 1974. Thresholds of pain sensitivity in workers of "vibration hazardous" occupations and in practically healthy persons of different age. *Uchenye zapiski Ukraninskii tsentralnyi institut gigieny truda, Professionalnykh zabolevanii* 4:10–12.

Ratloff, J. 1982. Occupational noise—the subtle pollutant. *Science News* 121:347–350.

Rohles, R. H. 1969. Preference for the thermal environment by the elderly. *Human Factors* 11:37–41.

Rosen, S., Bergman, M., Plester, D., El-Mofty, A., and Satti, M. H. 1962. Presbycusis study of a relatively noise-free population in the Sudan. *Annals of Otology, Rhinology, and Laryngology* 71:727–743.

Rosen, S., Plester, D., El-Mofty, A., and Rosen, H. V. 1964a. High frequency audiometry in presbycusis: A comparative study of the Mabaan tribe in the Sudan with urban populations. *Archives of Otolaryngology* 79:18–32.

Rosen, S., Plester, D., El-Mofty, A., and Rosen, H. V. 1964b. Relation of hearing loss to cardiovascular disease. *Transactions of the American Academy of Ophthalmology and Otology* 68:433–444.

Salthouse, T. A. 1980. Age differences in visual masking: A manifestation of decline in neural signal/noise ratio? Paper presented at the annual scientific meeting of the Gerontological Society, San Diego, CA.

Schiffman, S. 1977. Food recognition by the elderly. *Journal of Gerontology* 32:586–592.

Schuknecht, H. 1974. *Pathology of the Ear*. Cambridge, MA, Harvard University Press.

Sekuler, R., Kline, D., and Dismukes, K. 1982. *Aging and Human Visual Function*. New York, Alan R. Liss.

Smith, R., and Prather, W. F. 1971. Phoneme discrimination in older persons under varying signal-to-noise conditions. *Journal of Speech and Hearing Research* 14:630–635.

Spector, A. 1982. Aging of the lens and cataract formation. In Sekuler, R., Kline, D., and Dismukes, K. (Eds.), *Aging and Human Visual Function*. New York, Alan R. Liss, pp. 27–43.

Spoendlin, H. 1976. Anatomical changes following various noise exposures. In Henderson, D., Hamernik, R. P., Dosanjh, D. S., and Mills, J. H. (Eds.), *Effects of Noise on Hearing*. New York, Raven Press, pp. 69–87.

Spoor, A. 1967. Presbycusis values in relation to noise induced hearing loss. *International Audiology* 6:48–57.

Szanto, C., and Ionescu, M. 1983. Influence of age and sex on hearing threshold levels in workers exposed to different intensity levels of occupational noise. *Audiology* 22:339–356.

Tillman, T. W., Carhart, R., and Nicholls, S. 1973. Release from multiple maskers in elderly persons. *Journal of Speech and Hearing Research* 16:152–160.

Tripathi, R. C., and Tripathi, B. J. 1983. Lens morphology, aging and cataract. *Journal of Gerontology* 38:258–270.

von Gierke, H. E., and Johnson, D. L. 1976. Summary of present damage risk criteria. In Henderson, D., Hamernik, R. P., Dosanjh, D. S., and Mills, J. H. (Eds.), *Effects of Noise on Hearing*. New York, Raven Press, pp. 547–558.

Ward, W. D. 1976. A comparison of the effects of continuous, intermittent, and impulse noise. In Henderson, D., Hamernik, R. P., Dosanjh, D. S., and Mills, J. H. (Eds.), *Effects of Noise on Hearing*. New York, Raven Press, pp. 407–419.

Warren, L. R., Wagener, J. W., and Herman, G. E. 1978. Binaural analysis in the aging auditory system. *Journal of Gerontology* 33:731–736.

Weale, R. A. 1961. Retinal illumination and age. *Transactions of the Illuminating Engineering Society* 26:95–100.

Weale, R. A. 1965. On the eye. In Welford, A. T., and Birren, J. E. (Eds.),

Behavior, Aging, and the Nervous System. Springfield, IL, Charles C Thomas, pp. 307–325.

Weale, R. A. 1982. Senile ocular changes, cell death, and vision. In Sekuler, R., Kline, D., and Dismukes, K. (Eds.), *Aging and Human Visual Function.* New York, Alan R. Liss, pp. 161–171.

Wolf, E. 1967. Studies on the shrinkage of the visual field with age. *Highway Research Record* 167:1–7.

Index

Designed by Glen Burris
Set in Times Roman and Helvetica by Achorn Graphic Services, Inc.
Printed on 60-lb Glatfelter Hi-Brite and bound in Holliston Roxite
by The Maple Press Company